Explore more essential res~~ources~~ in the
NETTER BASIC SCIEN~~CE COLLECTION~~!

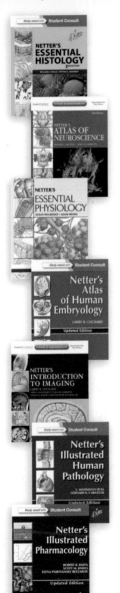

Netter's Essential Histology
With **Student Consult** Access
By William K. Ovalle, PhD and Patrick C. Nahirney, PhD
Bring histologic concepts to life through beautiful Netter illustrations!

Netter's Atlas of Neuroscience
With **Student Consult** Access
By David L. Felten, MD, PhD and Anil Shetty, PhD
Master the neuroscience fundamentals needed
for the classroom and beyond.

Netter's Essential Physiology
With **Student Consult** Access
By Susan Mulroney and Adam Myers, MD
Enhance your understanding of physiology the Netter way!

Netter's Atlas of Human Embryology
With **Student Consult** Access
By Larry R. Cochard, PhD
A rich pictorial review of normal and abnormal human
prenatal development.

Netter's Introduction to Imaging
With **Student Consult** Access
By Larry R. Cochard, PhD et al.
Finally...an accessible introduction to diagnostic imaging!

Netter's Illustrated Human Pathology
With **Student Consult** Access
By Maximilian L. Buja, MD and Gerhard R. F. Krueger
Gain critical insight into the structure-function relationships
and the pathological basis of human disease!

Netter's Illustrated Pharmacology
With **Student Consult** Access
*By Robert B. Raffa, PhD, Scott M. Rawls
and Elena Portyansky Beyzarov*
Take a distinct visual approach to understanding both
the basic science and clinical applications of pharmacology.

Learn more at MyNetter.com!

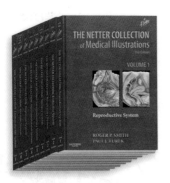
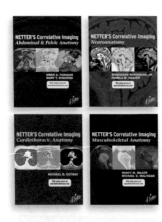

Netter's
Concise Radiologic Anatomy

SECOND EDITION

Edward C. Weber, DO
Radiologist, The Imaging Center
Fort Wayne, Indiana
Consultant, Medical Clinic of Big Sky
Big Sky, Montana
Adjunct Professor of Anatomy
and Cell Biology
Volunteer Clinical Professor of Radiology
and Imaging Sciences
Indiana University School of Medicine
Fort Wayne, Indiana

Joel A. Vilensky, PhD
Professor of Anatomy and Cell Biology
Indiana University School of Medicine
Fort Wayne, Indiana

Stephen W. Carmichael, PhD, DSc
Editor Emeritus, Clinical Anatomy
Professor Emeritus of Anatomy
Professor Emeritus of Orthopedic Surgery
Mayo Clinic
Rochester, Minnesota

Kenneth S. Lee, MD
Associate Professor of Radiology
Director, Musculoskeletal Ultrasound
Medical Director, Translational Imaging
University of Wisconsin School of
Medicine and Public Health
Madison, Wisconsin

Illustrations by **Frank H. Netter, MD**

Contributing Illustrator
Carlos A.G. Machado, MD

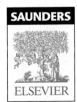

SAUNDERS

ELSEVIER

ELSEVIER
SAUNDERS

1600 John F. Kennedy Blvd.
Ste. 1800
Philadelphia, PA 19103-2899

NETTER'S CONCISE RADIOLOGIC ANATOMY,   ISBN: 978-1-4557-5323-9
SECOND EDITION

Notices

Knowledge and best practice in this field are constantly changing. As new research and experience broaden our understanding, changes in research methods, professional practices, or medical treatment may become necessary.

Practitioners and researchers must always rely on their own experience and knowledge in evaluating and using any information, methods, compounds, or experiments described herein. In using such information or methods they should be mindful of their own safety and the safety of others, including parties for whom they have a professional responsibility.

With respect to any drug or pharmaceutical products identified, readers are advised to check the most current information provided (i) on procedures featured or (ii) by the manufacturer of each product to be administered, to verify the recommended dose or formula, the method and duration of administration, and contraindications. It is the responsibility of practitioners, relying on their own experience and knowledge of their patients, to make diagnoses, to determine dosages and the best treatment for each individual patient, and to take all appropriate safety precautions.

To the fullest extent of the law, neither the Publisher nor the authors, contributors, or editors, assume any liability for any injury and/or damage to persons or property as a matter of products liability, negligence or otherwise, or from any use or operation of any methods, products, instructions, or ideas contained in the material herein.

ISBN: 978-1-4557-5323-9

Senior Content Strategist: Elyse O'Grady
Content Development Manager: Marybeth Thiel
Publishing Services Manager: Patricia Tannian
Senior Project Manager: John Casey
Senior Design Manager: Lou Forgione

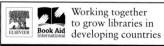

Working together
to grow libraries in
developing countries

www.elsevier.com • www.bookaid.org

Printed in China

Last digit is the print number: 9 8 7 6 5 4 3 2 1

Dedication

This book would not have been possible without the love and support of our wonderful wives, Ellen S. Weber, Deborah K. Meyer-Vilensky, Susan L. Stoddard, and Helen S. Lee, who graciously allowed us to spend countless weekends staring at radiographic images instead of spending time with them. We greatly appreciate all that they do for us and their tolerance of our many eccentricities.

Preface

Diagnostic medical images are now an integral component of contemporary courses in medical gross anatomy. This primarily reflects the steadily increasing teaching of clinical correlations within such courses. Accordingly, radiographic images are included in all gross anatomy atlases and textbooks. These images are typically plain radiographs, axial CT/MRI (computed tomography/magnetic resonance image) scans, and angiograms of various parts of the vascular system.

Although such images reflect the capabilities of diagnostic imaging technology of perhaps 25 years ago, they do not reflect the full integration of computer graphics capabilities into radiology. This integration has resulted in a tremendous expansion in the ability of radiology to represent human anatomy. The active process of reformatting imaging data into optimal planes and types of image reconstruction that best illustrate anatomic/pathologic features is not limited to academic centers. To the contrary, the graphics workstation is now a commonly used tool in the practice of diagnostic radiology. Special views and image reconstructions are currently part of the diagnostic process and are usually made available to all those participating in patient care, along with an interpretation by the radiologist that describes the pathology and relevant anatomy.

This situation led us to the realization that any student of anatomy would benefit from early exposure to the manner of appearance of key anatomic structures in diagnostic images, especially advanced CTs and MRIs. Thus, in 2007 we (a radiologist and two anatomists) chose to develop an atlas that illustrates how modern radiology portrays human anatomy. To accomplish this task, we decided to match modern diagnostic images with a subset of the anatomic drawings from the *Atlas of Human Anatomy* by Dr. Frank H. Netter. Netter's atlas has become the gold standard of human anatomy atlases. Its images are quite familiar to the vast majority of students who complete a course in human gross anatomy. By providing a bridge between the manner in which anatomic features appear in Netter's atlas to their appearance in radiographic images, this book enables the acquisition of comfortable familiarity with how human anatomy is typically viewed in clinical practice.

In this second edition of our atlas we welcome to our author team Dr. Kenneth S. Lee from the Department of Radiology at the University of Wisconsin School of Medicine and Public Health. Dr. Lee's area of specialty is diagnostic and therapeutic musculoskeletal ultrasound. We invited Dr. Lee to become an author of *Netter's Concise Radiologic Anatomy* because we have included in this edition approximately 10 new radiologic illustrations that match Netter plates with ultrasound images. We were reluctant to include ultrasound images in the first edition of this book because ultrasound, relative to radiographs, CT, and MRI, does not often provide a visual perspective on anatomy that is comparable to the Netter drawings. However, ultrasound anatomy is being incorporated into an increasing number of medical gross anatomy courses, and the utilization of ultrasound is now inherently part of many medical specialties. Therefore, with the help of Dr. Lee, we found examples of ultrasound images that could be matched with Netter drawings.

In addition to the incorporation of the ultrasound images, in this second edition we have improved the CT/MR matches for other plates, added a few new matches, and made corrections to errors we found in the first edition for which we apologize to any reader who was confused by our mistakes. We have also deleted a few illustrations that we felt did not portray as good a match as we initially thought and hopefully improved some of the clinical and anatomic notes we include with each plate.

In selecting and creating images for this atlas, we frequently had to choose between diagnostic images that are in very common use (axial, coronal, and sagittal slices) and images that result from more advanced reconstruction techniques, that is, images that are not commonly found in clinical practice but that more clearly depict anatomic structures and relationships. When a "routine" image was found that matched the *Netter Atlas* well and illustrated key anatomic points, it was selected. However, we decided to include many advanced image reconstructions, such as maximum intensity projection and volume rendered ("3-D") displays.

We understand that learning to interpret radiographic images requires reference to normal anatomy. Accordingly, we believe our atlas will facilitate this process by closing a common mental gap between how an anatomic feature looks in an anatomic atlas versus its appearance in clinical imaging.

**Edward C. Weber, Joel A. Vilensky,
Stephen W. Carmichael, Kenneth S. Lee**

Acknowledgments

We are very grateful to many individuals for assisting us in developing this atlas. We would like to thank Elsevier for accepting our book proposal and Madelene Hyde, Elyse O'Grady, and Marybeth Thiel for championing it and assisting us with every stage of the book's development. Among these three individuals, we had almost daily interactions with Ms. Thiel and were constantly impressed, amazed, and grateful for her diligence and efforts to make this atlas as good as it could be. Much of the credit for the final appearance of both editions of this this book belongs to her.

We would also like to thank the 2007 first- and second-year medical students at Indiana University School of Medicine–Fort Wayne for their suggestions to improve this book.

We extend our appreciation to Robert Conner, MD, who established The Imaging Center in Fort Wayne, Indiana, where so much of the work for this book was completed, and who was very supportive of this effort. The Imaging Center is staffed by nuclear medicine, mammography, general radiology, ultrasonography, CT, and MR technologists who not only conduct diagnostic procedures with superb technical skill but also (equally important) do so with great care for the personal needs of our patients.

As a final note, we would like to thank the patients whose images appear in this book and Drs. Frank Netter and Carlos Machado for their artistic insights into human anatomy.

About the Authors

Dr. Edward C. Weber was born and educated in Philadelphia. He has a BA from Temple University and a DO from the Philadelphia College of Osteopathic Medicine. Dr. Weber spent 4 years at the Albert Einstein Medical Center in Philadelphia in a 1-year surgical internship and a 3-year residency in diagnostic radiology. In 1980, the *Journal of the American Medical Association* published an article he wrote describing a new percutaneous interventional biliary procedure. After achieving certification by the American Board of Radiology, he began private practice in 1980 and in 1981 became a founding member of a radiology group based in Fort Wayne, Indiana. After 15 years of hospital radiology practice, Dr. Weber joined The Imaging Center, a private outpatient facility. At the Fort Wayne campus of the Indiana University School of Medicine, Dr. Weber presents radiology lectures within the medical gross anatomy course and is course director for the introduction to clinical medicine. He and his wife, Ellen, have a son who graduated from Brown University and obtained graduate degrees at City University of New York, and a daughter who graduated from Wellesley College and a received a master's degree in Human Computer Interaction at Carnegie Mellon University. Ellen and he celebrated his 50th birthday at the summit of Mt. Kilimanjaro, and they spend as much time as possible at their home in Big Sky, Montana, where he is Consultant Radiologist for The Medical Clinic of Big Sky.

Dr. Joel A. Vilensky is originally from Bayside, New York, but has been teaching medical gross anatomy at the Fort Wayne campus of Indiana University School of Medicine for more than 30 years. He graduated from Michigan State University in 1972 and received an MA from the University of Chicago in 1972 and a PhD from the University of Wisconsin in 1979. He has authored nearly 100 research papers on many topics, most recently on the 1920s worldwide epidemic of encephalitis lethargica, which also resulted in a book: *Encephalitis Lethargica: During and After the Epidemic*. In 2005 he published a book with Indiana University Press: *Dew of Death: The Story of Lewisite, America's World War I Weapon of Mass Destruction*. Dr. Vilensky is a coeditor of *Clinical Anatomy* for which he edits the *Compendium of Anatomical Variants*. Dr. Vilensky and his wife, Deborah, have two daughters, one a school administrator and the other a lawyer in Indianapolis. Dr. Vilensky is a contented workaholic but also enjoys watching television with his wife, traveling, and exercising.

Dr. Stephen W. Carmichael is originally from Modesto, California (featured in the movie *American Graffiti*) and was on the staff at the Mayo Clinic for 25 years, serving as Chair of the Department of Anatomy for 14 years. He graduated from Kenyon College, which honored him with a DSc degree in 1989. He earned a PhD degree in anatomy at Tulane University in 1971. He is author or coauthor of over 140 publications in peer-reviewed journals and 7 books, the majority relating to the adrenal medulla. He is a consulting editor of the fourth and fifth editions of the *Atlas of Human Anatomy* and was Editor-in-Chief of *Clinical Anatomy* from 2000-2012. Dr. Carmichael is married to Dr. Susan Stoddard and has a son who works for a newspaper in Boulder, Colorado. Dr. Carmichael is a certified scuba diver at the professional level, and he is challenged by underwater photography.

Dr. Kenneth S. Lee is originally from Ann Arbor, Michigan. He graduated from the University of Michigan in Ann Arbor with a degree in microbiology. He then matriculated at Tufts University School of Medicine's Dual-Degree Program, graduating in 2002 with both an MD and an MBA in Health Administration. During his residency at Henry Ford Hospital in Detroit, Michigan, he received the Howard P. Doub, MD Distinguished First Year Resident Award, the RSNA Introduction to Research Scholarship, the RSNA Roentgen Resident/Fellow Research Award, the William R. Eyler, MD Distinguished Senior Resident Award, was nominated for the Henry Ford Hospital-wide Outstanding Resident Award, and was Chief Resident from 2006-2007. He credits his mentors at Henry Ford Hospital, Dr. Marnix van Holsbeeck and Joseph Craig, for inspiring him to pursue academic medicine in the field of musculoskeletal (MSK) ultrasound. Dr. Lee joined the University of Wisconsin School of Medicine and Public Health as an MSK Radiology Fellow in 2007 and joined the faculty in 2008 as Director of MSK Ultrasound. In this capacity he directed the start-up of the new MSK Ultrasound Clinic, which has seen a 600% growth in service, providing quality-driven, patient-centered care in a unique environment.

Dr. Lee's research interests include basic science and clinical research. He has formed an MSK ultrasound multidisciplinary research team to develop and study ultrasound-based elastography techniques to quantitatively evaluate tendon elasticity of damaged tendons. He serves as both PI and co-PI on multiple prospective randomized control trials investigating the treatment outcomes of ultrasound-guided therapies, such as platelet-rich plasma, for sports injuries. Dr. Lee has made both national and international presentations of his research and serves on various national committees at the Radiological Society of North America (RNSA) and American Institute of Ultrasound in Medicine (AIUM).

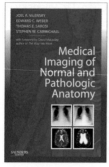

Drs. Vilensky, Weber, and Carmichael (with Dr. Thomas Sarosi) have also co-authored *Medical Imaging of Normal and Pathologic Anatomy*, and Drs. Weber and Vilensky (with Alysa Fog) have published *Practical Radiology: A Symptom-Based Approach*.

About the Artists

Frank H. Netter, MD

Frank H. Netter was born in 1906, in New York City. He studied art at the Art Students' League and the National Academy of Design before entering medical school at New York University, where he received his medical degree in 1931. During his student years, Dr. Netter's notebook sketches attracted the attention of the medical faculty and other physicians, allowing him to augment his income by illustrating articles and textbooks. He continued illustrating as a sideline after establishing a surgical practice in 1933, but he ultimately opted to give up his practice in favor of a full-time commitment to art. After service in the United States Army during World War II, Dr. Netter began his long collaboration with the CIBA Pharmaceutical Company (now Novartis Pharmaceuticals). This 45-year partnership resulted in the production of the extraordinary collection of medical art so familiar to physicians and other medical professionals worldwide.

In 2005, Elsevier, Inc., purchased the Netter Collection and all publications from Icon Learning Systems. More than 50 publications featuring the art of Dr. Netter are available through Elsevier, Inc. (in the US: www.us.elsevierhealth.com/Netter and outside the US: www.elsevierhealth.com).

Dr. Netter's works are among the finest examples of the use of illustration in the teaching of medical concepts. The 13-book *Netter Collection of Medical Illustrations*, which includes the greater part of the more than 20,000 paintings created by Dr. Netter, became and remains one of the most famous medical works ever published. *The Netter Atlas of Human Anatomy*, first published in 1989, presents the anatomic paintings from the Netter Collection. Now translated into 16 languages, it is the anatomy atlas of choice among medical and health professions students the world over.

The Netter illustrations are appreciated not only for their aesthetic qualities, but, more important, for their intellectual content. As Dr. Netter wrote in 1949, "… clarification of a subject is the aim and goal of illustration. No matter how beautifully painted, how delicately and subtly rendered a subject may be, it is of little value as a *medical illustration* if it does not serve to make clear some medical point." Dr. Netter's planning, conception, point of view, and approach are what inform his paintings and what make them so intellectually valuable.

Frank H. Netter, MD, physician and artist, died in 1991.

Learn more about the physician-artist whose work has inspired the Netter Reference collection: http://www.netterimages.com/artist/netter.htm

Carlos Machado, MD

Carlos Machado was chosen by Novartis to be Dr. Netter's successor. He continues to be the main artist who contributes to the Netter collection of medical illustrations.

Self-taught in medical illustration, cardiologist Carlos Machado has contributed meticulous updates to some of Dr. Netter's original plates and has created many paintings of his own in the style of Netter as an extension of the Netter collection. Dr. Machado's photorealistic expertise and his keen insight into the physician/patient relationship informs his vivid and unforgettable visual style. His dedication to researching each topic and subject he paints places him among the premier medical illustrators at work today.

Learn more about his background and see more of his art at: http://www.netterimages.com/artist/machado.htm.

Contents

Section 2 — Back and Spinal Cord

Section 3 — Thorax

Section 4   Abdomen

Section 5   Pelvis and Perineum

Section 6   Upper Limb

Section 7   **Lower Limb**

Introduction

Radiologic imaging technologies are the windows through which human anatomy is viewed hundreds of millions of times each year in the United States alone. We learn anatomy through lectures attended, reading text-based materials and web pages, studying drawings such as those in the Netter Atlas, and by performing dissection of cadavers. Occasionally, key features of human anatomy are exposed to our view during a surgical procedure. However, the increasing use of minimally invasive surgery, done through fiber-optic scopes and very small incisions, has limited even this opportunity to see internal structures. It is through the technology of medical imaging that anatomic structures are now seen by practicing clinicians on a regular basis. Therefore, the teaching and learning of human anatomy now includes these means of visualizing internal anatomic structures.

We do not present here a complete description of the physics underlying the various forms of medical imaging. An introductory text in radiology should be consulted for that information. Rather, we briefly present here some basic physical principles, the unique contribution each technology makes to clinical medicine and how each relates to the wonderful drawings of the Netter Atlas.

Radiography

Radiography, formerly done with film but now often with digital acquisition, is the foundation of diagnostic imaging. X-rays are produced in an x-ray tube by electrons striking a metallic target. The characteristics of the x-ray beam important for medical imaging include the number of photons used 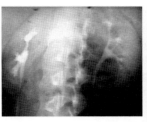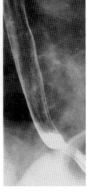 (measured by the milliamperage, "mA," of the current applied to the tube), and the distribution of energy among those photons (measured by the kilivoltage peak, "kVp"). The mA of the x-ray beam must be sufficient for adequate penetration of the body part imaged. The kVp of the beam affects the interaction of the x-ray photons with tissues containing varied quantities of atoms with different atomic weights. Atoms with larger nuclei are more likely to absorb or scatter photons in the x-ray beam. Therefore, the KvP affects the contrast resolution between different types of tissue. The x-ray beam that is directed toward the patient is shaped and limited geometrically or collimated to restrict exposure to a specific body part. The pattern of x-rays that passes through the patient and is not absorbed or scattered by tissues creates an image when it strikes either rare earth phosphor screens that expose a film or a variety of x-ray sensitive photoreceptors that create a digital radiograph. Characteristics of the receptors capturing the x-ray beam after it has passed through a patient are primarily responsible for the spatial resolution of an image.

In depicting anatomic features, this projectional technique may be limited by the overlap of structures along the path of an x-ray beam. This is rarely a problem if the anatomy needed for diagnosis is simple and intrinsic tissue contrast is high, as in most orthopedic imaging. A plain radiograph of a forearm, for example, to demonstrate a suspected or known fracture provides good visualization of the anatomic structures in question. Elaborate, even elegant, projections and patient positioning techniques have been developed to display anatomic structures clearly. Radiography provides very high spatial resolution and is still a critical part of imaging when such resolution is needed. The projectional images of radiography can provide an understandable image of a complex shape that is difficult to visualize upon viewing cross-sectional images.

If necessary, the contrast resolution of radiographs may be enhanced by the ingestion of a radiopaque substance and by injection of iodinated contrast media. Video fluoroscopy, the "real-time" version of radiography, enables observation of physiologic processes often not achievable by CT or MRI. For example, a swallowing study, done while a patient drinks a barium sulfate suspension under observation by video fluoroscopy, can provide the temporal resolution needed to visualize the surprisingly fast movement of swallowing. Similarly, injection of iodinated contrast material directly into a vessel being studied can provide high spatial, contrast, and temporal resolution. This technique can beautifully depict vascular anatomy but is considered an invasive procedure because of the need for arterial puncture and injection into the lumen of a deeply placed vessel. An imaging study requiring only injection into a peripheral intravenous line is considered a noninvasive study.

For some anatomic structures, projectional radiographic images, whether plain films, barium studies, or angiographic exams, may reveal anatomy in a way that best correlates with the drawings in the Netter Atlas.

Ultrasonography

High-frequency pulses of sound emerge from a transducer placed on a patient's skin surface or endoluminal mucosal surface and the returning echoes become bright pixels on a video image. The frame rate of image

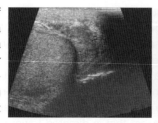 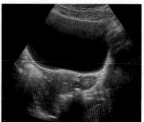

creation in sonography is rapid enough to be "real-time." With high-frequency trans-ducers, very high spatial resolution can be obtained with ultrasonography. Almost exclusively, diagnostic ultrasound images are made by freehand techniques not restricted to strict axial or sagittal planes. The almost infinite angulation and position of an ultrasound image in the hands of a skilled sonographer can often beautifully depict anatomic features. During real-time ultrasound examinations, curved ana-tomic structures can be "followed" and overlapping structures can be separated. Ultrasound images usually do not often reveal anatomic structures in ways that are visually comparable to the perspective on human anatomy provided by the Netter Atlas, although the Netter Atlas can be used to teach the anatomy needed to perform ultrasonography. Newer applications of computer graphics technology may advance the visual perspective offered by ultrasonography in the near future.

However, we present here examples of anatomic regions in which ultrasound scans can now be used to visualize key structures or relationships shown in the Netter illustrations. These plates were the basis for a significant part of this revised second edition.

Nuclear Medicine

Nuclear medicine uses unstable radioisotopes, emitters of ionizing radiation, that are "tagged" to pharmaceuticals that affect their biologic distribution. The pattern or distribution of emitted gamma radiation is detected, typically by a gamma camera. As a rule, nuclear medicine images provide func-tional information but do not provide high spatial resolution. In the detection and evaluation of disease, nuclear medicine imaging provides biochemical and physiologic information that is a critical component of modern diagnosis. For example, a radionuclide bone scan may demonstrate the extent of skeletal metastatic disease with high sensitivity for the detec-tion of tumor that remains radiographically occult. There is a growing importance of molecular imaging that can often tran-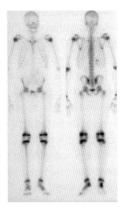scend the simple gross morphologic data acquired by traditional imaging. An example of extreme importance is the PET (positron emission tomography) scan, which can identify tumors not perceptible by even advanced CT or MRI. Further-more, PET scans can provide critically important metabolic information about a tumor that is not provided by simply seeing the size and shape of a tumor. The absence of nuclear medicine images such as radionuclide bone scans from this atlas does not signify any lack of importance of this technology for the practice of medi-cine; rather, it reflects that those images cannot be matched to the drawings in the Netter Atlas.

Computed Tomography

CT scanning uses x-ray tubes and detector arrays rotating around the patient. Measurements of x-ray absorption at a large number of positions and angles are treated mathematically 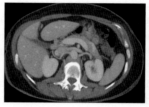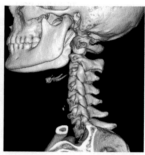 by a Fourier transformation, which calculates cross-sectional images. CT scanning not only provides the advantages of cross-sectional images compared to the projectional images of radiography, but also vastly improves tissue contrast resolution. A variety of oral and iodinated intravenous contrast agents are frequently administered to enhance contrast between different structures.

As new generations of CT scanners have become available, they have often leaped far beyond typical "model year changes" to quantum changes in imaging capability. During the past few decades, CT scanning has progressed from requiring over 2 minutes for the acquisition of a single 1 cm thick axial slice to commonly used scanners that can acquire 64 simultaneous sub-millimeter thick cross-sectional images within each third of a second. This vast improvement in temporal resolution enables CT angiography, because injected contrast material does not remain intravascular very long. The timing of optimal enhancement of different body tissues after contrast material injection varies with tissue characteristics such as composition and vascularity. Rapid CT scans allow for precise timing of CT acquisitions tailored to the organ being targeted. For example, the ideal time for imaging the liver is often approximately 65 seconds after initiating an intravenous injection of contrast material.

The processing of CT image data after the scan and after initial creation of cross-sectional images may be as crucial as the scanning itself. The range of tissue densities captured by a CT scanner far exceeds the human visual system's ability to perceive approximately 16 shades of grey. The selection of the width of the CT density spectrum that is presented in a range of visual densities perceptible by the human observer is referred to as the "window" and the mean CT density presented as a median shade of grey is the "level." A CT dataset viewed at a bone window (and level) may provide no useful representation of soft tissue structures. These window and level adjustments are the first stage of interactivity with image data that far surpasses the older "interactivity" with medical images that consisted of putting films on a view box.

Perhaps more relevant to this atlas is that current CT image data are acquired as a volumetric dataset in which each voxel—a specific volume within three dimensional space—of imaging information is isotropic, essentially cubic (this was not the case with older scanners). A variety of image reconstruction techniques can now map the CT data from each voxel to corresponding pixels on the workstation monitor in an increasing number of ways without geometric distortion. These techniques are discussed in the glossary of imaging terminology and techniques, but the important point is that image presentation has been extended well beyond routine axial CT slices to depicting anatomy in axial, coronal, and sagittal planes, oblique and curved planes, projectional techniques, and 3-D displays. Even holographic displays have become reality.

The graphics workstation, at which CT scans are interpreted, has become a medical instrument. This book demonstrates that with the current generation of CT scanners it has become common for physicians to view anatomic structures in ways that correspond with, or even match, the wonderful anatomic illustrations in the Netter Atlas.

Magnetic Resonance Imaging

Within static and gradient magnetic fields, a complex series of rapid radiofrequency (RF) pulses (radio waves) are applied to the patient and result in echoes of RF pulses detected by a receiver coil (essentially a radio antenna). In clinical MRI, it is the electromag-

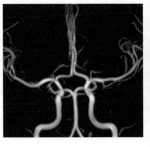 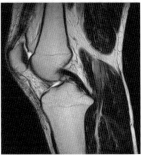

netic property of spin of water protons that is affected by the magnetic fields and RF pulses. To simplify, after an RF pulse tilts a proton out of alignment with the main magnetic field, it emits an RF pulse as it returns to its state before the applied pulse. The frequency and amplitude of the emitted signal depend on the physiochemical environment of that proton, strength of the magnetic field, timing of intervals between applied RF pulses, and time interval between an applied pulse and the measurement of the returning RF echo. A number of intravenous contrast agents containing gadolinium, which has strong paramagnetic properties, are used to enhance MR tissue contrast.

A variety of coils are available for the scanning of different body parts. The timing and character of MR pulse sequences affect tissue contrast. High MR signal in a returning RF echo is depicted as bright on the image reconstruction. A large variety of MR pulse sequences are available. Some of these sequences result in high signal from fluid. Some sequences specifically suppress the MR signal from fat. Most MRI protocols not only include imaging in several anatomic planes, but also a variety of specific MR pulse sequences that can ideally reveal tissue characteristics. These protocols are prescribed based on the body part being studied and the suspected pathology.

When CT images were still largely confined to the axial plane, MRI was a revolutionary way to view anatomic structures in all three orthogonal planes—axial, sagittal, and coronal. In some MRI applications, volumetric datasets are acquired, allowing the reformatting of images in ways comparable to CT. Although the multi-planar and volumetric capability of MRI is now matched by CT, MRI is still unequaled in its exquisite soft tissue contrast resolution. This often allows the detection of pathology not revealed by other diagnostic imaging technologies. Diseased tissues often have increased water content, and many MRI pulse sequences can show this clearly. Many MRI images in this atlas will clearly show how MRI can allow the viewing of anatomy that not long ago could be seen only in an anatomic atlas, the cadaver lab, or during open surgery. MRI is now also capable of providing astonishing spatial resolution, sometimes showing fine anatomy that is easily seen in vivo only with magnification. Many of the drawings in the Netter Atlas similarly show very fine anatomic details, for which our selected MR images comprise excellent matches.

Selection of Images for This Atlas

In selecting and creating images for this atlas, the authors frequently had to choose between diagnostic images that are in very common use (axial, coronal, and sagittal slices) or images that result from more advanced reconstruction techniques—images that are not commonly found in clinical practice but that more clearly depict anatomic structures and relationships. When a "routine" image was found that matched the Netter atlas well and illustrated key anatomic points, it was selected. However, we decided to include many advanced image reconstructions such as maximum intensity projection and volume rendered ("3-D") displays.

Another issue on image selection has to do with "the ideal." The idealized anatomy depicted in Netter plates is wonderful for teaching anatomic relationships; however, they can lead a student into not recognizing structures "in real life." A perfect example is the suprarenal (adrenal) gland. When a radiologist looks at a Netter plate showing the adrenal gland, he or she will likely think, "I've never seen an adrenal that looks like that." We felt it important to select images that showed such differences.

When previously published and annotated images were ideal for a particular Netter plate, we decided to use those for the sake of efficiency, as well as for recognition of work well done by others. Images in this atlas that are not credited to an outside source all came from The Imaging Center, Fort Wayne, Indiana and from radiologic facilities of the University of Wisconsin, Madison, Wisconsin.

The original imaging material used in this book was obtained from routine clinical scanning in a small, independent practice of diagnostic radiology. Because of concern about radiation exposure, no standard CT scan protocols were ever modified for the sake of producing an image. CT image data for the book were processed after patients had undergone routine scanning done appropriate to the medical reasons for which the scans were requested. None of these images came from a university or corporate imaging laboratory. They came from commercially available equipment in common use in the clinical practice of diagnostic radiology. The Imaging Center MRI scanner is an Infinion scanner from Philips Corporation. The

CT scanner used is a Brilliance 40, and the graphics workstation is the Extended Brilliance Workspace (EBW), both of these also manufactured by Philips.

Sonographic images of the musculoskeletal system presented in this atlas were obtained from routine clinical musculoskeletal ultrasound examinations that were performed at the University of Wisconsin Sports and Spine Imaging Center.

Often, the discovery of images useful for this atlas occurred while doing routine work in diagnostic radiology. The process of interpreting a CT scan, for example, is now one of clinical digital dissection, exposing views of a patient's anatomy with a computer mouse instead of a scalpel. It is hardly a coincidence when an ideal view for diagnosis is similar to a perspective on anatomic structures shown in the Netter Atlas.

Finally, our choices for "matching" a Netter plate were motivated primarily by an interest in teaching anatomy. In clinical practice, however, such decisions—should this patient have a CT or MR scan?—are usually driven by a motivation to reveal pathology that is suspected clinically. As imaging capabilities rapidly advance, it is often difficult to select the best diagnostic imaging procedure for each clinical problem. In making such decisions, patient care often benefits from consultation with an imaging specialist. As an excellent example of this decision making process, we recommend the "ACR Appropriateness Criteria" produced by The American College of Radiology.

Section 1   Head and Neck

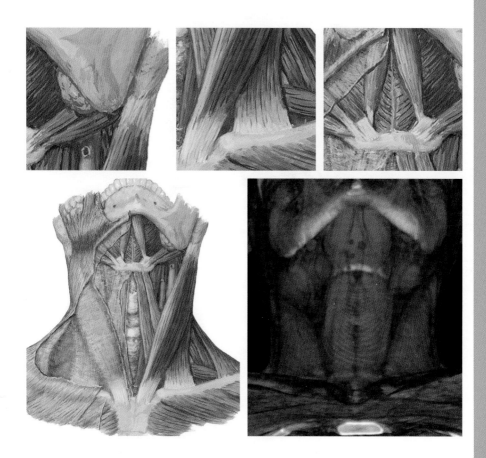

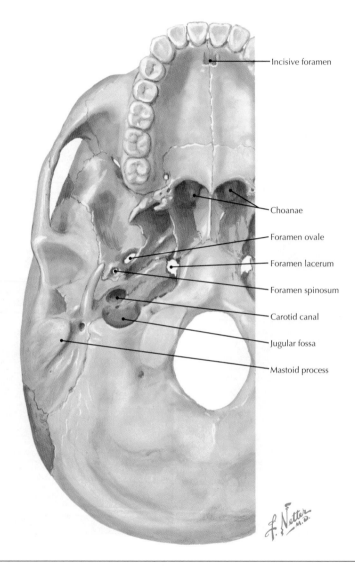

Incisive foramen

Choanae

Foramen ovale

Foramen lacerum

Foramen spinosum

Carotid canal

Jugular fossa

Mastoid process

Inferior view of the skull showing foramina *(Atlas of Human Anatomy, 6th edition, Plate 12)*

Clinical Note Maxillofacial three-dimensional (3-D) displays are very helpful in preoperative planning to correct deformities caused by trauma, tumor, or congenital malformations.

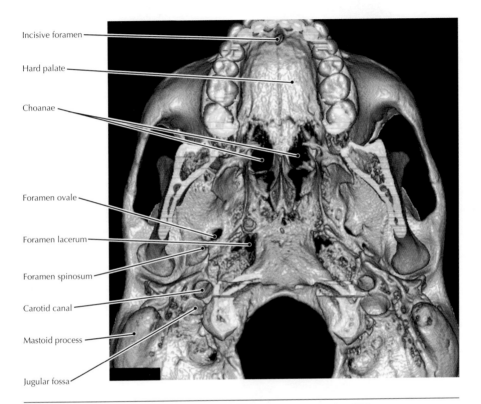

Incisive foramen
Hard palate
Choanae
Foramen ovale
Foramen lacerum
Foramen spinosum
Carotid canal
Mastoid process
Jugular fossa

Volume rendered display, maxillofacial computed tomography (CT)

- 3-D volume reconstructions have been shown to be useful for detecting the extent and exact nature of fractures of the skull base.
- The nasopalatine nerve is sensory to the anterior hard palate and may be anesthetized by injection into the incisive foramen.
- The mandibular branch of the trigeminal nerve (V_3) passes through the foramen ovale to innervate the muscles of mastication.

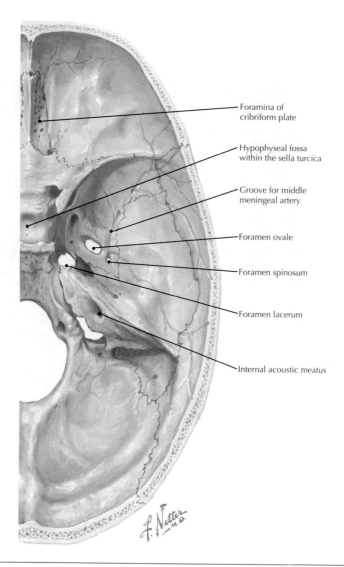

- Foramina of cribriform plate
- Hypophyseal fossa within the sella turcica
- Groove for middle meningeal artery
- Foramen ovale
- Foramen spinosum
- Foramen lacerum
- Internal acoustic meatus

Interior of skull showing foramina *(Atlas of Human Anatomy, 6th edition, Plate 13)*

Clinical Note The groove for the middle meningeal artery runs along the inner margin of the thinnest part of the lateral skull known as pterion; accordingly, a fracture of this region may result in an extradural hematoma.

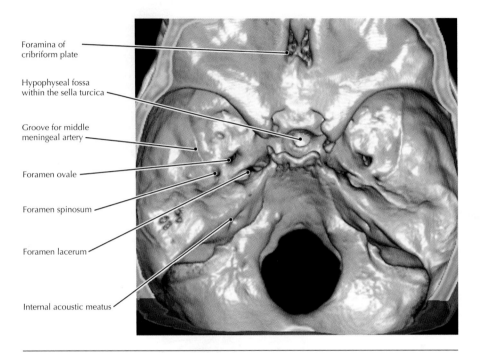

Foramina of
cribriform plate

Hypophyseal fossa
within the sella turcica

Groove for middle
meningeal artery

Foramen ovale

Foramen spinosum

Foramen lacerum

Internal acoustic meatus

Volume rendered display, CT of skull base

- The middle meningeal artery, a branch of the maxillary artery, enters the skull through the foramen spinosum.

- Foramina tend to be less apparent in radiographic images than in anatomic illustrations because of their obliquity.

- A volume rendered display may be useful in demonstrating tumor erosion of bone in the skull base because the skull base consists of many complex curved contours that are only partially shown in any single cross-sectional image. Scrolling through a series of such images may allow one to create a mental picture of bony involvement by tumor. A three-dimensional reconstruction, however, offers an accurate representation that is immediately comprehended.

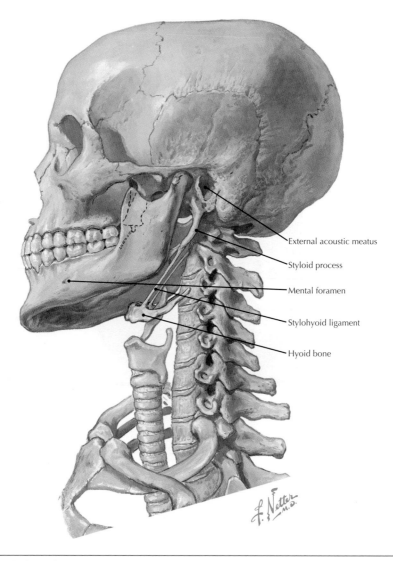

External acoustic meatus

Styloid process

Mental foramen

Stylohyoid ligament

Hyoid bone

Lateral view of the skeletal elements of the head and neck *(Atlas of Human Anatomy, 6th edition, Plate 15)*

Clinical Note In criminal proceedings, the finding of a fractured hyoid bone is considered to be strong evidence of strangulation.

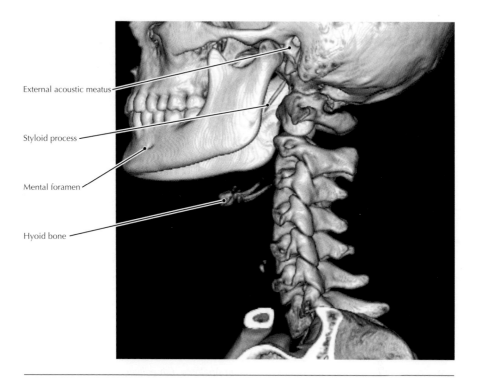

External acoustic meatus

Styloid process

Mental foramen

Hyoid bone

Volume rendered display, maxillofacial CT

- The lesser horn of the hyoid bone is attached to the stylohyoid ligament, which sometimes ossifies. An elongated styloid process in association with such an ossified ligament (or even without such ossification) can produce neck/swallowing pain and is known as Eagle's syndrome.

- In elderly patients who are edentulous, resorption of the alveolar process of the mandible exposes the mental nerve to pressure during chewing as it exits the foramen. Mastication then becomes a painful process for these patients.

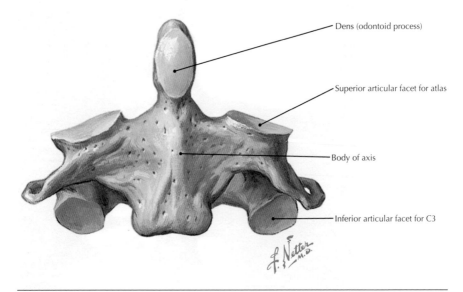

Dens (odontoid process)

Superior articular facet for atlas

Body of axis

Inferior articular facet for C3

Anterior view of the axis (C2) *(Atlas of Human Anatomy, 6th edition, Plate 19)*

Clinical Note The dens is susceptible to fracture that is classified by the level of the fracture site. The most common fracture occurs at the base of the dens (type II fracture).

Dens (odontoid process)

Superior articular facet for atlas

Body of axis

Inferior articular facet for C3

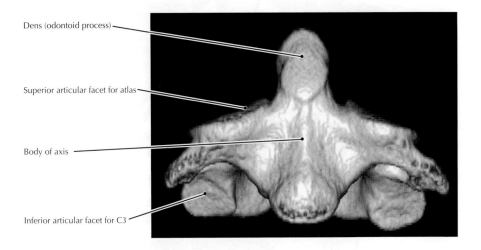

Volume rendered CT scan, axis

- The dens is embryologically the vertebral body of the atlas (C1).
- The articular facet on the dens articulates with the facet on the anterior arch of the atlas.
- In rare cases the dens does not appear on radiographs to be fused with the remainder of the vertebra. This condition, known as *os odontoideum,* may result in atlantoaxial instability.

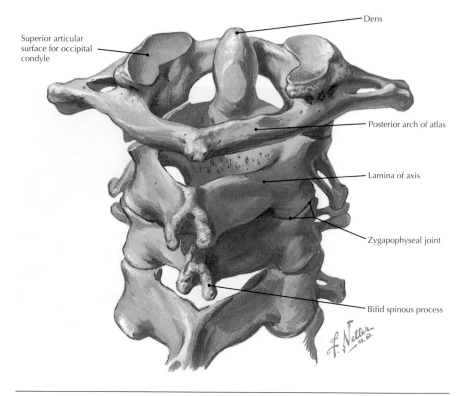

Dens

Superior articular surface for occipital condyle

Posterior arch of atlas

Lamina of axis

Zygapophyseal joint

Bifid spinous process

Posterior view of articulated C1-C4 vertebrae *(Atlas of Human Anatomy, 6th edition, Plate 19)*

Clinical Note   The hangman's fracture consists of bilateral pedicle or pars interarticularis fractures of the axis. Associated with this fracture is anterior subluxation or dislocation of the C2 vertebral body. It results from a severe extension injury, such as occurs from hanging.

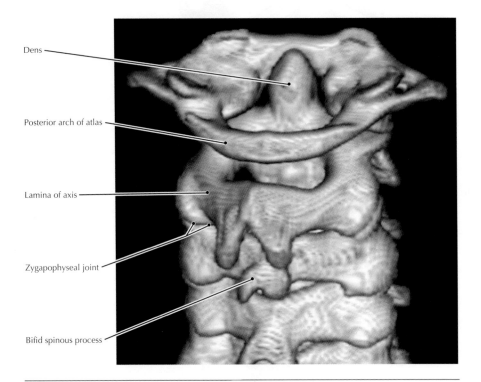

Dens

Posterior arch of atlas

Lamina of axis

Zygapophyseal joint

Bifid spinous process

Volume rendered display, cervical spine CT

- In the cervical region the articular facets of the zygapophyseal joints are oriented superiorly and inferiorly; thus, this is the only region of the vertebral column in which it is possible for adjoining vertebrae to dislocate (rotary) without fracture.

- The zygapophyseal joints are well innervated by medial branches from dorsal rami associated with both vertebral levels participating in the joint. To denervate a painful arthritic joint, the medial branches from both levels must be ablated.

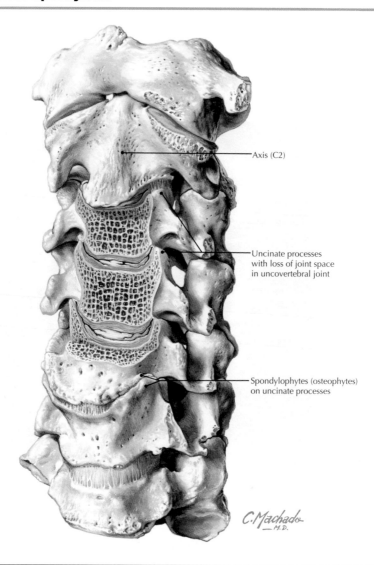

Axis (C2)

Uncinate processes with loss of joint space in uncovertebral joint

Spondylophytes (osteophytes) on uncinate processes

C. Machado
—M.D.

Degenerative changes in cervical vertebrae

Clinical Note Degenerative changes of the uncovertebral joints (of Luschka) typically occur with other degenerative changes such as the development of spondylophytes and the loss of intervertebral disc space. These changes reduce the size of the intervertebral foramina (neuroforamina) resulting in radiculopathy and associated pain, paresthesia, and numbness in the corresponding dermatomes.

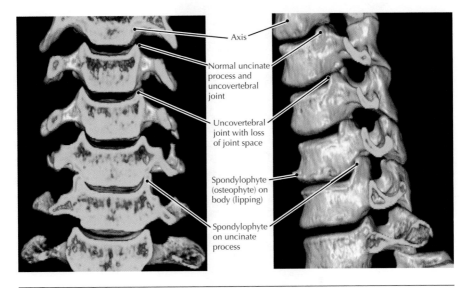

Volume rendered displays, cervical spine CT

- Surgeons may use an anterior or a posterior approach to address cervical spondylosis. A bone graft is inserted into the disc space to restore vertical spacing between segments and a metal plate is attached along the anterior margin of the spine to provide stability during the process of intervertebral bone fusion.

- The uncovertebral joints contribute to cervical spine stability and help to limit extension and lateral bending.

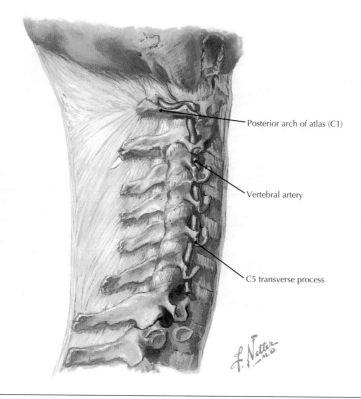

Posterior arch of atlas (C1)

Vertebral artery

C5 transverse process

Lateral view of the cervical spine and vertebral artery *(Atlas of Human Anatomy, 6th edition, Plate 22)*

Clinical Note Vertebral artery dissection, a subintimal hematoma, may cause cerebellar or brain infarction; occurrence may be idiopathic or secondary to trauma.

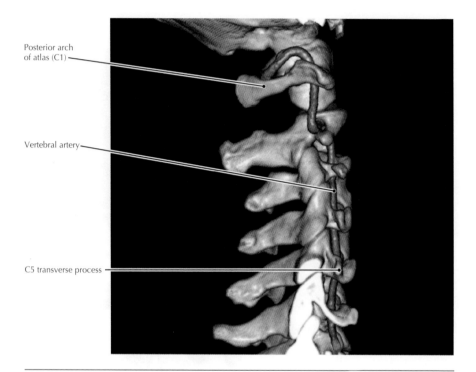

Posterior arch
of atlas (C1)

Vertebral artery

C5 transverse process

Volume rendered display, CTA of the neck

- The intimate association of the vertebral artery to the cervical spine makes it
  susceptible to injury during cervical spine trauma.
- The vertebral artery is typically the first branch of the subclavian artery, although it
  can arise directly from the arch of the aorta.
- Most commonly, the vertebral artery enters the foramina of the transverse
  processes of the cervical vertebrae at C6.

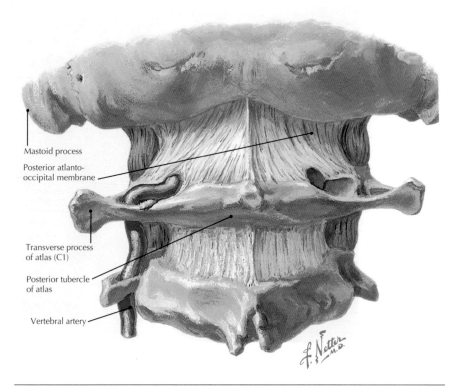

Mastoid process

Posterior atlanto-
occipital membrane

Transverse process
of atlas (C1)

Posterior tubercle
of atlas

Vertebral artery

Vertebral artery on the posterior arch of the atlas *(Atlas of Human Anatomy, 6th edition, Plate 22)*

Clinical Note This is the most tortuous segment of the vertebral artery; increases in tortuosity are associated with atherosclerotic changes.

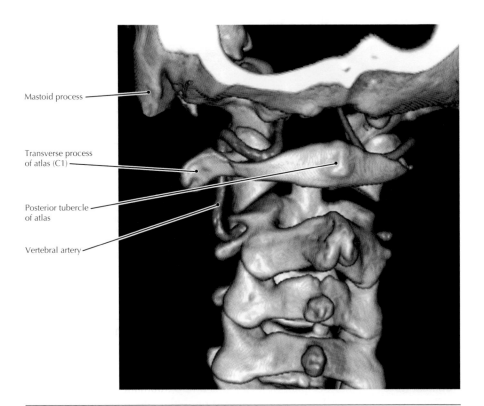

Mastoid process

Transverse process
of atlas (C1)

Posterior tubercle
of atlas

Vertebral artery

Volume rendered display, CTA of the neck

- The vertebral artery pierces the dura and arachnoid mater and ascends anterior to the medulla to unite with the contralateral vessel to form the basilar artery.
- The vertebral artery supplies the muscles of the suboccipital triangle before entering the cranial cavity.

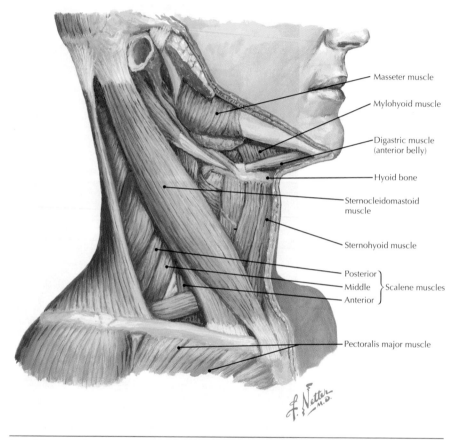

Masseter muscle

Mylohyoid muscle

Digastric muscle
(anterior belly)

Hyoid bone

Sternocleidomastoid
muscle

Sternohyoid muscle

Posterior ⎫
Middle ⎬ Scalene muscles
Anterior ⎭

Pectoralis major muscle

Lateral view of the superficial muscles of the neck *(Atlas of Human Anatomy, 6th edition, Plate 29)*

Clinical Note Congenital torticollis (wryneck) is typically associated with a birth injury to the sternocleidomastoid muscle that results in a unilateral shortening of the muscle, and the associated rotated and tilted head position.

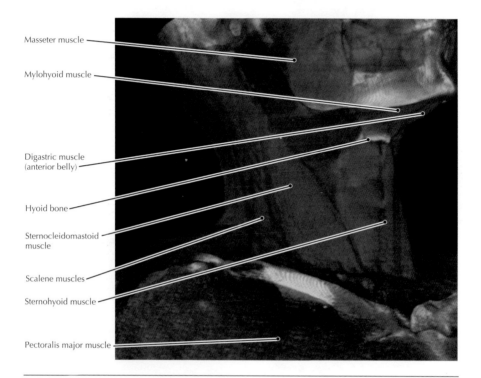

Masseter muscle

Mylohyoid muscle

Digastric muscle
(anterior belly)

Hyoid bone

Sternocleidomastoid
muscle

Scalene muscles

Sternohyoid muscle

Pectoralis major muscle

Volume rendered display, CT of the neck

- The sternocleidomastoid is a large and consistent anatomic structure that is easily identifiable and is used to divide the neck into anterior and posterior triangles.

- The hyoid bone provides an anchor for many neck muscles and is suspended solely by these muscles (it has no bony articulation).

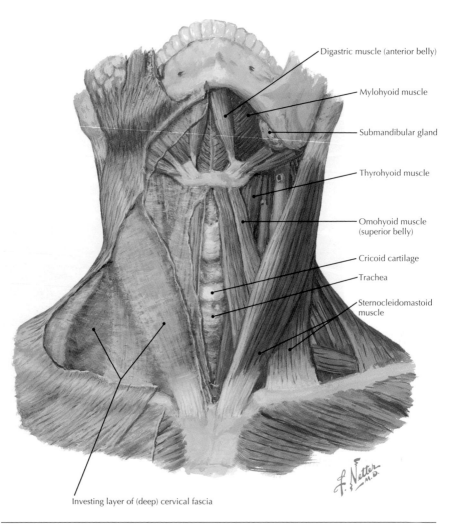

Digastric muscle (anterior belly)

Mylohyoid muscle

Submandibular gland

Thyrohyoid muscle

Omohyoid muscle (superior belly)

Cricoid cartilage

Trachea

Sternocleidomastoid muscle

Investing layer of (deep) cervical fascia

Anterior view of the superficial muscles of the neck (*Atlas of Human Anatomy, 6th edition, Plate 27*)

Clinical Note When a tracheostomy is performed, the trachea is entered inferior to the cricoid cartilage in the midline, between the right and left groups of strap (infrahyoid) muscles.

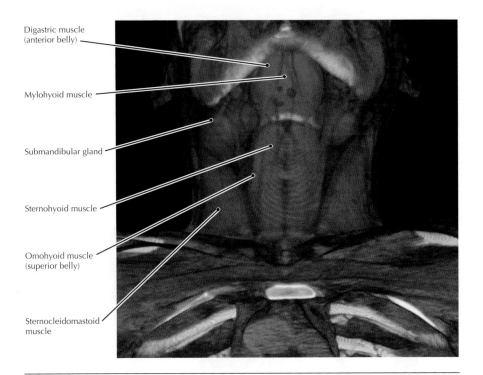

Digastric muscle
(anterior belly)

Mylohyoid muscle

Submandibular gland

Sternohyoid muscle

Omohyoid muscle
(superior belly)

Sternocleidomastoid
muscle

Volume rendered display, CT of the neck

- All of the strap muscles (sternohyoid, sternothyroid, thyrohyoid, and omohyoid) are innervated by the ansa cervicalis, which is made up of fibers from the ventral rami of C1-C3.
- The strap muscles are covered by the investing layer of the deep cervical fascia.

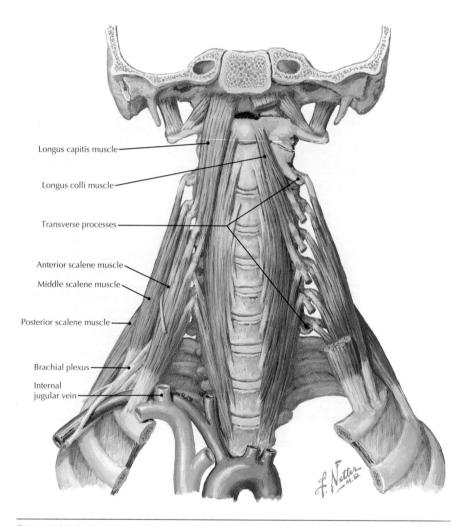

Longus capitis muscle

Longus colli muscle

Transverse processes

Anterior scalene muscle

Middle scalene muscle

Posterior scalene muscle

Brachial plexus

Internal
jugular vein

Prevertebral muscles and the three scalene muscles *(Atlas of Human Anatomy, 6th edition, Plate 30)*

Clinical Note Compression of the structures within the scalene triangle (bordered by the anterior and middle scalene muscles, and the first rib) can produce a complex of vascular and neurologic signs and symptoms commonly referred to as thoracic outlet syndrome.

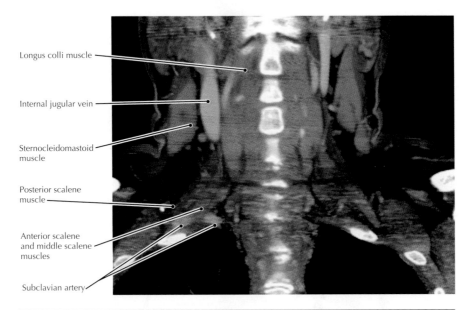

Longus colli muscle

Internal jugular vein

Sternocleidomastoid muscle

Posterior scalene muscle

Anterior scalene and middle scalene muscles

Subclavian artery

Coronal thin slab, volume rendered display, contrast-enhanced (CE) CT scan of the neck

- The longus colli and capitis muscles flex the head and neck.

- The scalene muscles originate from the cervical transverse processes; the anterior and middle scalenes insert onto the first rib whereas the posterior scalene inserts onto the second rib.

- Because the brachial plexus emerges posterior to the anterior scalene muscle, that muscle is a good landmark for finding the brachial plexus in coronal MR images.

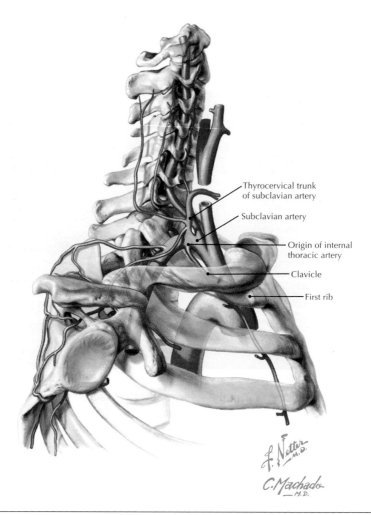

Thyrocervical trunk
of subclavian artery

Subclavian artery

Origin of internal
thoracic artery

Clavicle

First rib

Lateral view of the origin, path, and branches of the right subclavian artery

Clinical Note   The internal thoracic (mammary) artery (usually the left) is often used in coronary bypass operations. Lateral thoracic and intercostal arteries then supply the chest wall structures normally supplied by the internal thoracic artery.

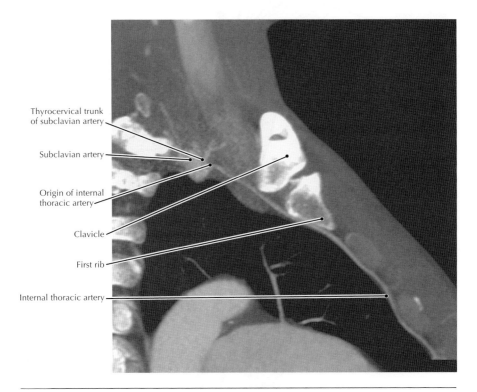

Thyrocervical trunk of subclavian artery

Subclavian artery

Origin of internal thoracic artery

Clavicle

First rib

Internal thoracic artery

Oblique sagittal maximum intensity projection (MIP), CE CTA of the lower neck and upper chest

- The internal thoracic (mammary) artery arises from the subclavian artery near the thyrocervical trunk.

- The branches of the thyrocervical trunk are the suprascapular, transverse cervical (superficial cervical), and inferior thyroid arteries.

- This type of image may be used to document the patency of an internal thoracic artery coronary bypass graft.

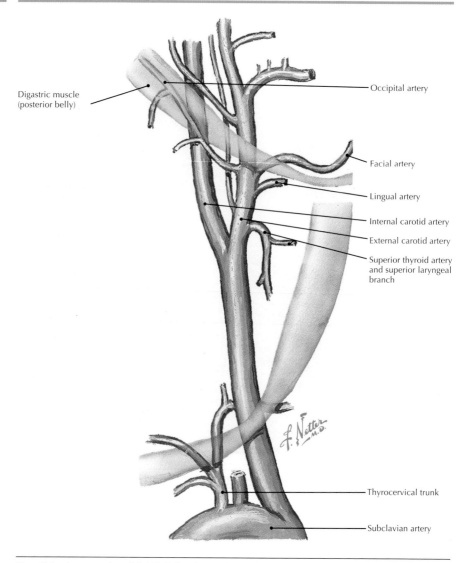

Digastric muscle
(posterior belly)

Occipital artery

Facial artery

Lingual artery

Internal carotid artery

External carotid artery

Superior thyroid artery
and superior laryngeal
branch

Thyrocervical trunk

Subclavian artery

Carotid artery system highlighting branches of the external carotid *(Atlas of Human Anatomy, 6th edition, Plate 34)*

Clinical Note   Ligation of the external carotid artery is sometimes necessary to control hemorrhage from one of its branches (e.g., in cases of otherwise uncontrollable epistaxis). Some blood continues to reach the structures served by the ligated vessel via collateral circulation from the contralateral external carotid artery.

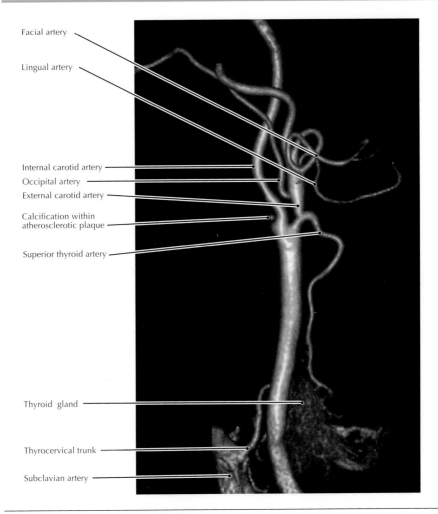

Facial artery

Lingual artery

Internal carotid artery

Occipital artery

External carotid artery

Calcification within
atherosclerotic plaque

Superior thyroid artery

Thyroid gland

Thyrocervical trunk

Subclavian artery

Volume rendered display, carotid CTA

- The thyroid gland would be the same density as shown here in a CT scan done without intravenous (IV) contrast because of its high iodine content, a "natural" contrast agent.

- A "dot" of calcification within atherosclerotic plaque in the most caudal part of the internal carotid artery (directly superior to the bifurcation) is visible.

- Often the lingual and facial arteries arise from a single stem, known as the linguofacial trunk.

- The occipital artery travels with the greater occipital nerve to supply the posterior aspect of the scalp.

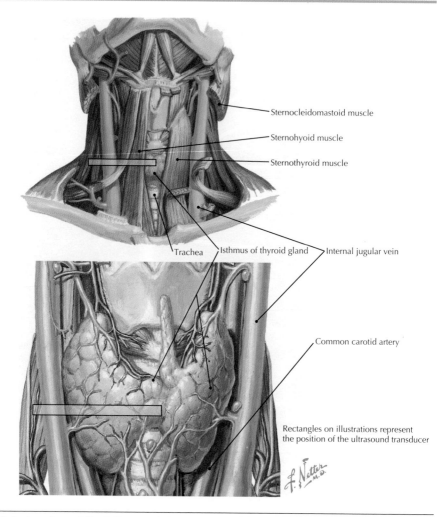

- Sternocleidomastoid muscle
- Sternohyoid muscle
- Sternothyroid muscle
- Trachea
- Isthmus of thyroid gland
- Internal jugular vein
- Common carotid artery

Rectangles on illustrations represent the position of the ultrasound transducer

Anterior view of the isthmus of the thyroid gland *(Atlas of Human Anatomy, 6th edition, Plates 28, 76)*

Clinical Note Ultrasound (US) is the primary imaging modality for examining morphologic abnormalities of the thyroid gland. Because of the intimate relationship between the common carotid artery and the thyroid gland, carotid sonography often reveals unsuspected, incidental thyroid nodules. A standard procedure to evaluate thyroid nodules that are suspicious for cancer is US-guided fine-needle aspiration. A radionuclide scan and radioiodine uptake measurement, along with serum chemistries, are used to evaluate thyroid function.

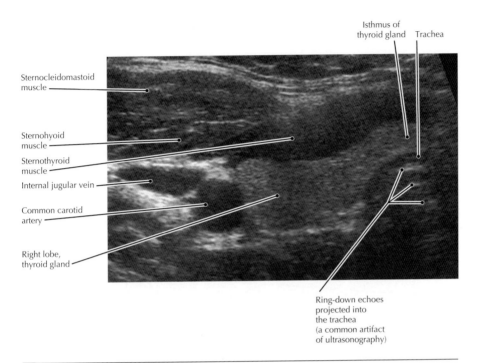

Isthmus of
thyroid gland   Trachea

Sternocleidomastoid
muscle

Sternohyoid
muscle

Sternothyroid
muscle

Internal jugular vein

Common carotid
artery

Right lobe,
thyroid gland

Ring-down echoes
projected into
the trachea
(a common artifact
of ultrasonography)

Axial US at the level of the thyroid isthmus

- Approximately half of all people have a pyramidal lobe of the thyroid gland that may reach the hyoid bone via connective tissue.

- A normal parathyroid gland is occasionally seen on thyroid US scans as a small hypoechoic nodule at the posterior margin of the thyroid, but this usually is not apparent. The number and size of parathyroid glands are extremely variable.

- The shape of the thin-walled internal jugular vein depends on intraluminal pressure, may vary with the patient's state of hydration and cardiac status (distended with elevated right cardiac pressures), and can be observed to vary with respiration.

Neck, Axial Section at Thyroid Gland

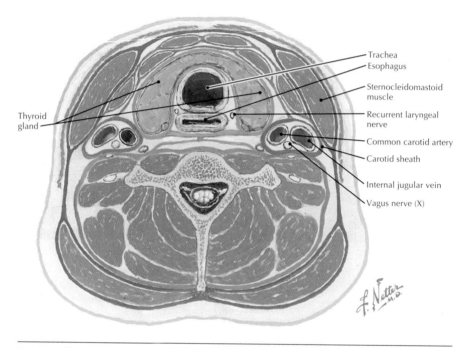

Trachea
Esophagus
Sternocleidomastoid muscle
Thyroid gland
Recurrent laryngeal nerve
Common carotid artery
Carotid sheath
Internal jugular vein
Vagus nerve (X)

Axial section of the neck at C7 showing fascial layers *(Atlas of Human Anatomy, 6th edition, Plate 26)*

Clinical Note The location of the vagus nerve within the carotid sheath renders it susceptible to injury during carotid endarterectomy. Also, the recurrent laryngeal nerve innervates most of the muscles of the larynx and may be injured during surgery on the thyroid gland.

Head and Neck

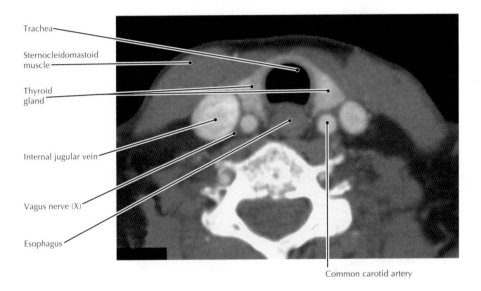

Trachea
Sternocleidomastoid muscle
Thyroid gland
Internal jugular vein
Vagus nerve (X)
Esophagus
Common carotid artery

Axial CE CT of the neck

- The asymmetry in the diameters of the left and right internal jugular veins, shown here, is typical.

- The esophagus is normally collapsed so its lumen is not typically apparent in CT images. Occasionally air just swallowed by a patient (or an eructation) may expand the lumen so that it becomes evident.

Nasal Conchae

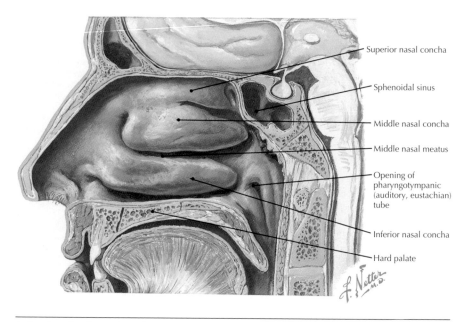

Superior nasal concha

Sphenoidal sinus

Middle nasal concha

Middle nasal meatus

Opening of
pharyngotympanic
(auditory, eustachian)
tube

Inferior nasal concha

Hard palate

Lateral wall of nasal cavity highlighting conchae (turbinates) *(Atlas of Human Anatomy, 6th edition, Plate 36)*

Clinical Note Inferior concha (turbinate) enlargement associated with chronic rhinitis or nasal septum deviation may compromise respiratory function (nasal breathing) in some patients. Surgical reduction or removal of the concha often provides relief in these cases.

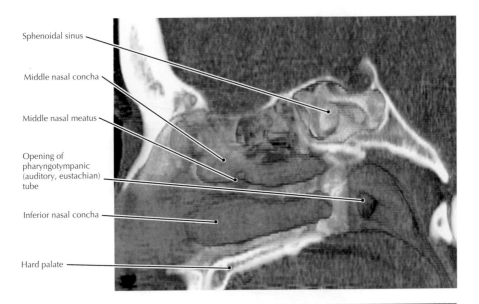

Sphenoidal sinus

Middle nasal concha

Middle nasal meatus

Opening of
pharyngotympanic
(auditory, eustachian)
tube

Inferior nasal concha

Hard palate

Volume rendered display, CT scan of paranasal sinuses

- The nasal conchae provide increased surface area in the airway in order to warm and moisturize the inspired air and to filter out particulate matter.

- Each concha has a space inferior and lateral to it (meati). The nasolacrimal duct drains into the inferior meatus, and paranasal sinuses drain into the superior and middle meati.

- The location of the opening of the pharyngotympanic (auditory, eustachian) tube directly posterior to the inferior concha explains how severe nasal congestion can occlude the opening and thus reduce hearing efficacy.

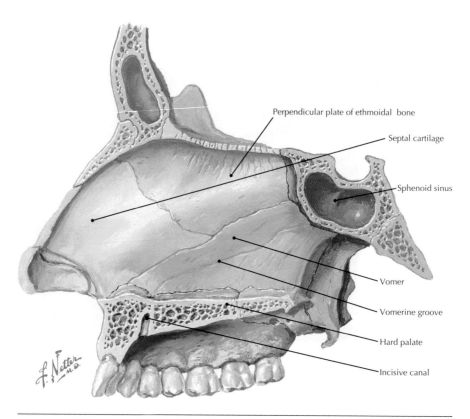

Perpendicular plate of ethmoidal bone

Septal cartilage

Sphenoid sinus

Vomer

Vomerine groove

Hard palate

Incisive canal

Medial wall of nasal cavity (nasal septum) *(Atlas of Human Anatomy, 6th edition, Plate 38)*

Clinical Note Approximately 80% of all nasal septums are off-center, a condition that is generally unsymptomatic. A "deviated septum" occurs when the septum is severely shifted away from the midline. The most common symptom associated with a highly deviated septum is difficulty with nasal breathing. The symptoms are usually worse on one side. In some cases, the crooked septum can interfere with sinus drainage, resulting in chronic nasal infections. Septoplasty is the preferred surgical treatment to correct a deviated septum.

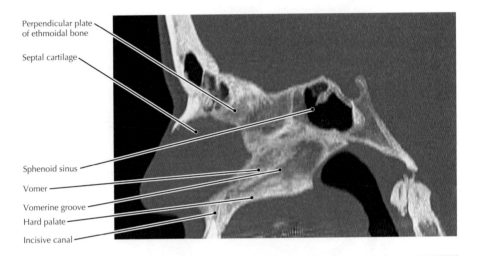

Perpendicular plate
of ethmoidal bone

Septal cartilage

Sphenoid sinus

Vomer

Vomerine groove

Hard palate

Incisive canal

Sagittal thin slab MIP, CT scan of paranasal sinuses

- The vomerine groove is for the nasopalatine nerve and vessels, which are branches of the maxillary nerve (V_2) and artery. These structures pass through the incisive foramen to supply the most anterior part of the hard palate.

- The hard palate is formed by the palatine process of the maxilla and the horizontal plate of the palatine bone.

- Small parts of the maxilla and palatine bones also contribute to the formation of the nasal septum.

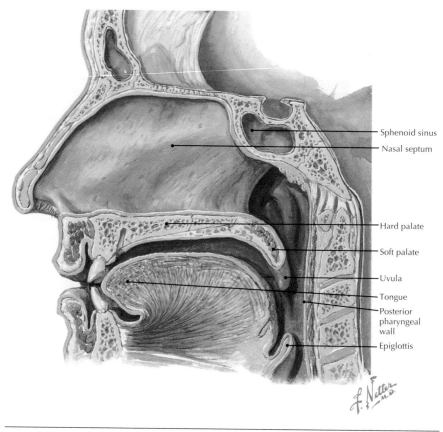

Medial view of the nasal septum and sagittal section through oral cavity and pharynx *(Atlas of Human Anatomy, 6th edition, Plate 38)*

Clinical Note Uvulopalatoplasty is a surgical procedure that reshapes the soft palate and uvula to reduce airflow resistance and thereby reduce sleep apnea and snoring.

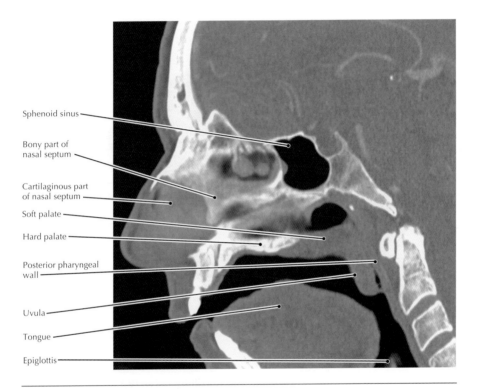

Sphenoid sinus

Bony part of
nasal septum

Cartilaginous part
of nasal septum

Soft palate

Hard palate

Posterior pharyngeal
wall

Uvula

Tongue

Epiglottis

Sagittal reconstruction, maxillofacial CT

- During swallowing and the production of certain sounds (e.g., whistling) the soft palate is approximated to the posterior pharyngeal wall.

- The tongue is composed of both intrinsic and extrinsic muscles, all but one of which are innervated by the hypoglossal nerve (XII).

Pterygopalatine Fossa

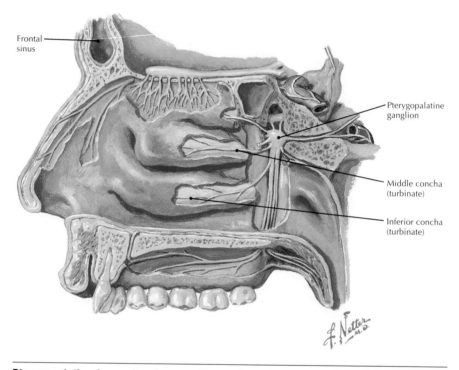

Frontal sinus

Pterygopalatine ganglion

Middle concha (turbinate)

Inferior concha (turbinate)

Pterygopalatine fossa showing ganglion and maxillary nerve (V₂) *(Atlas of Human Anatomy, 6th edition, Plate 39)*

Clinical Note Cluster headache, a unilateral headache with the pain typically occurring around the eyes, temple, and forehead, may be related to irritation of the ipsilateral pterygopalatine ganglion.

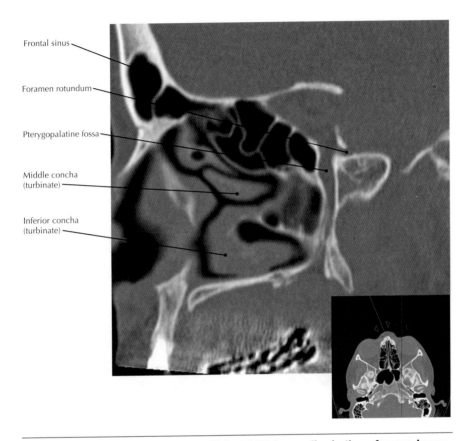

Frontal sinus

Foramen rotundum

Pterygopalatine fossa

Middle concha
(turbinate)

Inferior concha
(turbinate)

Oblique sagittal reconstruction, maxillofacial CT (*green line* in the reference image indicates the position and orientation of the main image)

- To obtain an image through the foramen rotundum, the plane of section had to be rotated away from a midsagittal plane (see *green line* in axial reference image).
- The pterygopalatine ganglion receives preganglionic parasympathetic fibers from the facial nerve via the nerve of the pterygoid canal (Vidian nerve).
- Posterior superior lateral nasal branches from maxillary nerve (V_2) innervate the mucosa of the middle turbinate.
- Posterior inferior lateral nasal branch from maxillary nerve (V_2) innervates the mucosa of the inferior turbinate.

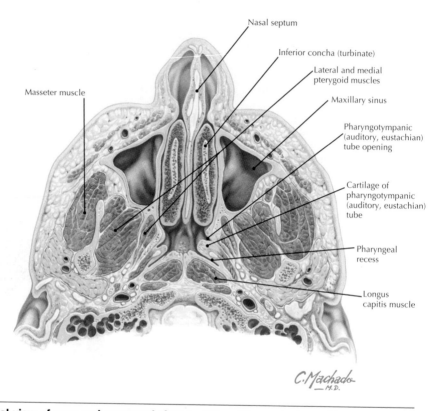

Axial view of nose and paranasal sinuses *(Atlas of Human Anatomy, 6th edition, Plate 42)*

Clinical Note Children are more susceptible to middle ear infections than adults because the pharyngotympanic (auditory, eustachian) tube is shorter and straighter, thus more easily allowing invasion of bacteria from the nasopharynx.

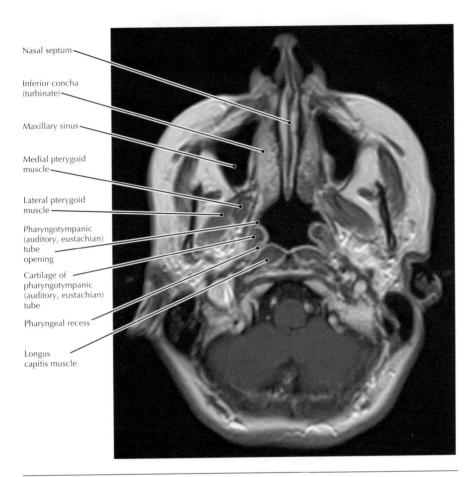

Nasal septum

Inferior concha
(turbinate)

Maxillary sinus

Medial pterygoid
muscle

Lateral pterygoid
muscle

Pharyngotympanic
(auditory, eustachian)
tube
opening

Cartilage of
pharyngotympanic
(auditory, eustachian)
tube

Pharyngeal recess

Longus
capitis muscle

Axial CE T1 MR image of the nasopharynx

- The MR image illustrates how the high MR signal (brightness) of fat on T1 images may clearly outline and separate nonfatty structures.

- The mucosa of the nasopharynx shows high signal (lighter shade of gray on image) on this gadolinium-enhanced T1 MR image. This is normal and can be helpful in displaying mucosal tumors that may interrupt the smooth, contrast-enhanced mucosa.

Olfactory Bulbs

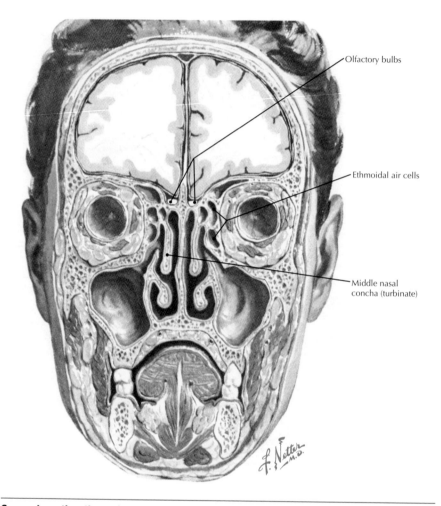

Olfactory bulbs

Ethmoidal air cells

Middle nasal
concha (turbinate)

Coronal section through anterior head *(Atlas of Human Anatomy, 6th edition, Plate 43)*

Clinical Note Anosmia may result from head injury because the olfactory nerves are delicate and are easily torn along their path to the olfactory bulb; anosmia may be the presenting symptom of a tumor of olfactory tissue (esthesioneuroblastoma).

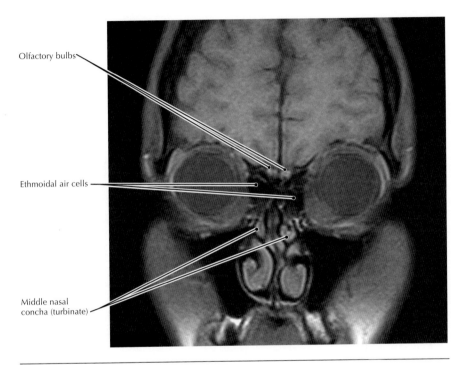

Olfactory bulbs

Ethmoidal air cells

Middle nasal
concha (turbinate)

Coronal fat-suppressed (FS) T1, maxillofacial MR image

- The olfactory bulbs receive the bipolar olfactory nerves that are stimulated by odors detected in the nasal cavity. These nerves pass through the foramina in the cribriform plate of the ethmoid bone.

- From the olfactory bulbs, the olfactory impulses are conducted via the olfactory tract to the temporal lobe of the brain.

- Compact bone and air have no signal in this or any MR image.

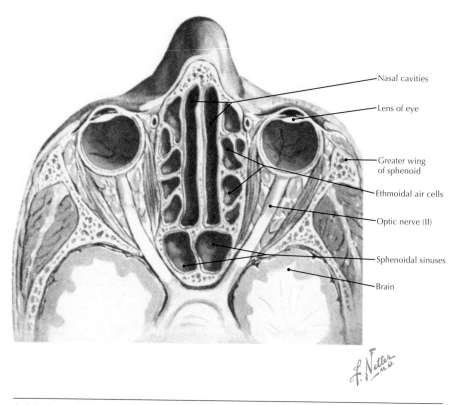

- Nasal cavities
- Lens of eye
- Greater wing of sphenoid
- Ethmoidal air cells
- Optic nerve (II)
- Sphenoidal sinuses
- Brain

Axial view of nasal cavity and paranasal sinuses *(Atlas of Human Anatomy, 6th edition, Plate 43)*

Clinical Note   Infections may spread from the ethmoidal air cells (labyrinth) causing inflammation of the optic nerve (optic neuritis).

Nasal cavities

Lens of eye

Greater wing of
sphenoid

Ethmoidal air cells

Optic nerve (II)

Sphenoidal sinuses

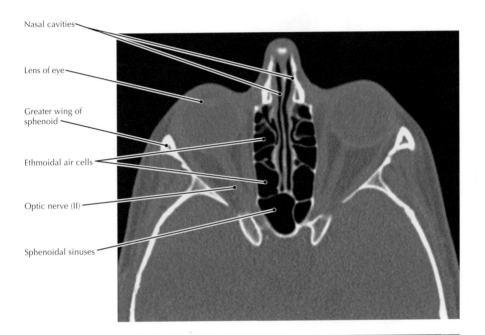

Axial CT, paranasal sinuses

- Anatomic variations in the drainage pathways of the ethmoid air cells and sphenoid sinus can lead to sinusitis.
- The ethmoid cells drain into both the middle and superior meati whereas the sphenoid sinus drains into the sphenoethmoidal recess.

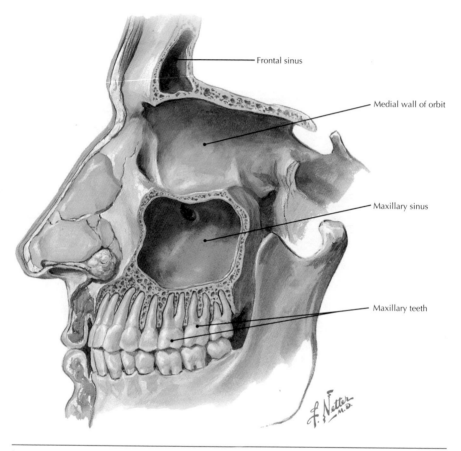

Frontal sinus

Medial wall of orbit

Maxillary sinus

Maxillary teeth

Lateral dissection of maxillary sinus *(Atlas of Human Anatomy, 6th edition, Plate 44)*

Clinical Note During the extraction of a maxillary tooth a dentist may inadvertently force a root into the maxillary sinus, forming a lumen between the oral cavity and the sinus. This may lead to chronic inflammation in the sinus.

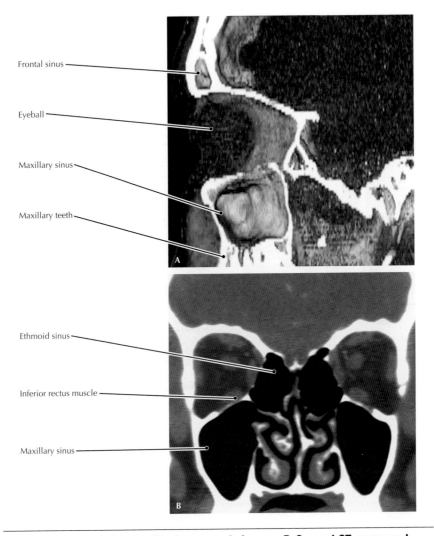

Frontal sinus

Eyeball

Maxillary sinus

Maxillary teeth

Ethmoid sinus

Inferior rectus muscle

Maxillary sinus

A, Volume rendered display, CT of paranasal sinuses; *B,* Coronal CT, paranasal sinuses

- A blowout fracture of the orbit may result in the herniation of orbital contents (e.g., inferior rectus muscle) into the maxillary sinus through the orbit's very thin floor.
- The posterior, middle, and anterior superior alveolar nerves (branches of V_2) pass through and along the walls of the maxillary sinus to innervate the maxillary teeth.

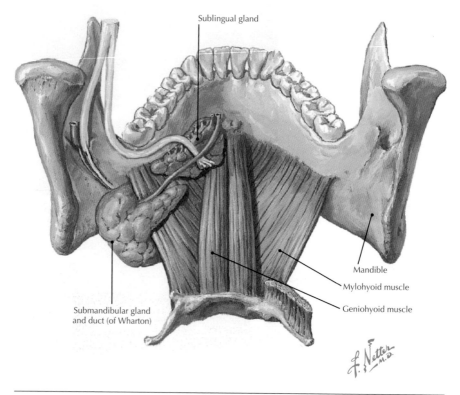

Sublingual gland

Mandible

Mylohyoid muscle

Geniohyoid muscle

Submandibular gland
and duct (of Wharton)

Superior view of the floor of the mouth *(Atlas of Human Anatomy, 6th edition, Plate 58)*

Clinical Note Ludwig's angina can involve swelling (cellulitis) of the portion of the submandibular gland superior to the mylohyoid, resulting in a potentially fatal obstruction of the airway. Swelling of the gland inferior to the mylohyoid presents as a lump in the neck.

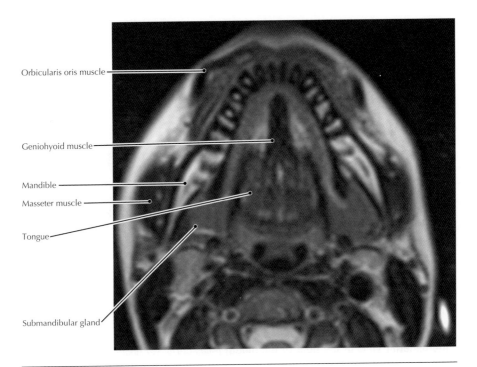

Orbicularis oris muscle

Geniohyoid muscle

Mandible

Masseter muscle

Tongue

Submandibular gland

Axial T2 MR image of the floor of the mouth

- The geniohyoid muscle is innervated by a branch from the ventral ramus of C1.
- The orbicularis oris is a muscle of facial expression that protrudes the lips and brings them together.
- The high signal of fatty marrow within the trabeculae (bright) of the mandible may be contrasted with the adjacent thick markedly hypodense cortical bone (dark).

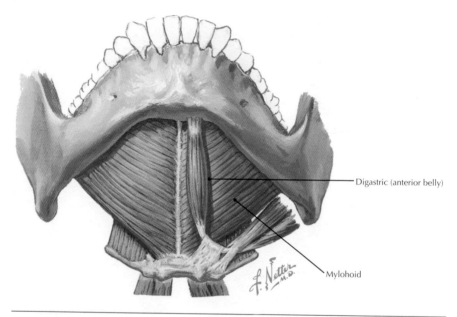

Digastric (anterior belly)

Mylohoid

Anteroinferior view of the floor of the mouth *(Atlas of Human Anatomy, 6th edition, Plate 58)*

Clinical Note Submental US is used to evaluate the aging neck to assess the relative contribution of various components of this region to age-related ptosis before cosmetic surgery. Submental US is also used to evaluate breastfeeding difficulties in infants.

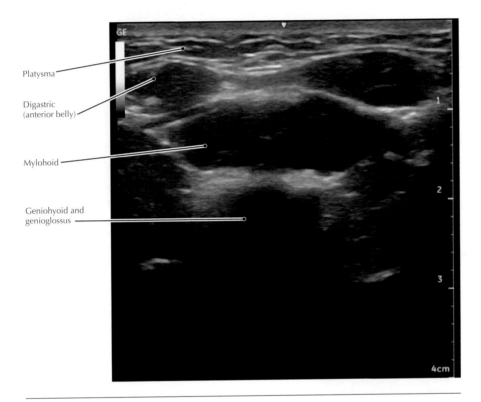

Platysma

Digastric
(anterior belly)

Mylohoid

Geniohyoid and
genioglossus

Axial US of the submental region

- The US transducer for evaluation of the submental region is placed under the chin so that the digastric muscle appears on "top" the mylohyoid muscle in this image, whereas the digastric is actually inferior to the mylohyoid, as shown in the illustration.
- The anterior belly of the digastric muscle is innervated by the mylohyoid nerve, a branch of the mandibular nerve, whereas the posterior belly is innervated by the facial nerve, which also innervates the platysma muscle.

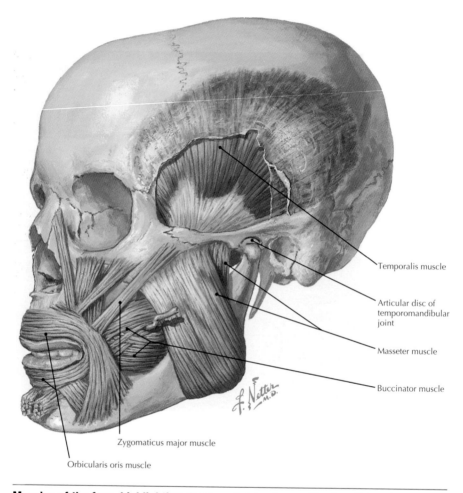

Temporalis muscle

Articular disc of temporomandibular joint

Masseter muscle

Buccinator muscle

Zygomaticus major muscle

Orbicularis oris muscle

Muscles of the face, highlighting those pertaining to mastication *(Atlas of Human Anatomy, 6th edition, Plate 48)*

Clinical Note An imbalance in the forces of the muscles of mastication can disturb the temporomandibular joint (TMJ). Excessive grinding of the teeth, especially during sleep, is known as bruxism. Both of these conditions can cause TMJ pain.

Temporalis muscle

Superficial temporal artery

Masseter muscle

Zygomaticus major muscle

Orbicularis oris muscle

Buccinator muscle

Facial vein

External jugular vein

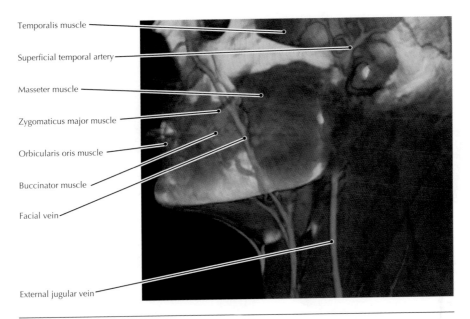

Volume rendered display, CE maxillofacial CT

- The buccinator muscle lies within the cheek and during chewing acts to keep food out of the vestibule. It, similar to all the muscles of facial expression, is innervated by the facial nerve (VII).

- The facial artery (adjacent to the facial vein but not visible in this CT display) crosses the body of the mandible at the anterior border of the masseter where it can be palpated and used to register a pulse.

Temporomandibular Joint

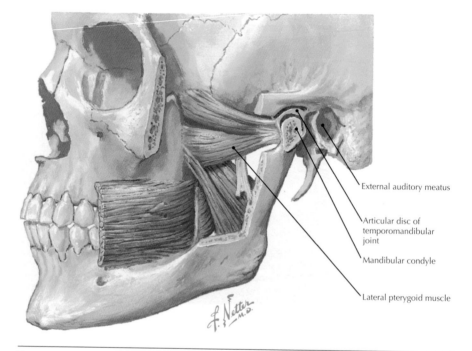

External auditory meatus

Articular disc of temporomandibular joint

Mandibular condyle

Lateral pterygoid muscle

Temporomandibular joint and muscles of mastication *(Atlas of Human Anatomy, 6th edition, Plate 49)*

Clinical Note Temporomandibular joint (TMJ) dysfunction is common after whiplash injuries. Presenting symptoms are pain and clicking during chewing.

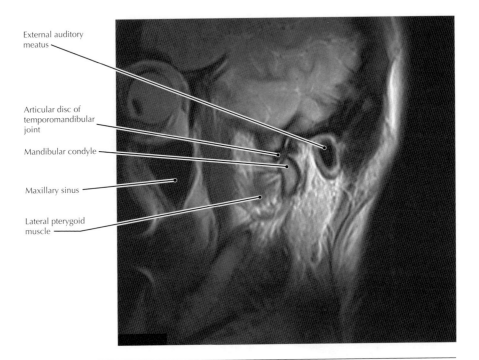

External auditory meatus

Articular disc of temporomandibular joint

Mandibular condyle

Maxillary sinus

Lateral pterygoid muscle

Sagittal T1 MR image, temporomandibular joint

- The articular disc divides the TMJ into two compartments. Protrusion and retrusion of the mandible occur in the superior compartment; elevation and depression occur in the inferior compartment.
- The lateral pterygoid muscle is the only major muscle of mastication that can assist gravity in opening the mouth (depressing the mandible).

Pterygoid Muscles

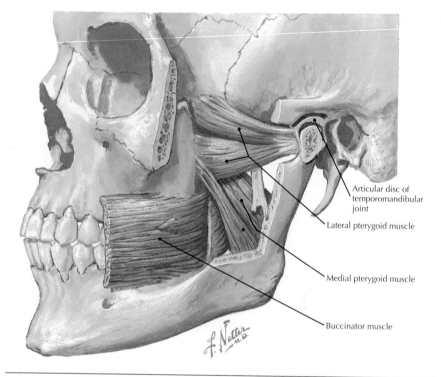

Articular disc of
temporomandibular
joint

Lateral pterygoid muscle

Medial pterygoid muscle

Buccinator muscle

Pterygoid muscles and buccinators *(Atlas of Human Anatomy, 6th edition, Plate 49)*

> **Clinical Note** Because of its insertion into the disc within the TMJ, abnormal
> lateral pterygoid muscle activity has been implicated in TMJ disorders.
> However, there is no firm evidence supporting this implication.

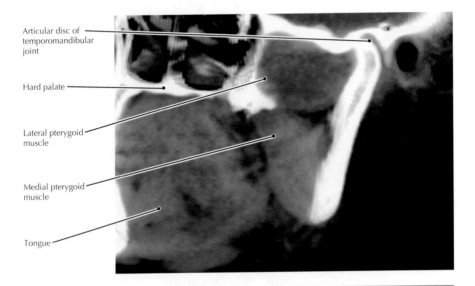

Articular disc of
temporomandibular
joint

Hard palate

Lateral pterygoid
muscle

Medial pterygoid
muscle

Tongue

Volume rendered display, maxillofacial CT

- Both pterygoid muscles arise primarily from the lateral pterygoid plate of the sphenoid bone, the lateral from its lateral surface and the medial from its medial surface.

- Alternate action of the pterygoids of each side produces a rotary (grinding) movement of the mandible that is important for effective mastication.

- Both pterygoid muscles are innervated by the mandibular division of the trigeminal nerve (V_3).

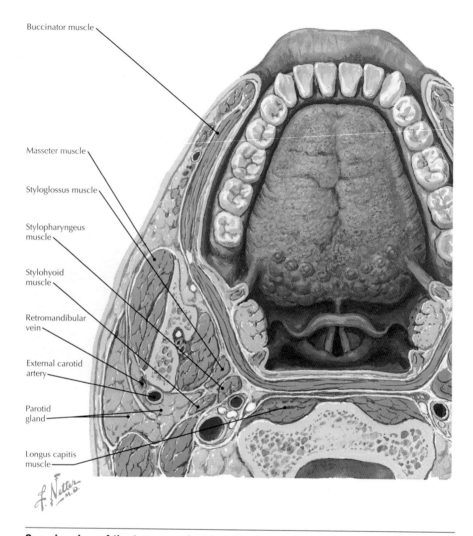

Buccinator muscle

Masseter muscle

Styloglossus muscle

Stylopharyngeus muscle

Stylohyoid muscle

Retromandibular vein

External carotid artery

Parotid gland

Longus capitis muscle

Superior view of the tongue and oral cavity *(Atlas of Human Anatomy, 6th edition, Plate 47)*

Clinical Note Taste buds are located in papillae on the surface of the tongue. Because of this superficial location taste buds are subject to direct attack from viral infections, chemicals, and drugs. In addition, many medical disorders such as facial nerve (Bell's) palsy, gingivitis, pernicious anemia, and Parkinson's disease may be associated with dysfunction in the sense of taste.

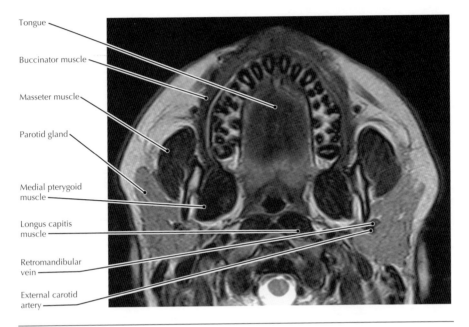

Tongue

Buccinator muscle

Masseter muscle

Parotid gland

Medial pterygoid muscle

Longus capitis muscle

Retromandibular vein

External carotid artery

Axial T1 maxillofacial MR image

- The chorda tympani nerve, which is a branch of the facial nerve (VII), carries most of the taste sensation from the tongue, although some taste sensation is carried by the glossopharyngeal (IX) and vagus (X) nerves.

- Tongue piercing has grown in popularity among young people and is associated with oral lesions, teeth chipping, and teeth breakage, especially in the lower four front teeth.

- Tongue piercing may also prevent satisfactory maxillofacial magnetic resonance imaging (MRI) because metal distorts the magnetic field.

- The buccinator is a muscle contained within the cheek that keeps food out of the vestibule of the mouth during chewing.

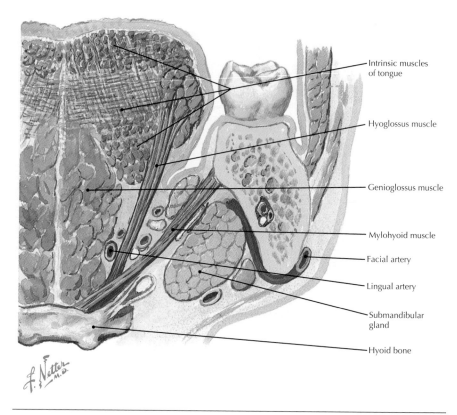

Intrinsic muscles of tongue

Hyoglossus muscle

Genioglossus muscle

Mylohyoid muscle

Facial artery

Lingual artery

Submandibular gland

Hyoid bone

Coronal section of the tongue posterior to first molar *(Atlas of Human Anatomy, 6th edition, Plate 47)*

Clinical Note Tongue lacerations are common, especially in children after falls or collisions. Because of a rich vascular supply, tongue lacerations generally heal well. However, surgical intervention may still sometimes be required because lacerations that do not heal normally may compromise speech or swallowing.

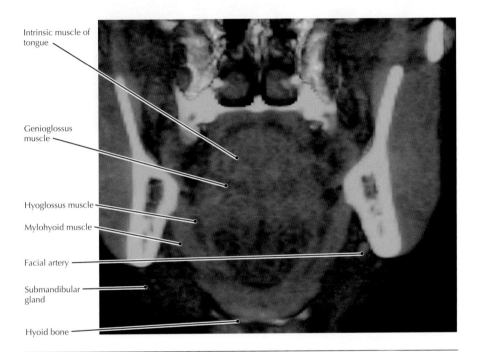

Intrinsic muscle of tongue

Genioglossus muscle

Hyoglossus muscle

Mylohyoid muscle

Facial artery

Submandibular gland

Hyoid bone

Coronal volume rendered CE CT of the soft tissues of the neck

- Lateral tongue bites are a classic sign of epilepsy, whereas bites at the tip of the tongue are more likely to be associated with syncope.
- The lingual artery is the only major structure that passes medial to the hyoglossus muscle.
- The mylohyoid muscle supports the floor of the mouth and is innervated by the mylohyoid nerve, which is a branch of V_3.

Head and Neck 63

Parotid and Submandibular Salivary Glands

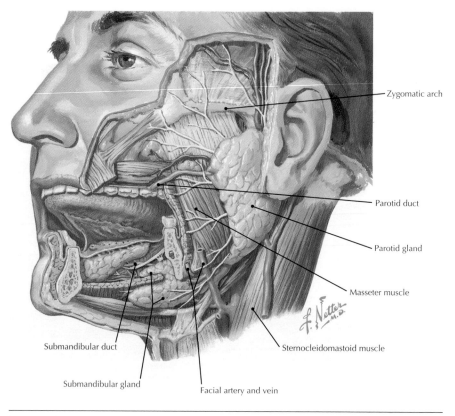

Zygomatic arch

Parotid duct

Parotid gland

Masseter muscle

Sternocleidomastoid muscle

Submandibular duct

Submandibular gland

Facial artery and vein

Lateral view of the three major salivary glands *(Atlas of Human Anatomy, 6th edition, Plate 46)*

Clinical Note Gustatory sweating (Frey's syndrome) is a condition that may follow parotidectomy or damage to the parotid gland and can be very troublesome to the patient. Ingestion of food or thoughts of food result in warmth and perspiration in the skin overlying the position of the parotid gland. Presumably, with removal of or damage to the gland, the parasympathetic fibers that previously innervated the parotid gland develop novel synapses with the sweat glands in the skin.

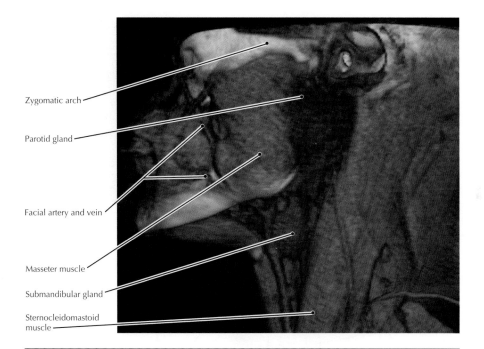

Zygomatic arch

Parotid gland

Facial artery and vein

Masseter muscle

Submandibular gland

Sternocleidomastoid
muscle

Volume rendered CE CT of the soft tissues of the neck

- The parotid gland drains via the parotid duct, which opens opposite the upper second molar. The submandibular and sublingual salivary glands drain primarily via the submandibular duct, which opens onto the floor of the mouth adjacent to the lingual frenulum. These ducts may be examined radiographically via injection of contrast into their openings (sialogram).

- The parotid gland is the most common location of salivary gland tumors, accounting for 70% to 85% of cases. As a general rule, the smaller the salivary gland in adults, the higher the probability that a neoplasm arising in that gland will be malignant.

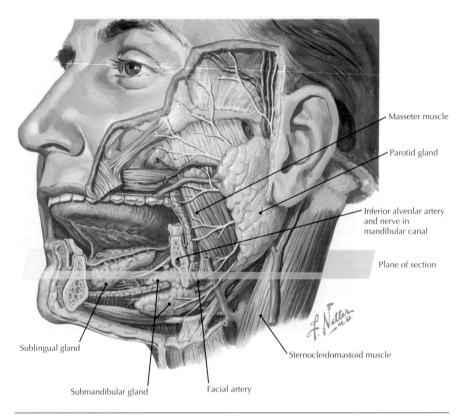

Masseter muscle

Parotid gland

Inferior alveolar artery
and nerve in
mandibular canal

Plane of section

Sternocleidomastoid muscle

Sublingual gland

Submandibular gland

Facial artery

Parotid, submandibular, and sublingual salivary glands and associated ducts *(Atlas of Human Anatomy, 6th edition, Plate 46)*

> **Clinical Note** Salivary calculi cause pain and swelling of salivary glands when they obstruct a salivary duct. Most salivary gland disease results from such obstruction.

Facial artery

Mandibular canal

Tongue

Masseter muscle

Submandibular gland

Oral pharynx

Sternocleidomastoid muscle

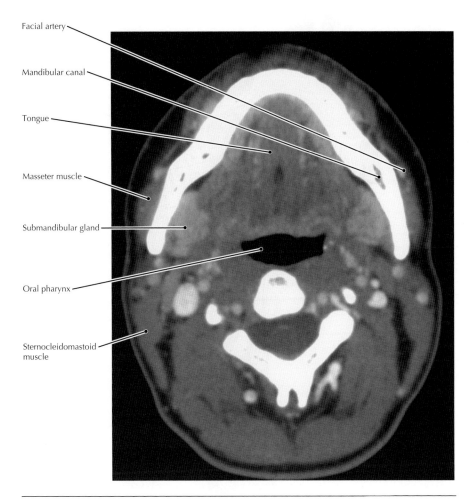

Axial CE CT of the neck

- CT scanning is the procedure of choice for sialolithiasis because a calculus does not have any magnetic resonance signal and will be invisible on MR images.
- The facial artery enters the face at the anterior border of the masseter muscle and can be palpated there.
- The inferior alveolar nerve and artery, which run in the mandibular canal, supply the mandibular teeth, and a branch exits the canal through the mental foramen.

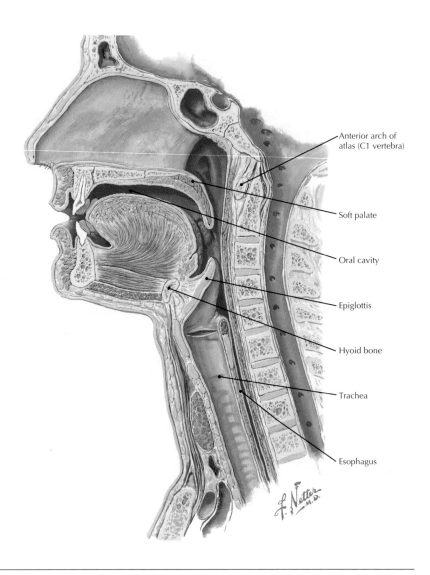

Anterior arch of
atlas (C1 vertebra)

Soft palate

Oral cavity

Epiglottis

Hyoid bone

Trachea

Esophagus

Median sagittal section of the head and neck, emphasizing the pharynx *(Atlas of Human Anatomy, 6th edition, Plate 64)*

Clinical Note Esophageal cancer causes difficulty in swallowing (dysphagia), which is typically progressive in nature. Invasion of the airway may occur in advanced cases of esophageal cancer.

Anterior arch of
atlas (C1 vertebra)

Soft palate

Epiglottis

Hyoid bone

Trachea

Esophagus

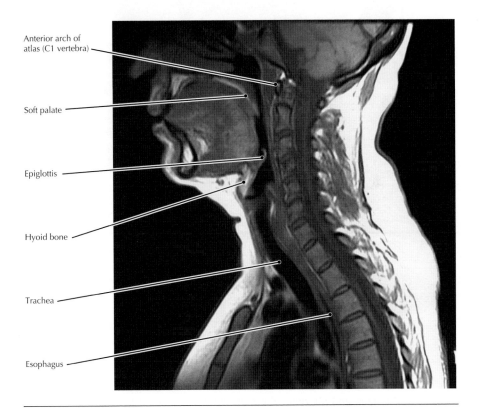

Sagittal T1 MR image of the head and neck

- The oral cavity is a potential space when the tongue is elevated against the palate. Similarly, the esophagus is a potential space.
- The tracheal lumen is always air-filled because it is maintained by incomplete cartilaginous rings.

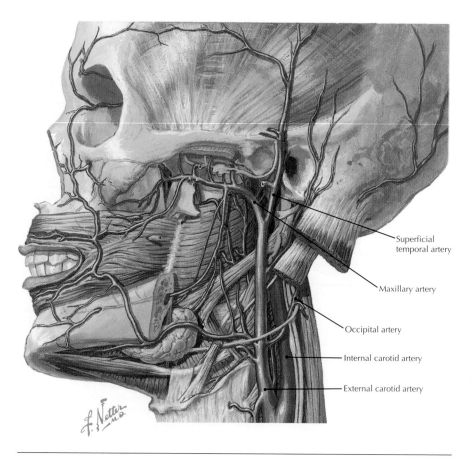

Superficial temporal artery

Maxillary artery

Occipital artery

Internal carotid artery

External carotid artery

Arteries of the neck and pharyngeal region *(Atlas of Human Anatomy, 6th edition, Plate 72)*

Clinical Note Stroke, due to atherothrombosis of the extracranial carotid arteries, results from a combination of factors involving the blood vessels, the clotting system, and hemodynamics. Carotid atherosclerosis is usually most severe within 2 cm of the bifurcation of the common carotid artery and predominantly involves the posterior wall of the internal carotid artery. The plaque decreases the vessel's lumen and frequently extends inferiorly into the common carotid artery.

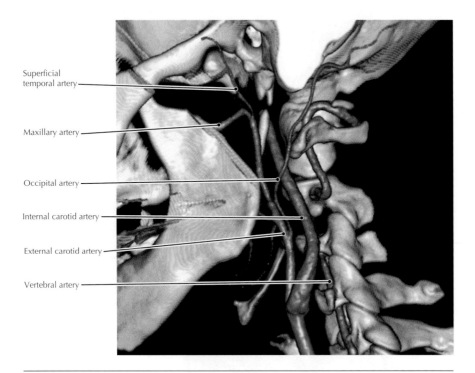

Superficial temporal artery —

Maxillary artery —

Occipital artery —

Internal carotid artery —

External carotid artery —

Vertebral artery —

Volume rendered carotid CTA

- The superficial temporal and maxillary arteries are the terminal branches of the external carotid artery. The former supplies the temporal region of the skull, and the latter crosses the infratemporal fossa to eventually enter the skull through the pterygomaxillary fissure and supply the nasal cavity.

- The internal carotid artery does not have any extracranial branches; it enters the skull using the carotid foramen in the temporal bone and eventually ascends and passes through the cavernous sinus to supply, along with the vertebral artery, all of the cerebral arteries.

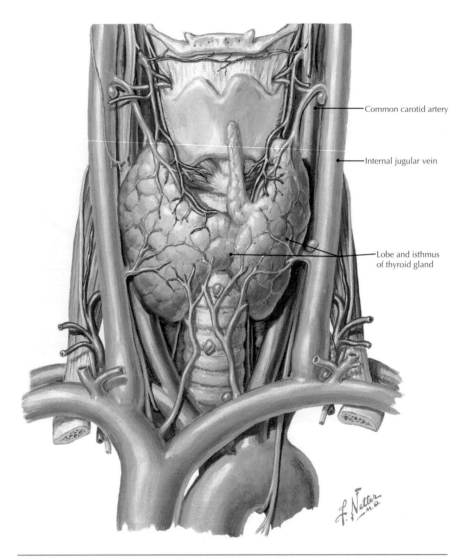

Common carotid artery

Internal jugular vein

Lobe and isthmus
of thyroid gland

Thyroid gland, vasculature supply; and common carotid artery and internal jugular vein *(Atlas of Human Anatomy, 6th edition, Plate 76)*

Clinical Note Ectopic thyroid tissue may be present anywhere along the embryologic line of descent of the thyroid gland, which begins at the foramen cecum of the tongue.

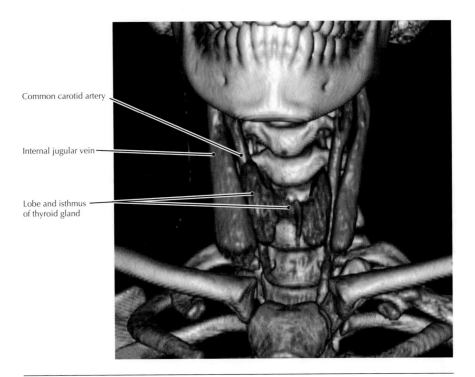

Common carotid artery

Internal jugular vein

Lobe and isthmus
of thyroid gland

Coronal volume rendered CE CT of the neck

- The rounded end at the inferior aspect of the internal jugular veins shown in this CT image occurred because the scan was done just when the contrast bolus had reached this level in the veins as it was quickly moving downward.
- In addition to the superior and inferior thyroid arteries, the thyroid gland may receive a thyroid ima artery that arises directly from the arch of the aorta and ascends on the trachea.
- The superior and middle thyroid veins drain to the internal jugular veins, and the inferior thyroid veins drain to the brachiocephalic veins.

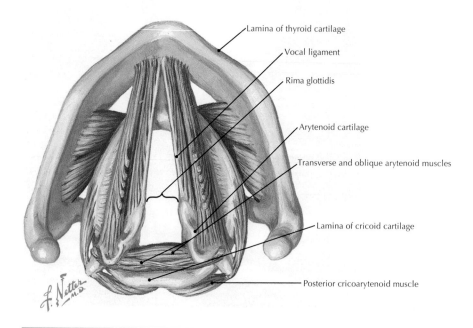

Lamina of thyroid cartilage

Vocal ligament

Rima glottidis

Arytenoid cartilage

Transverse and oblique arytenoid muscles

Lamina of cricoid cartilage

Posterior cricoarytenoid muscle

Downward-looking view of the laryngeal skeleton and selected muscles *(Atlas of Human Anatomy, 6th edition, Plate 80)*

Clinical Note The rima glottidis (space between the vocal folds) is usually the most narrow portion of the upper airway, so any instrument passed into the airway (bronchoscope, etc.) must fit through the rima.

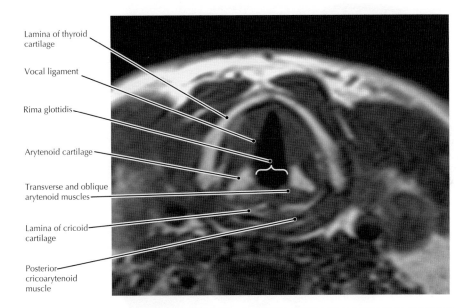

Lamina of thyroid
cartilage

Vocal ligament

Rima glottidis

Arytenoid cartilage

Transverse and oblique
arytenoid muscles

Lamina of cricoid
cartilage

Posterior
cricoarytenoid
muscle

Axial T1 MR image of the neck

- The thyroid, cricoid, and arytenoid cartilages are the main components of the skeleton of the larynx.

- The cricoid cartilage is the only skeletal structure that completely encircles the upper airway.

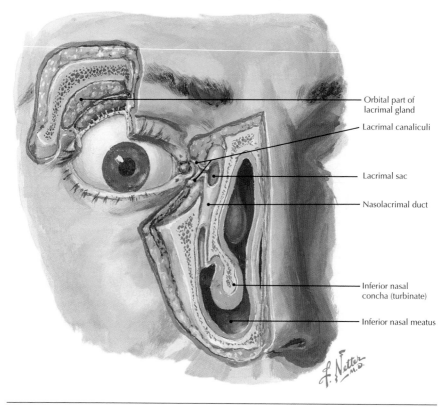

Orbital part of
lacrimal gland

Lacrimal canaliculi

Lacrimal sac

Nasolacrimal duct

Inferior nasal
concha (turbinate)

Inferior nasal meatus

Lacrimal apparatus *(Atlas of Human Anatomy, 6th edition, Plate 84)*

Clinical Note   Nasolacrimal duct obstruction can be congenital (occurs in infants) or acquired (often due to inflammation or fibrosis). The primary sign is an overflow of tears.

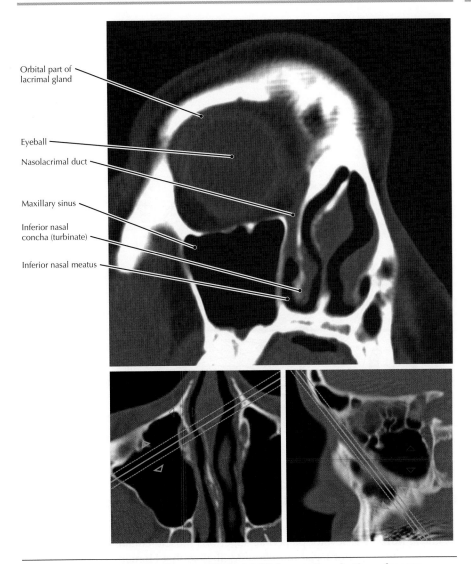

Orbital part of lacrimal gland

Eyeball

Nasolacrimal duct

Maxillary sinus

Inferior nasal concha (turbinate)

Inferior nasal meatus

Oblique coronal reconstruction, maxillofacial CT (*green lines* in the reference images indicate the position and orientation of the main image)

- The lacrimal apparatus consists of the following structures:
  - Lacrimal glands—secrete tears
  - Lacrimal ducts—convey tears to sclera
  - Lacrimal canaliculi—convey tears to lacrimal sac
  - Nasolacrimal duct—drains tears to the inferior nasal meatus

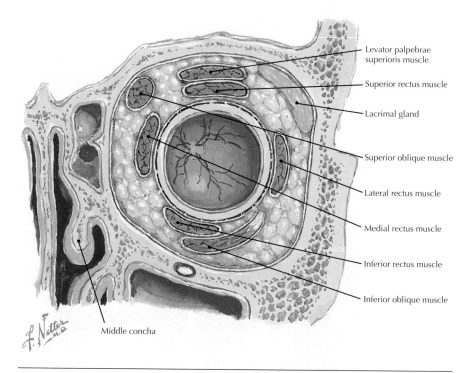

Levator palpebrae
superioris muscle

Superior rectus muscle

Lacrimal gland

Superior oblique muscle

Lateral rectus muscle

Medial rectus muscle

Inferior rectus muscle

Inferior oblique muscle

Middle concha

Coronal section through the orbit *(Atlas of Human Anatomy, 6th edition, Plate 85)*

Clinical Note The levator palpebrae superioris muscle contains some smooth muscle cells (superior tarsal muscle of Müller) so that Horner's syndrome is associated with some drooping of the upper eyelid (ptosis).

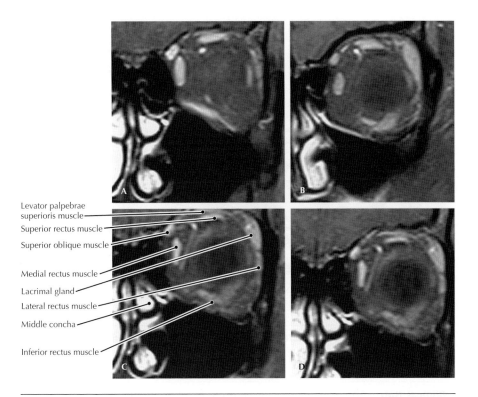

Levator palpebrae
superioris muscle

Superior rectus muscle

Superior oblique muscle

Medial rectus muscle

Lacrimal gland

Lateral rectus muscle

Middle concha

Inferior rectus muscle

Sequential coronal CE, FS T1 MR images of the orbit (*A-D,* posterior to anterior)

- The fine detail revealed by MRI is evident in the differentiation between the levator palpebrae superioris and the superior rectus muscles.
- As the extraocular muscles fuse with the eyeball anteriorly, they become indistinguishable on MRI.

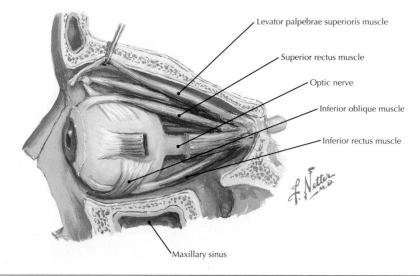

Levator palpebrae superioris muscle

Superior rectus muscle

Optic nerve

Inferior oblique muscle

Inferior rectus muscle

Maxillary sinus

Lateral aspect of the orbit (lateral rectus has been cut) *(Atlas of Human Anatomy, 6th edition, Plate 86)*

Clinical Note Abnormal extraocular muscle function, which results in specific limitations in eye movement, can often help localize an underlying intracranial lesion because of the different innervations of the muscles: lateral rectus by cranial nerve VI, superior oblique by IV, and the remainder by III.

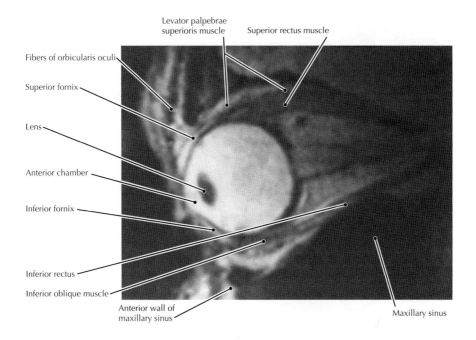

Levator palpebrae superioris muscle

Superior rectus muscle

Fibers of orbicularis oculi

Superior fornix

Lens

Anterior chamber

Inferior fornix

Inferior rectus

Inferior oblique muscle

Anterior wall of maxillary sinus

Maxillary sinus

Sagittal T2 fast spin echo (FSE) MR image of the orbit *(From Mafee MF, Karimi A, Shah J, et al: Anatomy and pathology of the eye: Role of MR imaging and CT. Radiol Clin North Am 44(1):135-157, 2006)*

- A retinal tumor, which causes progressive loss of vision, may be well revealed by MRI.
- The inferior oblique muscle works with the superior rectus muscle to produce upward gaze.

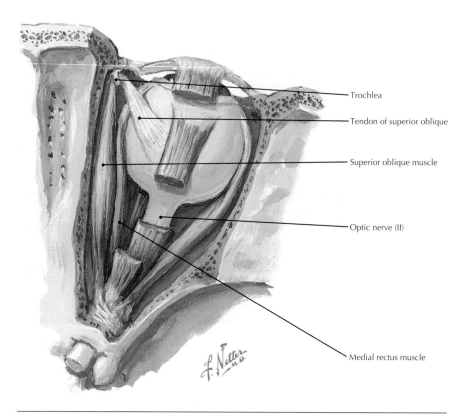

Trochlea

Tendon of superior oblique

Superior oblique muscle

Optic nerve (II)

Medial rectus muscle

Superior view of the orbit showing all of the superior oblique muscle *(Atlas of Human Anatomy, 6th edition, Plate 86)*

Clinical Note Paralysis of the trochlear nerve (IV), which innervates the superior oblique muscle, impairs the patient's ability to look down and thus the patient has difficulty descending stairs.

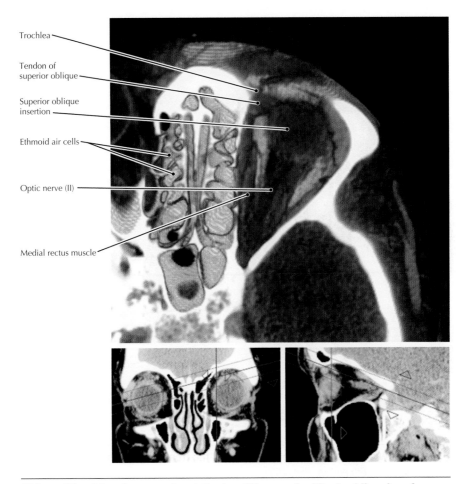

Trochlea

Tendon of superior oblique

Superior oblique insertion

Ethmoid air cells

Optic nerve (II)

Medial rectus muscle

Oblique thin slab volume rendered display, CT scan of orbits (*red lines* in reference images indicate position and orientation of the main image)

- Head trauma is the most typical cause of an isolated lesion of the trochlear nerve, resulting in superior oblique paralysis.
- The superior oblique muscle works with the inferior rectus muscle to produce downward gaze.

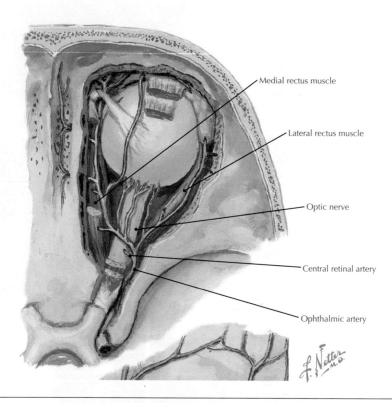

Medial rectus muscle

Lateral rectus muscle

Optic nerve

Central retinal artery

Ophthalmic artery

Superior view of the orbit with orbital plate of the frontal bone removed *(Atlas of Human Anatomy, 6th edition, Plate 87)*

Clinical Note The extremely thin lamina papyracea may be penetrated by an untreated and severe infectious ethmoid sinusitis, resulting in orbital disease.

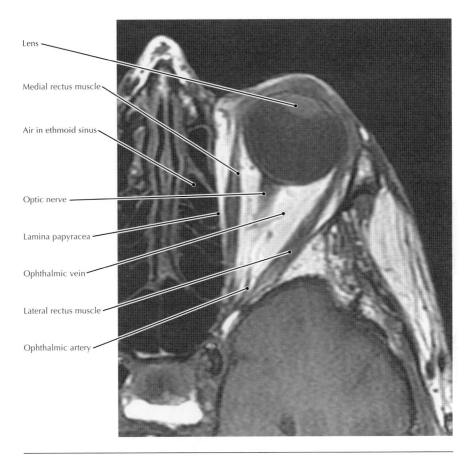

Lens

Medial rectus muscle

Air in ethmoid sinus

Optic nerve

Lamina papyracea

Ophthalmic vein

Lateral rectus muscle

Ophthalmic artery

Axial T1 FSE MR image of the orbit *(From Mafee MF, Karimi A, Shah J, et al: Anatomy and pathology of the eye: Role of MR imaging and CT. Radiol Clin North Am 44(1):135-157, 2006)*

- The extensive orbital fat, which is T1 hyperintense (bright) and appears white in the MR image, cushions and supports the eyeball.

- The thin medial bony wall (lamina papyracea), which separates the orbit from the ethmoidal sinus, is difficult to see on MRI, as evident in the image above.
  To visualize such thin bony structures more clearly, CT is the preferred imaging modality.

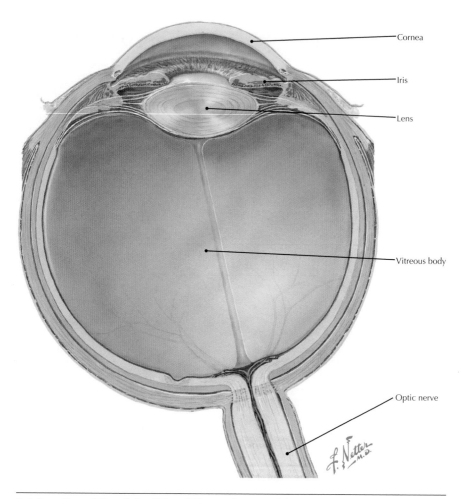

Cornea

Iris

Lens

Vitreous body

Optic nerve

Axial section of the globe *(Atlas of Human Anatomy, 6th edition, Plate 89)*

> **Clinical Note** A *cataract* is a clouding of the lens. Cataracts are more common with aging; by age 80, more than half of all Americans either have a cataract or have had cataract surgery. Also associated with aging is *presbyopia,* the loss of the ability to focus actively on near (vs. far) objects. Presbyopia results from a loss of elasticity in the lens.

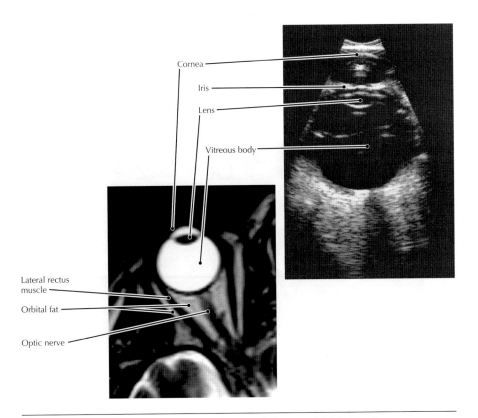

Cornea

Iris

Lens

Vitreous body

Lateral rectus
muscle

Orbital fat

Optic nerve

Axial T2 MR image *(left)* **and axial US image of the eye** *(right)* *(Courtesy Roger P. Harrie, MD, Clinical Professor of Ophthalmology, University of Utah Moran Eye Center)*

- Because the eye is composed of fluid chambers, echogenic structures such as the surfaces of the lens are easily seen on US images.

- Note the brightly echogenic orbital fat in the US image.

- Orbital fat is important for supporting and cushioning the eye. The "shrunken eye" appearance of emaciated people, with backward displacement of the globe (enophthalmos), results from loss of orbital fat.

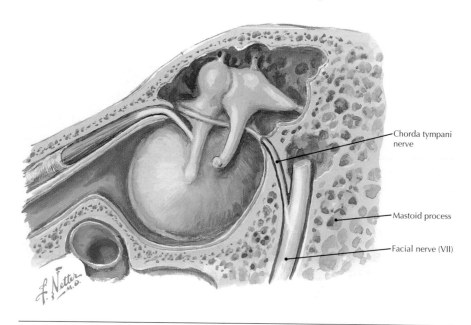

Chorda tympani nerve

Mastoid process

Facial nerve (VII)

Sagittal section of facial nerve in the facial canal *(Atlas of Human Anatomy, 6th edition, Plate 96)*

Clinical Note Bell's palsy, a usually temporary unilateral facial paralysis, may frequently be caused by a viral infection triggering an inflammatory response in the facial nerve (VII).

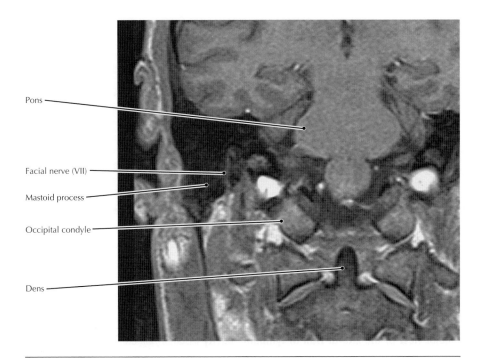

Pons

Facial nerve (VII)

Mastoid process

Occipital condyle

Dens

Coronal CE FS T1 MR image through the mastoid process

- The mastoid process is markedly hypodense (dark) because it is composed of compact cortical bone and mastoid air cells, which have no signal on MRI.
- Because the mastoid process is not developed at birth, the facial nerve is very susceptible to injury in infants.

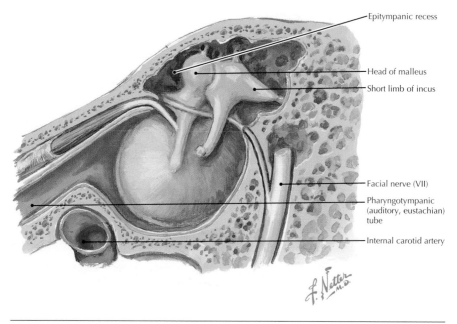

Epitympanic recess

Head of malleus

Short limb of incus

Facial nerve (VII)

Pharyngotympanic (auditory, eustachian) tube

Internal carotid artery

Medial view of the lateral wall of tympanic cavity *(Atlas of Human Anatomy, 6th edition, Plate 96)*

Clinical Note Otitis media refers to inflammation of the tympanic cavity; it is common in children because of the easy spread of infectious agents from the nasopharynx to the cavity via the pharyngotympanic (auditory, eustachian) tube, which is shorter and straighter in children than in adults.

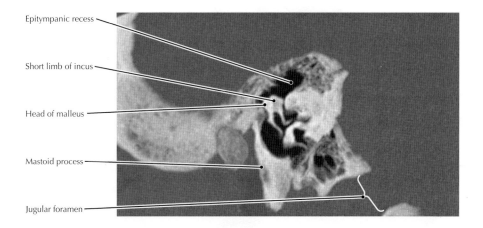

Epitympanic recess

Short limb of incus

Head of malleus

Mastoid process

Jugular foramen

Oblique coronal CT of the tympanic cavity *(Courtesy the Philips Corporation)*

- The epitympanic recess connects via the mastoid antrum to the air cells within the mastoid process. Accordingly, infections of the middle ear cavity can lead to mastoiditis if left untreated.

- The pharyngotympanic (auditory, eustachian) tube allows for equalization of air pressure on both sides of the tympanic membrane, thus facilitating free movement. The tube is normally closed but is opened by the actions of the salpingopharyngeus and the tensor and levator veli palatini during swallowing or yawning.

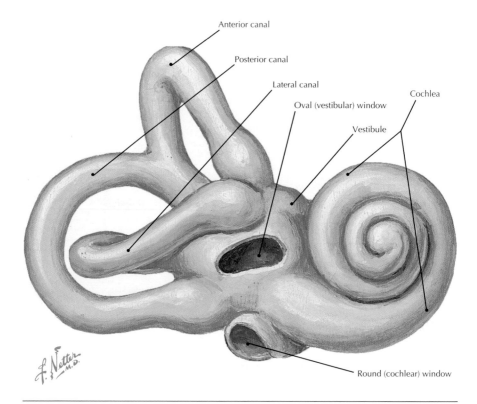

Anterior canal

Posterior canal

Lateral canal

Oval (vestibular) window

Cochlea

Vestibule

Round (cochlear) window

Anterolateral view of right bony labyrinth *(Atlas of Human Anatomy, 6th edition, Plate 97)*

Clinical Note The semicircular canals provide the central nervous system with information about rotary (circular) motion. Disorders of the endolymphatic system may lead to vertigo (spinning sensation) such as occurs in benign paroxysmal positional vertigo (BPPV), which is a brief sensation of vertigo occurring with specific changes in head position.

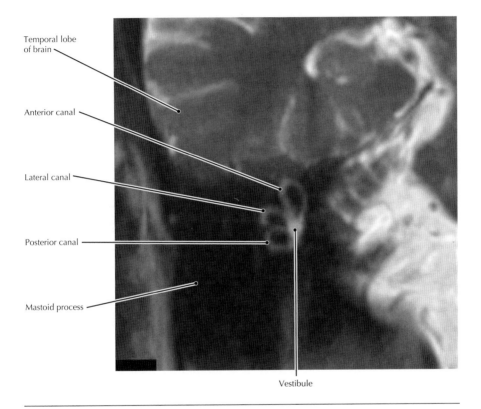

Temporal lobe of brain

Anterior canal

Lateral canal

Posterior canal

Mastoid process

Vestibule

Slightly oblique coronal T2 MR image of the inner ear

- The utricle and saccule are organs within the vestibule that detect linear acceleration (movement in a straight line) and static equilibrium (position of the head).
- The semicircular canals detect rotation of the head in the plane of its respective duct.

Superior Sagittal Sinus

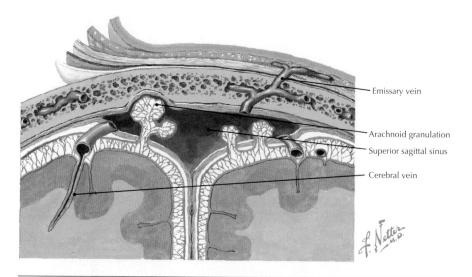

- Emissary vein
- Arachnoid granulation
- Superior sagittal sinus
- Cerebral vein

Coronal view of superior sagittal sinus *(Atlas of Human Anatomy, 6th edition, Plate 101)*

> **Clinical Note** Large cerebral sinuses, such as the superior sagittal sinus, are most frequently involved in venous sinus thrombosis that is often associated with systemic inflammatory diseases and coagulation disorders.

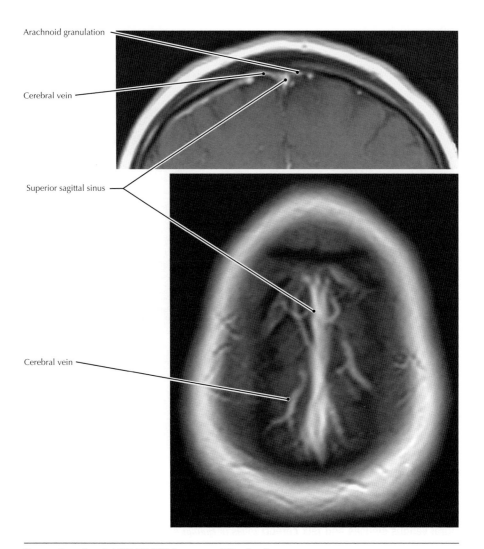

Arachnoid granulation

Cerebral vein

Superior sagittal sinus

Cerebral vein

Coronal and axial CE T1 MR images of the brain

- Emissary veins permit the spread of infection from the scalp to the superior sagittal sinus.
- Cerebrospinal fluid (CSF) returns to the venous circulation via arachnoid granulations within the superior sagittal sinus.

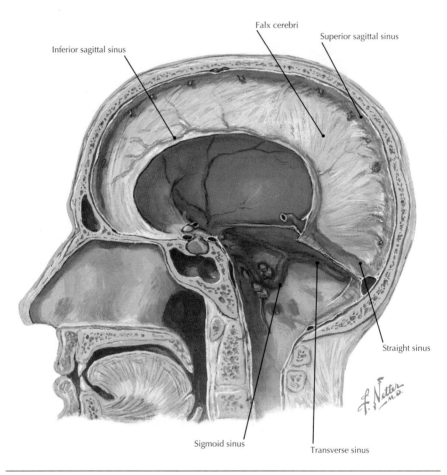

Dural venous sinuses and falx cerebri *(Atlas of Human Anatomy, 6th edition, Plate 104)*

Clinical Note Absence or hypoplasia of a venous sinus may occur and can be mistaken radiologically for a thrombosed sinus.

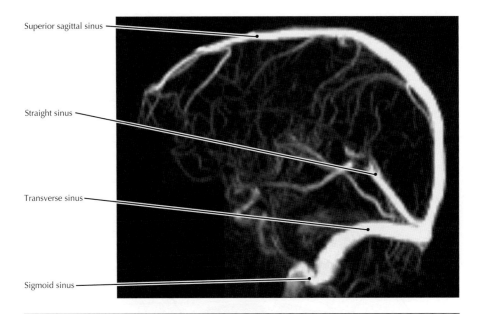

Superior sagittal sinus

Straight sinus

Transverse sinus

Sigmoid sinus

Venous 3-D phase contrast MRA *(Image courtesy of Wendy Hopkins, Philips Clinical Education Specialist)*

- Both phase contrast and time-of-flight (TOF) magnetic resonance pulse sequences are flow-sensitive sequences that do not require injection of contrast material for visualization of veins or arteries. Phase contrast angiography (PCA) acquisitions can be encoded for sensitivity to flow within a certain range of velocities, thus highlighting venous or arterial flow.

- In CT, the phrase "3-D" is often used to describe a shaded surface or volume rendered display. In MRI, "3-D" refers to the technique of image data acquisition, as is the case here.

- The superior sagittal sinus drains to the internal jugular vein via the transverse and sigmoid sinuses.

- Some dural sinuses not shown in these images include the petrosal, cavernous, and marginal sinuses.

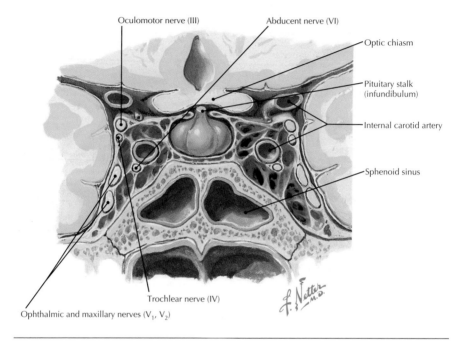

Oculomotor nerve (III)
Abducent nerve (VI)
Optic chiasm
Pituitary stalk (infundibulum)
Internal carotid artery
Sphenoid sinus
Trochlear nerve (IV)
Ophthalmic and maxillary nerves (V_1, V_2)

Coronal section of the cavernous sinus and adjacent structures *(Atlas of Human Anatomy, 6th edition, Plate 105)*

> **Clinical Note** Atherosclerosis of the internal carotid artery within the cavernous sinus can cause pressure on the abducent nerve (VI) because of the very close relationship between these two structures.

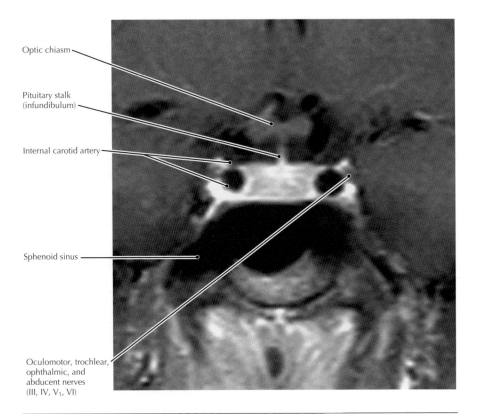

Optic chiasm

Pituitary stalk
(infundibulum)

Internal carotid artery

Sphenoid sinus

Oculomotor, trochlear,
ophthalmic, and
abducent nerves
(III, IV, V$_1$, VI)

Coronal CE FS T1 MR image

- The looping of the internal carotid artery siphon results in the vessel passing through the plane of this MR image twice.
- On the CE MR image, the cavernous sinus is bright because it is a venous structure. Although the entire endovascular space within the sinus may contain the injected gadolinium (including the internal carotid artery), the rapid arterial flow in artery results in a signal (flow) void.
- The MR image is slightly anterior to the drawing so that all the cranial nerves are bundled into the superolateral corner of the sinus as they are about to traverse the superior orbital fissure.

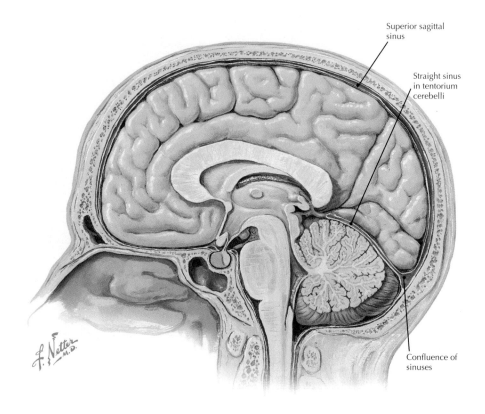

Superior sagittal
sinus

Straight sinus
in tentorium
cerebelli

Confluence of
sinuses

Sagittal view of the head and brain showing some of the cerebral venous sinuses
(Atlas of Human Anatomy, 6th edition, Plate 107)

Clinical Note   The clinical presentation of cerebral venous thrombosis is
nonspecific. Therefore, clinical diagnosis may be elusive. Predisposing
conditions include hypercoagulable states, adjacent tumor or infection, and
dehydration. However, it is idiopathic in up to 25% of cases.

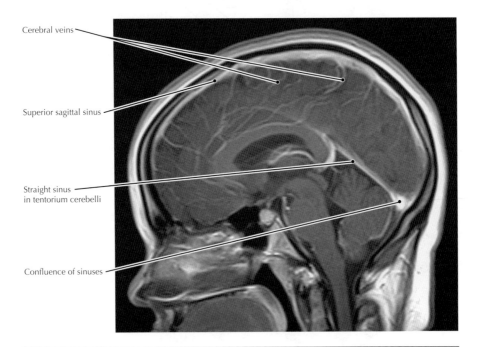

Cerebral veins

Superior sagittal sinus

Straight sinus
in tentorium cerebelli

Confluence of sinuses

Sagittal CE T1 MR image of the brain

- The drainage of the cerebral veins to the superior sagittal sinus is visible in this MR image.
- The dural venous sinuses are contained within spaces found between the endosteal and meningeal layers of dura.

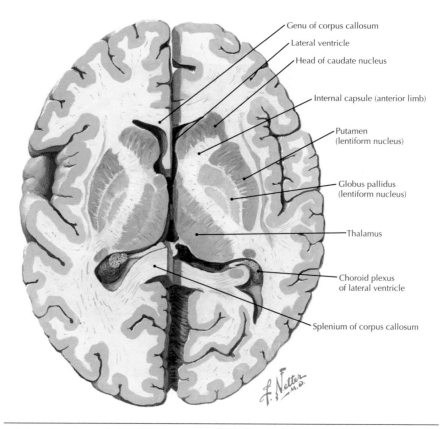

Genu of corpus callosum

Lateral ventricle

Head of caudate nucleus

Internal capsule (anterior limb)

Putamen (lentiform nucleus)

Globus pallidus (lentiform nucleus)

Thalamus

Choroid plexus of lateral ventricle

Splenium of corpus callosum

Axial section through the basal ganglia; the left and right sections are at slightly different transverse planes *(Atlas of Human Anatomy, 6th edition, Plate 111)*

Clinical Note Lesions of the basal ganglia are often associated with movement disorders such as Huntington's and Parkinson's diseases, and Tourette's syndrome.

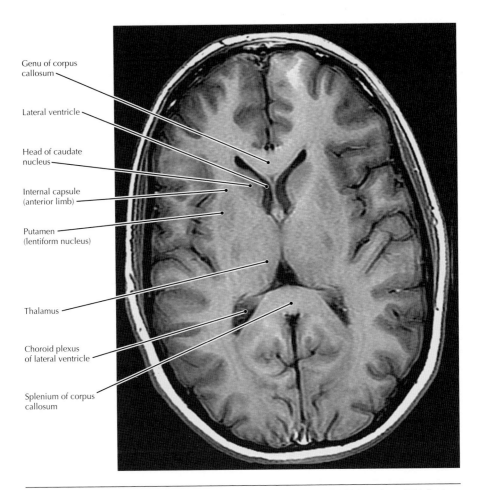

Genu of corpus callosum

Lateral ventricle

Head of caudate nucleus

Internal capsule (anterior limb)

Putamen (lentiform nucleus)

Thalamus

Choroid plexus of lateral ventricle

Splenium of corpus callosum

Axial T1 MR image of the brain *(From DeLano M, Fisher C: 3T MR imaging of the brain. Magn Reson Imaging Clin N Am 14(1):77-88, 2006)*

- This image shows good distinction between white and gray matter.
- The anterior limb of the internal capsule separates the caudate nucleus from the putamen and globus pallidus (together called the lentiform nucleus).

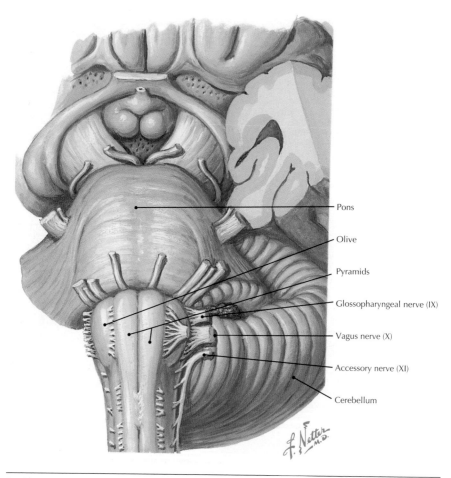

- Pons
- Olive
- Pyramids
- Glossopharyngeal nerve (IX)
- Vagus nerve (X)
- Accessory nerve (XI)
- Cerebellum

Brainstem (pons and medulla) *(Atlas of Human Anatomy, 6th edition, Plate 115)*

Clinical Note Cranial nerves IX, X, and XI all exit the skull through the jugular foramen, and any pathologic process (e.g., tumor) that compresses these nerves within this foramen may compromise their function (jugular foramen syndrome).

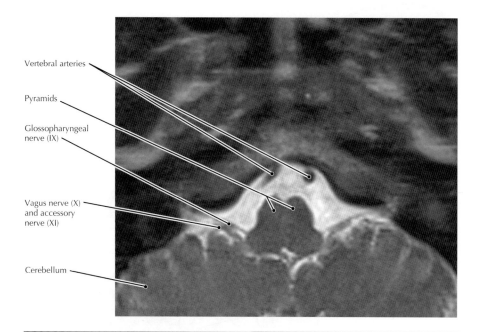

Vertebral arteries

Pyramids

Glossopharyngeal
nerve (IX)

Vagus nerve (X)
and accessory
nerve (XI)

Cerebellum

Axial T2 MR image of the brain

- Cerebrospinal fluid (CSF) is hyperdense (white) in this MR image.
- The vertebral arteries unite to form the basilar artery on the pons.
- The absence of signal (black) within the lumen of arteries in this MR image is known as a signal or flow void.

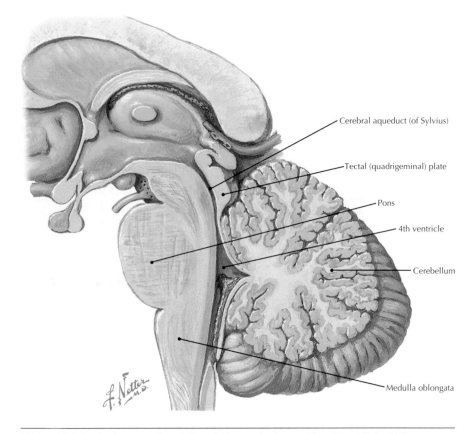

Cerebral aqueduct (of Sylvius)

Tectal (quadrigeminal) plate

Pons

4th ventricle

Cerebellum

Medulla oblongata

Midsagittal brainstem section *(Atlas of Human Anatomy, 6th edition, Plate 116)*

Clinical Note Diseases of the cerebellum typically present with ataxia, which is a complex of symptoms and signs involving a lack of coordination.

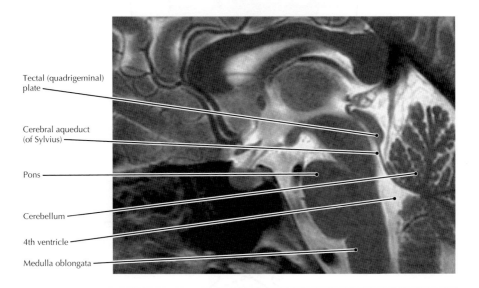

Tectal (quadrigeminal) plate

Cerebral aqueduct (of Sylvius)

Pons

Cerebellum

4th ventricle

Medulla oblongata

Sagittal T2 MR image of the brain *(From DeLano M, Fisher C: 3T MR imaging of the brain. Magn Reson Imaging Clin N Am 14(1):77-88, 2006)*

- Note the close relationship of the cerebellum to the medulla, pons, and mesencephalon.

- The cerebrospinal fluid (CSF)–containing fourth ventricle lies between the cerebellum, medulla, and pons; it communicates with CSF spaces in the spinal cord caudally and those in the mesencephalon and brain rostrally.

- The CSF-containing third ventricle communicates with the fourth ventricle via a narrow passageway (the cerebral aqueduct, or aqueduct of Sylvius) in the dorsal portion of the mesencephalon, beneath the quadrigeminal (tectal) plate.

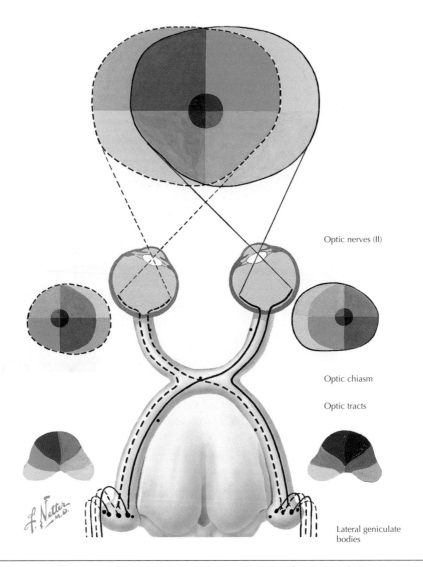

Optic nerves (II)

Optic chiasm

Optic tracts

Lateral geniculate bodies

Optic pathway schema from eye to lateral geniculate bodies *(Atlas of Human Anatomy, 6th edition, Plate 121)*

Clinical Note Visual field deficits result from lesions along the visual pathway, with the specific deficit dependent on the anatomic site of the lesion.

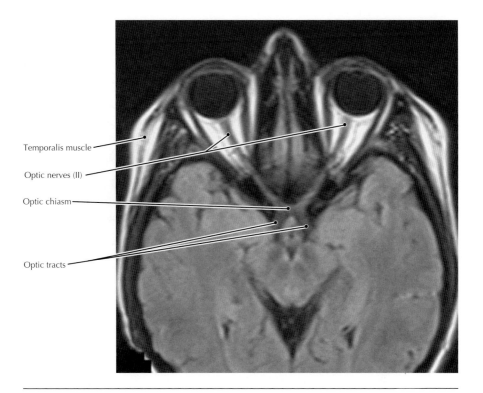

Temporalis muscle

Optic nerves (II)

Optic chiasm

Optic tracts

Axial fluid-attenuated inversion recovery (FLAIR) MR image of the brain

- The FLAIR sequence is T2 sensitive, although the signal from simple serous fluid (such as CSF) is suppressed. Therefore, T2 hyperintense acute lesions (bright) are conspicuous even when adjacent to CSF.

- In this MR image, the optic chiasm is clearly seen because the surrounding fluid is dark. However, unlike the FLAIR sequence, pathology may be isointense with normal brain on unenhanced T1 images.

- The FLAIR sequence has become fundamental in brain MRI; it is especially helpful in detecting the white matter lesions of multiple sclerosis.

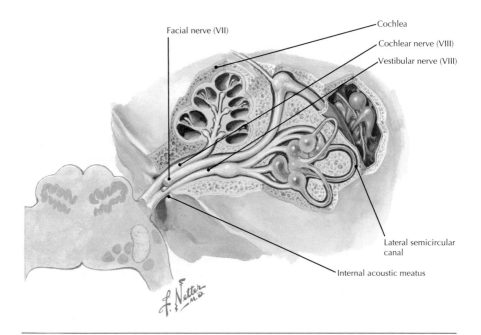

Schema of nerves entering internal acoustic meatus (*Atlas of Human Anatomy, 6th edition, Plate 125*)

Clinical Note An acoustic neuroma (neurofibroma) usually begins in the vestibular nerve in the internal acoustic meatus, but the first symptom is often a decrease in hearing acuity.

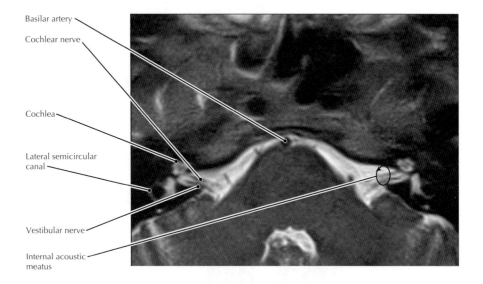

Basilar artery

Cochlear nerve

Cochlea

Lateral semicircular
canal

Vestibular nerve

Internal acoustic
meatus

Axial T2 single shot FSE MR image through the internal auditory meatus

- The vestibular nerve carries sensation from the utricle, saccule, and semicircular canals, and the cochlear nerve carries sensation from the spiral ganglion of the cochlea.

- Vertigo is a hallucination of movement that may result from a lesion of the vestibular nerve.

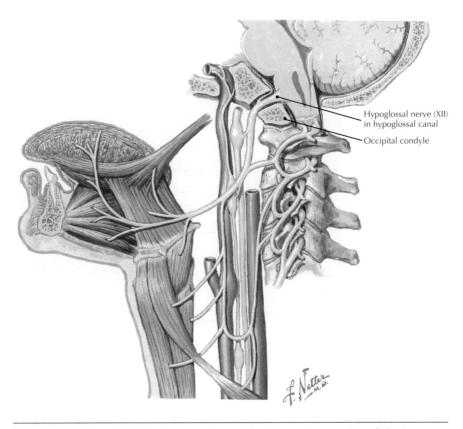

Hypoglossal nerve (XII) in hypoglossal canal

Occipital condyle

Hypoglossal nerve (XII) passing through canal to innervate muscles of the tongue
(Atlas of Human Anatomy, 6th edition, Plate 129)

Clinical Note Impaired function of the hypoglossal nerve (XII) typically results in deviation of the tongue to the side of the lesion on protrusion.

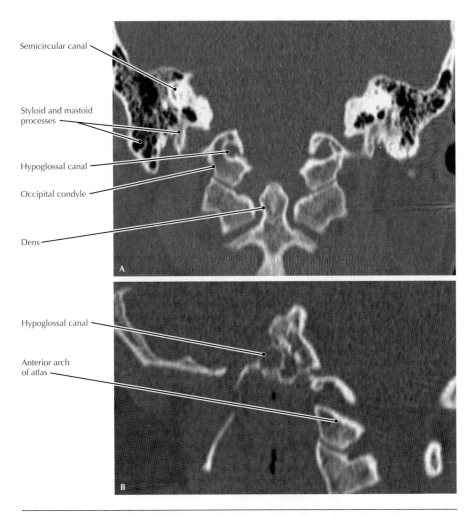

Semicircular canal

Styloid and mastoid processes

Hypoglossal canal

Occipital condyle

Dens

A

Hypoglossal canal

Anterior arch of atlas

B

Coronal *(A)* and sagittal *(B)* CT reconstructions of the hypoglossal canal

- The hypoglossal nerve (XII) innervates all the muscles of the tongue (intrinsic and extrinsic) except the palatoglossus.
- Multiplanar CT reconstructions similar to those shown above are critically important in the evaluation of fractures and congenital abnormalities involving the craniovertebral junction.

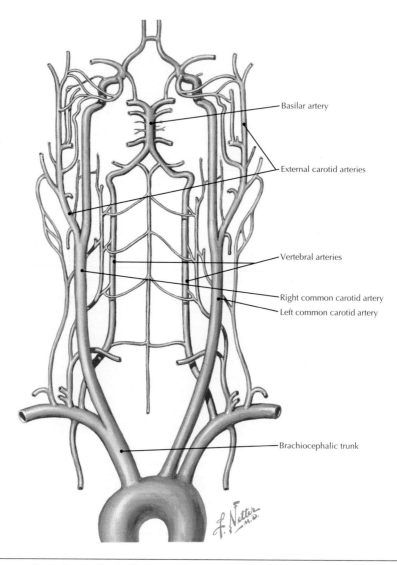

- Basilar artery
- External carotid arteries
- Vertebral arteries
- Right common carotid artery
- Left common carotid artery
- Brachiocephalic trunk

Schema of arteries to the brain *(Atlas of Human Anatomy, 6th edition, Plate 139)*

Clinical Note Partial or complete occlusion of the arteries that supply the brain can cause minor or major strokes. Typically, such occlusion is caused by arteriosclerotic plaque or an embolus.

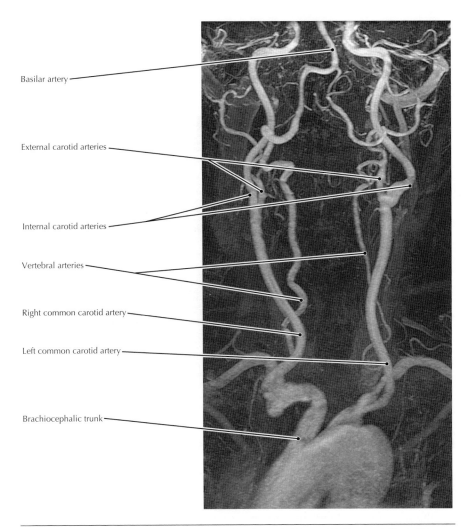

Basilar artery

External carotid arteries

Internal carotid arteries

Vertebral arteries

Right common carotid artery

Left common carotid artery

Brachiocephalic trunk

CE MRA of the arteries supplying the brain *(From DeMarco JK, Huston J, Nash AK: Extracranial carotid MR imaging at 3T. Magn Reson Imaging Clin N Am 14(1):109-121, 2006)*

- The vertebral arteries typically branch from the subclavian arteries and ascend through the transverse foramina of the cervical vertebrae, and then enter the skull through the foramen magnum to join and form the basilar artery.
- The asymmetry in the diameter of the vertebral arteries, shown in this MRA, is common and is not pathologic.

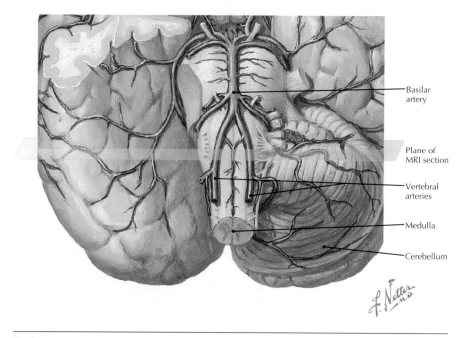

- Basilar artery
- Plane of MRI section
- Vertebral arteries
- Medulla
- Cerebellum

Brainstem and vertebral arteries *(Atlas of Human Anatomy, 6th edition, Plate 140)*

Clinical Note   The absence of a flow void (indicating blood flow) on the MR image may be direct evidence of arterial occlusion. Significant discrepancy in the size of normal vertebral arteries is common and of no clinical significance. Vertebrobasilar artery insufficiency often presents with neurologic dysfunction that is clinically distinct from the more common carotid artery disease.

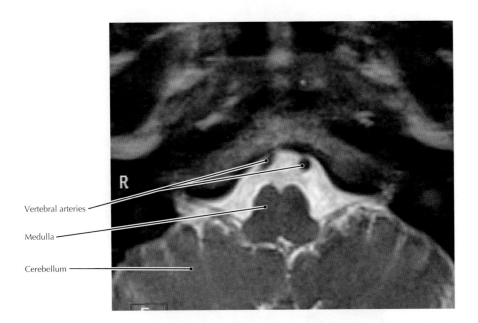

Vertebral arteries

Medulla

Cerebellum

R

Axial T2 MR image of the brain

- Cerebrospinal fluid (CSF) is hyperintense (bright) in this image.
- The vertebral arteries converge at the level of the pons to form the basilar artery.
- The absence of MR signal (black) within the artery lumen is called a "flow void," indicating that the artery is patent.

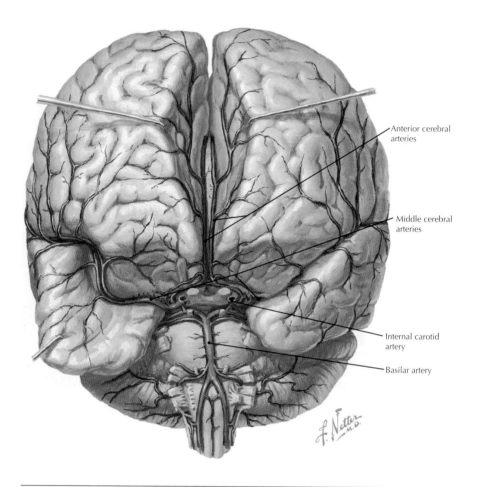

Anterior cerebral arteries

Middle cerebral arteries

Internal carotid artery

Basilar artery

Anterior view of the arteries supplying the brain *(Atlas of Human Anatomy, 6th edition, Plate 142)*

Clinical Note A stroke is associated with impaired blood flow to specific regions of the brain resulting either from a blockage (embolic) or rupture (hemorrhagic) of a cerebral artery.

Anterior cerebral
arteries

Middle cerebral arteries

Internal carotid
arteries

Basilar artery

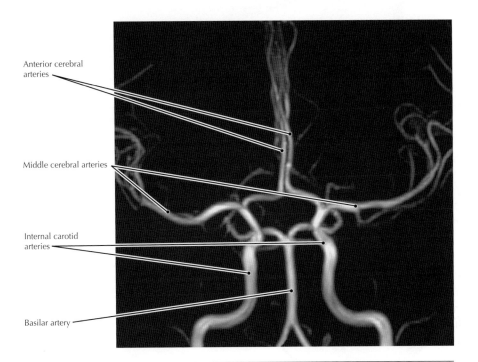

MIP, unenhanced MRA using TOF sequence

- Intracranial MRA is a noninvasive screening test commonly used in patients who are at high risk for intracranial aneurysm.
- Whereas the cerebral arterial circle (of Willis) theoretically permits compensatory blood flow in cases of occlusion of a contributory vessel, often the communicating arteries are very small and compensatory flow is inadequate.

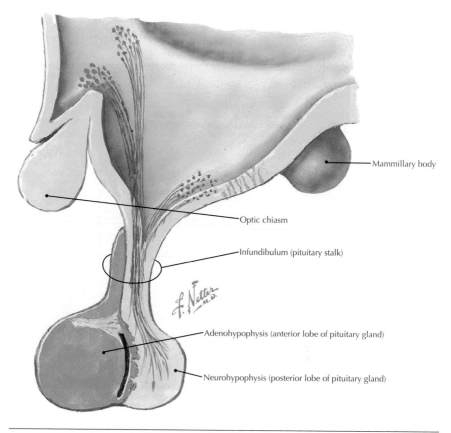

Mammillary body

Optic chiasm

Infundibulum (pituitary stalk)

Adenohypophysis (anterior lobe of pituitary gland)

Neurohypophysis (posterior lobe of pituitary gland)

Hypophysis (pituitary gland) *(Atlas of Human Anatomy, 6th edition, Plate 148)*

Clinical Note Acromegaly (enlargement of the extremities) results from overproduction of growth hormone by the pituitary (adenohypophysis). It typically affects middle-aged adults and can result in serious illness and premature death. In over 90% of acromegaly patients, the excessive production of growth hormone is caused by a benign tumor of the pituitary gland called an adenoma.

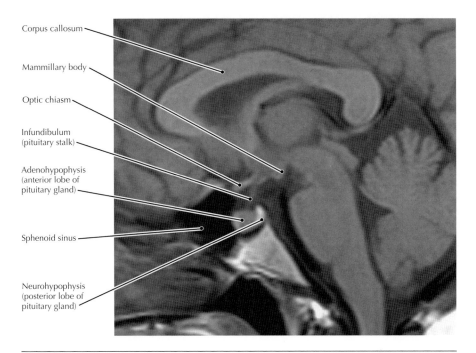

Corpus callosum

Mammillary body

Optic chiasm

Infundibulum
(pituitary stalk)

Adenohypophysis
(anterior lobe of
pituitary gland)

Sphenoid sinus

Neurohypophysis
(posterior lobe of
pituitary gland)

Sagittal T1 MR image of the brain

- Note the close relationship between the pituitary gland and the optic chiasm. Large pituitary lesions may impinge on the chiasm, causing a visual field deficit to be the earliest symptom.

- Growth hormone deficiency is a disorder in children resulting from insufficient production of growth hormone by the anterior lobe of the pituitary. The children do not grow taller at a typical rate, although their body proportions remain normal.

- Vasopressin and oxytocin granules within the neurohypophysis explain the strong differentiation between the two pituitary regions in this image. The high signal inferior to the pituitary results from fatty marrow in the clivus.

Section 2   **Back and Spinal Cord**

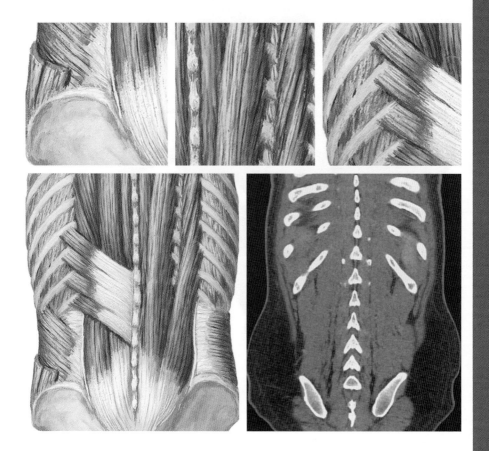

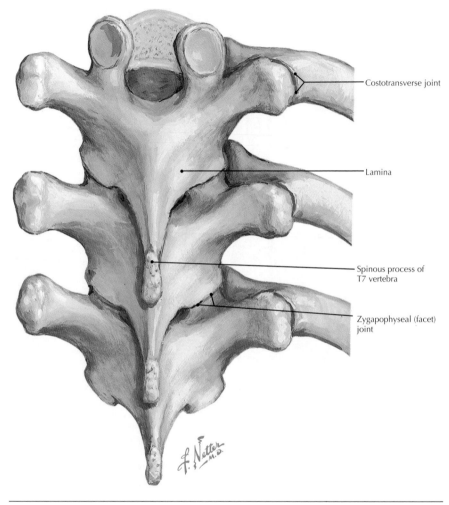

Costotransverse joint

Lamina

Spinous process of T7 vertebra

Zygapophyseal (facet) joint

Posterior view of the thoracic spine *(Atlas of Human Anatomy, 6th edition, Plate 154)*

Clinical Note Excessive kyphosis is an abnormal increase in the thoracic curvature. This occurs frequently in osteoporotic women who develop anterior wedging–type compression fractures of thoracic vertebrae.

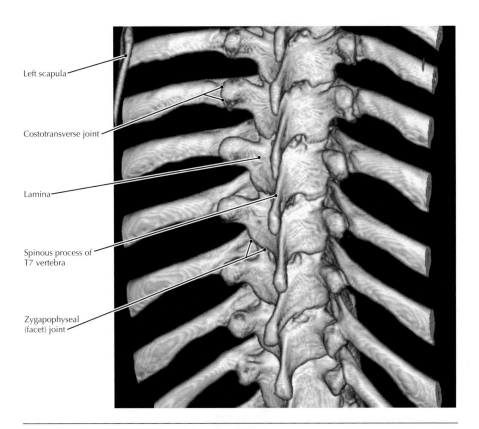

Left scapula

Costotransverse joint

Lamina

Spinous process of
T7 vertebra

Zygapophyseal
(facet) joint

Volume rendered display, thoracic spine CT

- The thoracic region of the vertebral column is the least mobile of the presacral vertebral column because of thin intervertebral discs, overlapping spinous processes, and the presence of ribs. This minimizes the potential for disruption of respiratory processes and maximizes stability of the thoracic spine.

- The normal thoracic curvature (kyphosis) is due almost entirely to the bony configuration of the vertebrae, whereas in the cervical and lumbar regions thicker discs also contribute to the respective curvatures in these regions.

- The overlapping of angled osseous structures of the thoracic spine's posterior elements and costovertebral junctions may result in confusion pertaining to bone changes caused by trauma or tumors on radiographs or cross-sectional images. Volume rendered displays can, in such cases, provide anatomic clarity not easily perceived on other image displays.

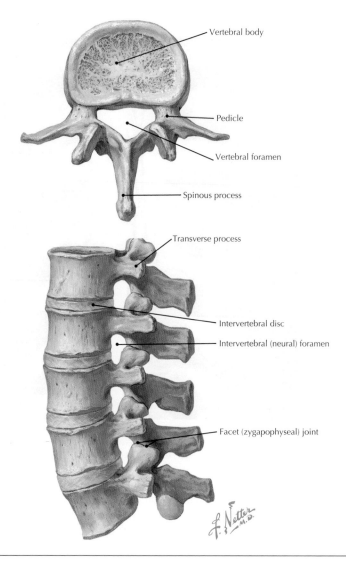

Vertebral body

Pedicle

Vertebral foramen

Spinous process

Transverse process

Intervertebral disc

Intervertebral (neural) foramen

Facet (zygapophyseal) joint

Superior and lateral views of lumbar vertebrae *(Atlas of Human Anatomy, 6th edition, Plate 155)*

Clinical Note Lumbar spinal stenosis may be congenital or acquired. Symptoms include pain, numbness, or weakness in the lower back or lower limbs; the symptoms may be temporally variable and are often worse after prolonged standing or walking.

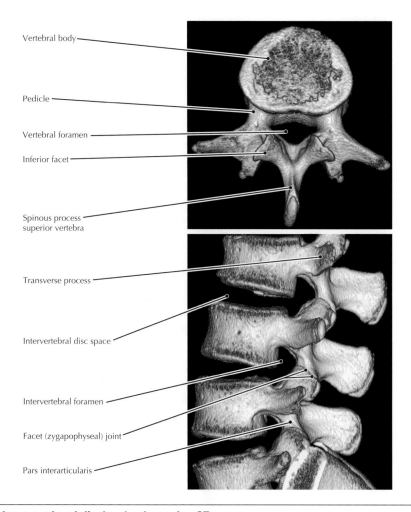

Vertebral body

Pedicle

Vertebral foramen

Inferior facet

Spinous process
superior vertebra

Transverse process

Intervertebral disc space

Intervertebral foramen

Facet (zygapophyseal) joint

Pars interarticularis

Volume rendered display, lumbar spine CT

- Spondylolisthesis refers to the anterior displacement of a vertebra in relation to the inferior vertebra; it is most commonly found at L5/S1because of a defect or non-united fracture at the pars interarticularis (the segment of the vertebral arch between the superior and inferior facets).

- There are typically five lumbar vertebrae, but the fifth lumbar may become fused with the sacrum (sacralization of L5) or the first sacral vertebrae may not be fused with the remaining sacral vertebrae (lumbarization of S1).

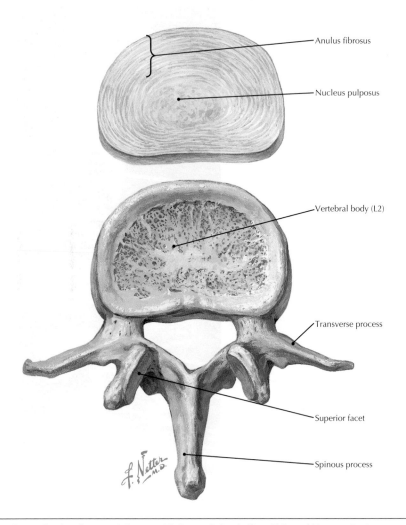

Anulus fibrosus

Nucleus pulposus

Vertebral body (L2)

Transverse process

Superior facet

Spinous process

Structure of a lumbar vertebra and intervertebral disc *(Atlas of Human Anatomy, 6th edition, Plate 155)*

Clinical Note Degenerative disc disease is associated with dehydration of the nucleus pulposus, which typically occurs with aging.

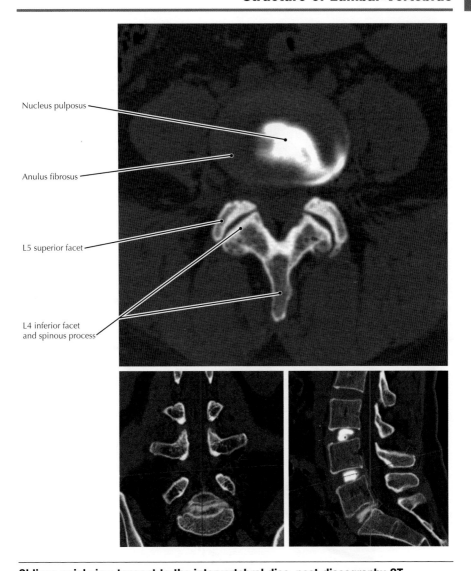

Nucleus pulposus

Anulus fibrosus

L5 superior facet

L4 inferior facet and spinous process

Oblique axial view tangent to the intervertebral disc, post-discography CT (*red lines* in the reference images indicate the position and orientation of the main image)

- Contrast material that had been injected into the nucleus pulposus has extravasated through a tear in the anulus fibrosus in this CT scan.
- Note that the main (axial) section shows the spinous process, lamina, and inferior facets of the vertebra above and the superior facets of the segment below.
- The vertebral arch is composed of the two (right and left) pedicles and lamina.

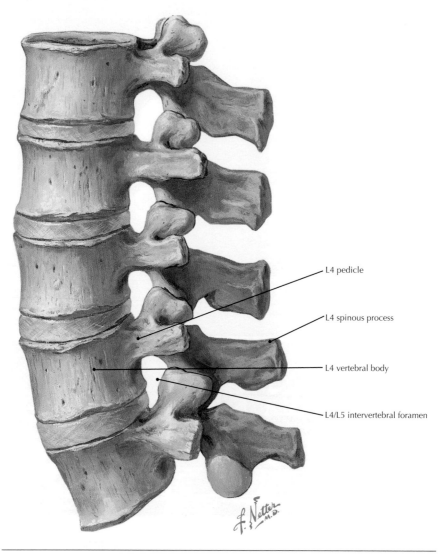

L4 pedicle

L4 spinous process

L4 vertebral body

L4/L5 intervertebral foramen

Sagittal view of the lumbar vertebral column *(Atlas of Human Anatomy, 6th edition, Plate 155)*

Clinical Note Vertebral bodies are most frequently fractured by excessive flexion (compression) forces, whereas the vertebral arches tend to fracture when the vertebral column is excessively extended.

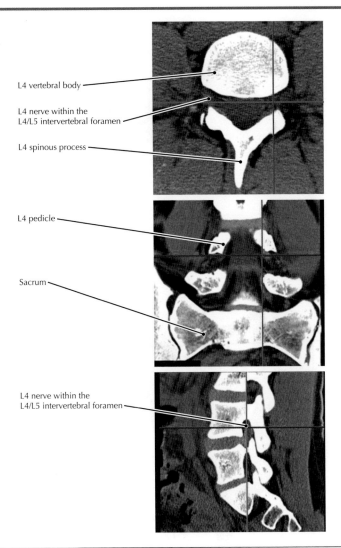

L4 vertebral body

L4 nerve within the
L4/L5 intervertebral foramen

L4 spinous process

L4 pedicle

Sacrum

L4 nerve within the
L4/L5 intervertebral foramen

Multiplanar reconstructions, lumbar CT

- The parasagittal CT image is at the level of the *blue lines* in the coronal and axial views. The axial section is at the level indicated by the *red line*. The coronal reconstruction is at the level of the *green line*.

- It is clinically important that the lumbar intervertebral foramina (also called neuroforamina or nerve root canals) extend superior to the associated disc. Herniated L4/5 disc fragments that extend upward and laterally may impinge on the exiting L4 root within the L4/5 intervertebral foramen, whereas herniation of an L4/5 disc fragment posteriorly and inferiorly may impinge on the L5 nerve root.

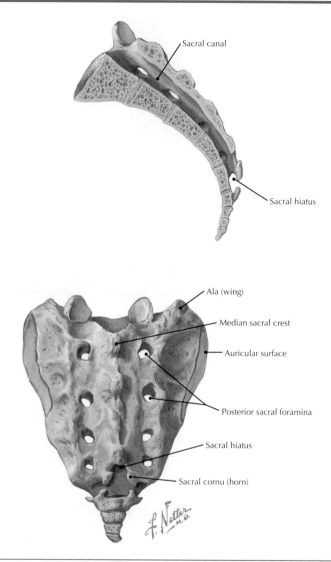

Midsagittal and posterior views of the sacrum (Atlas of Human Anatomy, 6th edition, Plate 157)

Clinical Note A caudal epidural block, often used during parturition, is administered by inserting an indwelling catheter into the sacral hiatus to release an anesthetic agent that eliminates sensation primarily from the S2-S4 spinal nerves. These nerves carry sensations from the uterine cervix, vagina, and perineum.

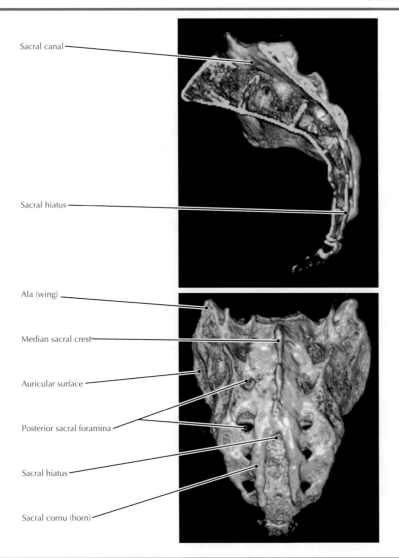

Sacral canal

Sacral hiatus

Ala (wing)

Median sacral crest

Auricular surface

Posterior sacral foramina

Sacral hiatus

Sacral cornu (horn)

Volume rendered display, lumbosacral CT

- The division of spinal nerves into dorsal and ventral rami occurs within the sacral canal so that the primary rami exit the sacrum via the anterior and posterior sacral foramina.

- The auricular surface of the sacrum is for articulation with the ilium forming the complicated sacroiliac joint (SIJ). Arthritis in this joint may be a source of lumbago.

- In osteoporotic patients, the sacrum is less able to resist the shearing force associated with the transfer of upper body weight to the pelvis; this may result in a vertical "insufficiency" fracture.

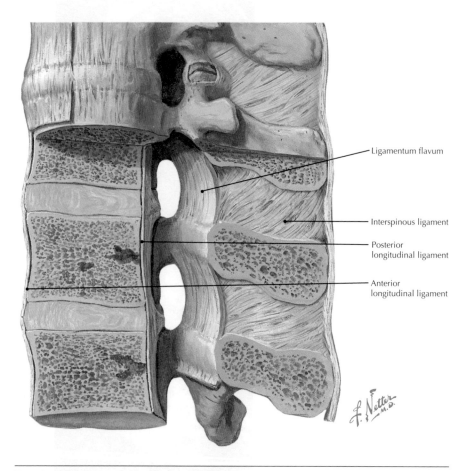

Ligamentum flavum

Interspinous ligament

Posterior longitudinal ligament

Anterior longitudinal ligament

Vertebral ligaments in the lumbar region *(Atlas of Human Anatomy, 6th edition, Plate 159)*

Clinical Note The posterior longitudinal ligament is well innervated with nociceptive fibers and is thought to be the origin of some of the pain associated with intervertebral disc herniation.

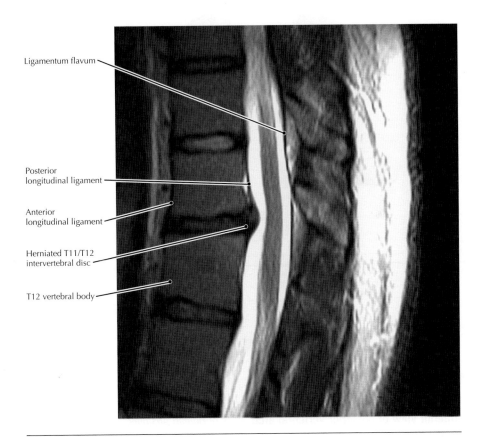

Ligamentum flavum

Posterior longitudinal ligament

Anterior longitudinal ligament

Herniated T11/T12 intervertebral disc

T12 vertebral body

Sagittal T2 MR image of the thoracolumbar spine

- The anterior longitudinal ligament tends to limit extension of the vertebral column, whereas the posterior ligament tends to limit flexion.
- Herniation of intervertebral discs at the thoracic/lumbar junction is common because the thoracic region of the spine is relatively immobile compared to the lumbar and cervical regions.

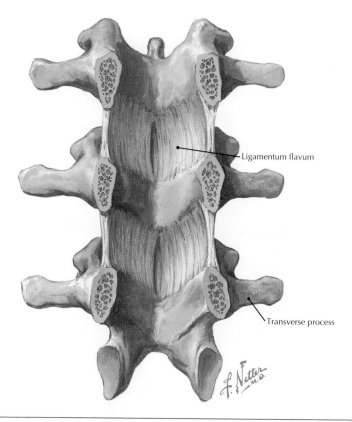

Ligamentum flavum

Transverse process

Anterior view of posterior vertebral arch *(Atlas of Human Anatomy, 6th edition, Plate 159)*

Clinical Note In addition to posterior disc bulging and hypertrophic arthritic facet joints, thickening of the ligamentum flavum is often a major component of degenerative spinal canal stenosis. Symptoms of spinal stenosis are usually worse in extension and improved in flexion, presumably because of infolding of the ligament in extension and stretching out and thinning of the ligament in flexion.

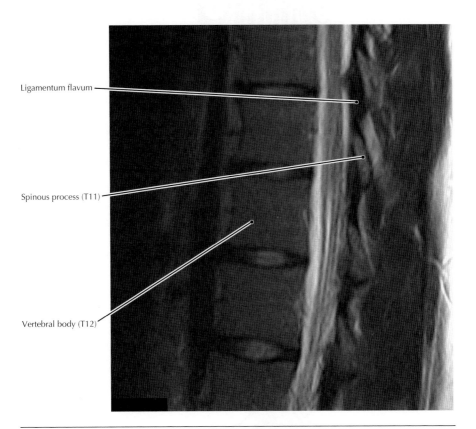

Ligamentum flavum

Spinous process (T11)

Vertebral body (T12)

Sagittal T2 MR image of thoracic spine, just off midline

- The ligamentum flavum contains elastic tissue that prevents the ligament from being pinched between the lamina when the vertebral column is hyperextended.
- Anesthesiologists use penetration of the ligamentum flavum as an indicator that the needle has reached the epidural space for epidural anesthesia.

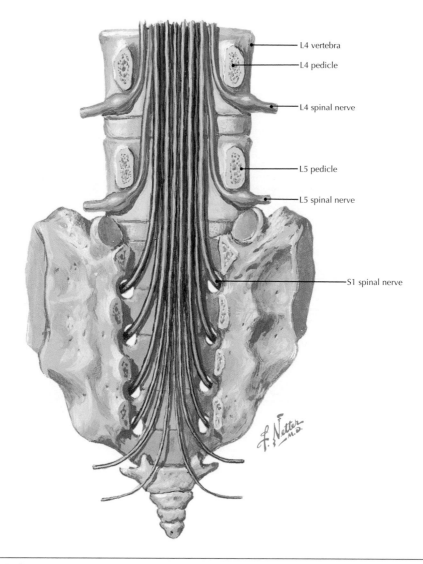

L4 vertebra

L4 pedicle

L4 spinal nerve

L5 pedicle

L5 spinal nerve

S1 spinal nerve

Relationship between the lower spinal nerves and their respective neuroforamina (intervertebral foramina) *(Atlas of Human Anatomy, 6th edition, Plate 161)*

Clinical Note Lower lumbar disc herniation may produce sciatica, which is pain along the path of the sciatic nerve. This occurs because the sciatic nerve consists of components from L4-S2 spinal segments.

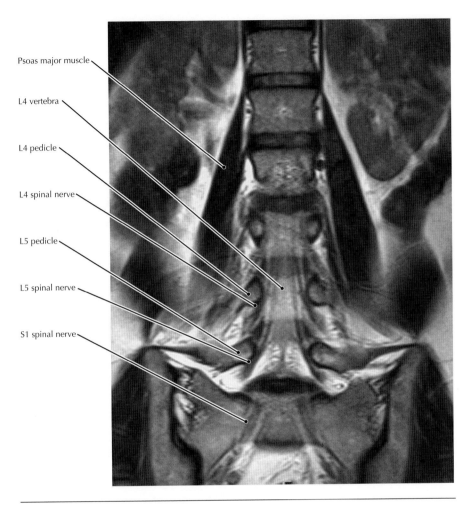

Psoas major muscle

L4 vertebra

L4 pedicle

L4 spinal nerve

L5 pedicle

L5 spinal nerve

S1 spinal nerve

Coronal T2 MR image of the lower spine

- The L4 spinal nerve passes caudal to the L4 pedicle to exit the spinal canal through the L4/L5 neuroforamen (intervertebral foramen).
- Similarly, the L5 nerve passes caudal to the L5 pedicle to exit the spinal canal through the L5/S1 neuroforamen.
- Coronal MR images may clearly show disc fragments that have herniated laterally and how they potentially affect nerve roots within or lateral to the neuroforamen.

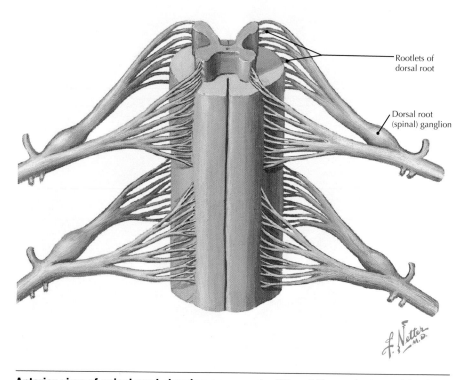

Rootlets of
dorsal root

Dorsal root
(spinal) ganglion

Anterior view of spinal cord showing nerve roots *(Atlas of Human Anatomy, 6th edition, Plate 165)*

Clinical Note The dorsal root (spinal) ganglia contain the cell bodies of the sensory neurons entering the spinal cord at a particular level. These cell bodies may be specifically targeted in certain disease states (e.g., herpes zoster infection, "shingles") resulting in a sensory neuropathy.

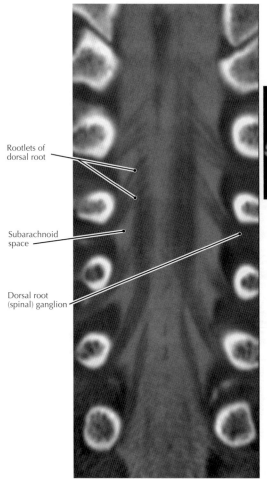
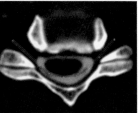

Rootlets of
dorsal root

Subarachnoid
space

Dorsal root
(spinal) ganglion

Curved coronal reconstruction at the level of the posterior rootlets, CT cervical myelogram (curved *green line* in the reference axial image shows the plane of section for the coronal image)

- In this CT image the rootlets of the dorsal roots are represented by the delicate black inclined lines; the gray material represents opacified (contrast-enhanced) cerebrospinal fluid (CSF) within the subarachnoid space. The CSF was opacified by an intradural injection of iodinated contrast material that was injected with a very fine needle during a simple outpatient procedure.
- For patients who cannot undergo MRI—for example, those with a pacemaker— CT myelography is an alternative imaging procedure that is capable of showing very delicate anatomy (e.g., spinal nerve rootlets).

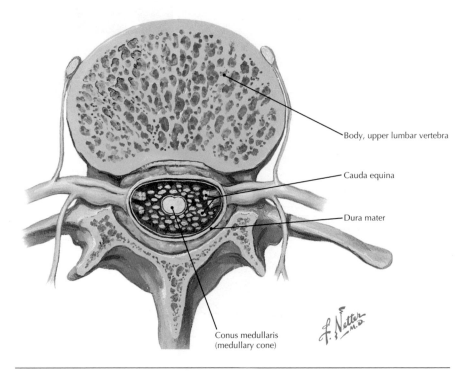

Body, upper lumbar vertebra

Cauda equina

Dura mater

Conus medullaris
(medullary cone)

Axial section through an upper lumbar vertebra *(Atlas of Human Anatomy, 6th edition, Plate 166)*

Clinical Note Lumbar puncture to obtain cerebrospinal fluid (CSF) is done inferior to L3 because the conus medullaris typically terminates at L1/L2, allowing for needle penetration below this level with little risk of injury to the freely floating spinal nerve roots that are suspended in the lumbar cistern.

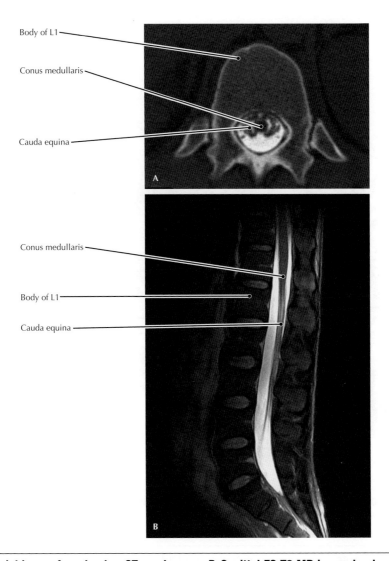

Body of L1

Conus medullaris

Cauda equina

A

Conus medullaris

Body of L1

Cauda equina

B

A, Axial image from lumbar CT myelogram; *B,* Sagittal FS T2 MR image lumbar spine

- The conus medullaris may terminate as high as T12 or as low as L3.
- The cauda equina consists primarily of the spinal nerve roots that innervate the lower limbs.

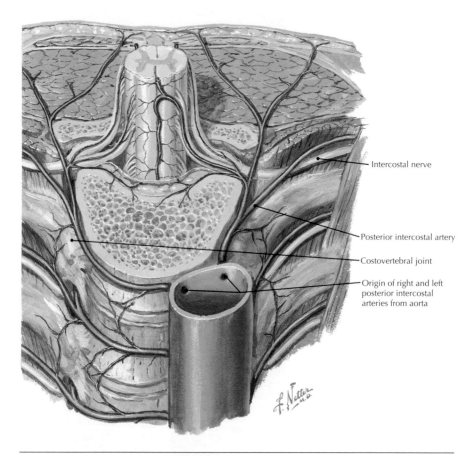

Intercostal nerve

Posterior intercostal artery

Costovertebral joint

Origin of right and left posterior intercostal arteries from aorta

Posterior thoracic wall showing origin of posterior intercostal arteries *(Atlas of Human Anatomy, 6th edition, Plate 168)*

Clinical Note The intercostal neurovascular bundle usually traverses the subcostal groove under the superior rib of the intercostal space. When a surgical incision or procedure (thoracotomy, thoracocentesis) is performed, the superior aspect of the intercostal space is avoided.

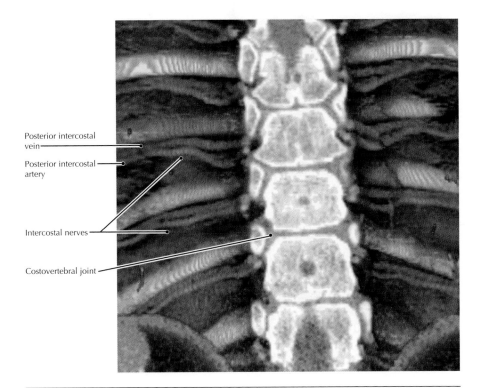

Posterior intercostal vein

Posterior intercostal artery

Intercostal nerves

Costovertebral joint

Curved coronal 10-mm slab, volume rendered display, CE CT of the chest

- The intercostal nerves and vessels traverse the potential space between the internal and innermost intercostal muscles.
- From superior to inferior the typical order of structures in an intercostal space is vein, artery, and nerve (VAN).

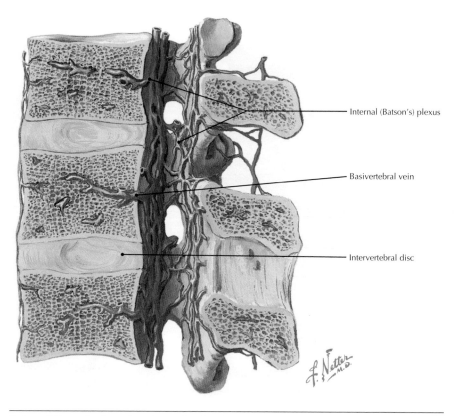

Internal (Batson's) plexus

Basivertebral vein

Intervertebral disc

Veins of the spinal cord and vertebral column *(Atlas of Human Anatomy, 6th edition, Plate 169)*

Clinical Note The absence of valves in the vertebral venous plexus allows retrograde flow, with the result that prostatic or breast cancer cells may metastasize to the spine, which explains the high prevalence of spinal metastatic disease in prostate and breast carcinoma.

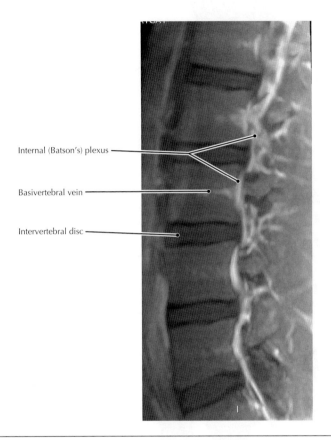

Internal (Batson's) plexus —

Basivertebral vein —

Intervertebral disc —

Parasagittal 8-mm MIP, contrast-enhanced FS T1 MR image

- The internal (Batson's) vertebral venous plexus is within the spinal canal whereas the external venous plexus surrounds the vertebrae.
- The veins of these plexuses are valveless and connect to segmental intervertebral veins and to the cerebral venous sinuses.

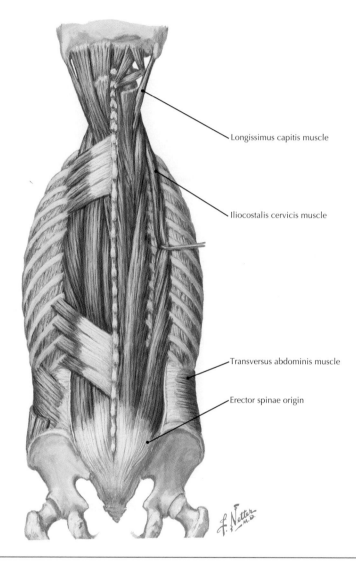

Longissimus capitis muscle

Iliocostalis cervicis muscle

Transversus abdominis muscle

Erector spinae origin

Intermediate muscle layer of the back *(Atlas of Human Anatomy, 6th edition, Plate 172)*

Clinical Note Disease or degenerative processes that result in the generation of abnormal activation patterns of the different components of the erector spinae can produce a functional scoliosis.

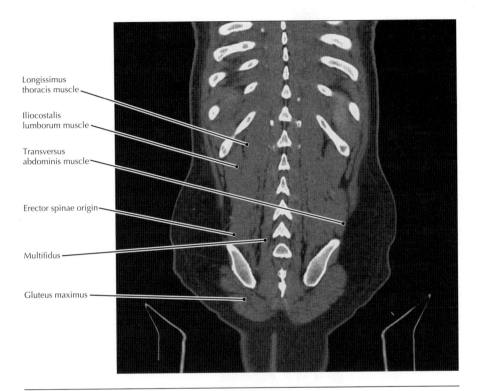

Longissimus
thoracis muscle

Iliocostalis
lumborum muscle

Transversus
abdominis muscle

Erector spinae origin

Multifidus

Gluteus maximus

Curved coronal reconstruction, CT lumbar spine

- Spasm in the erector spinae is associated with lumbago as the muscles spastically contract to reduce spinal movements.
- The erector spinae muscle group is entirely innervated by segmental dorsal rami.
- The three longitudinal components of the erector spinae (from lateral to medial) are the iliocostalis, longissimus, and spinalis.

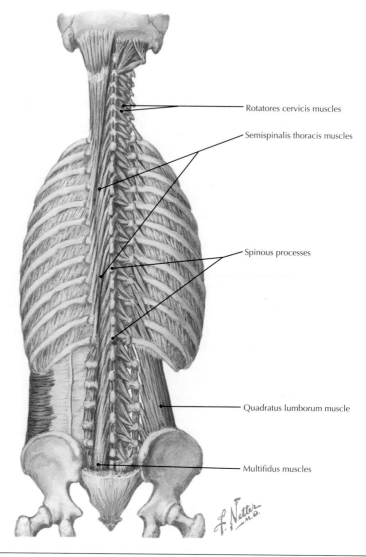

Rotatores cervicis muscles

Semispinalis thoracis muscles

Spinous processes

Quadratus lumborum muscle

Multifidus muscles

Multifidus, rotatores, and other deep back muscles *(Atlas of Human Anatomy, 6th edition, Plate 173)*

Clinical Note   Although often not considered important clinically, spasms in the deep back muscles (especially multifidus) may be associated with radiculopathy and pain.

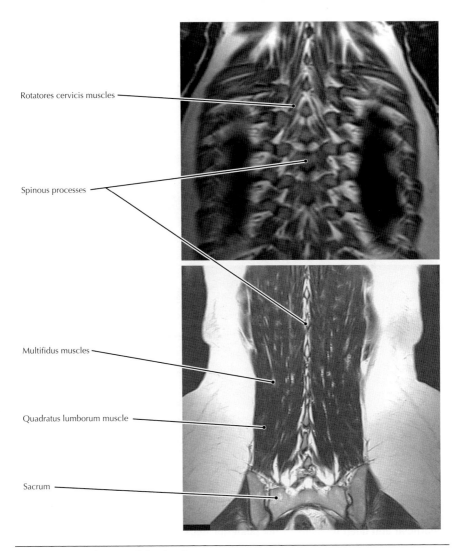

Rotatores cervicis muscles

Spinous processes

Multifidus muscles

Quadratus lumborum muscle

Sacrum

Coronal T1 MR image of the back

- The deep back muscles are primarily responsible for delicate adjustments between individual vertebrae that correlate with changes in posture.
- The three components of the transversospinalis muscle group are semispinalis, multifidus, and rotatores, but they are not equally developed in all regions (multifidus is best developed in the lumbar region).
- The deep back muscles are all innervated by segmental dorsal rami.

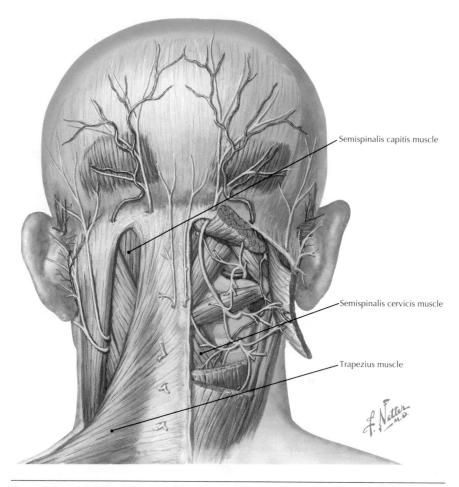

Semispinalis capitis muscle

Semispinalis cervicis muscle

Trapezius muscle

Superficial and deep muscles of the posterior neck *(Atlas of Human Anatomy, 6th edition, Plate 175)*

Clinical Note The insertion of the semispinal capitis is a reliable indicator of the location of the transverse sinus and thus can be used by neurosurgeons to avoid damaging this structure in surgical approaches to the posterior fossa and craniovertebral junction.

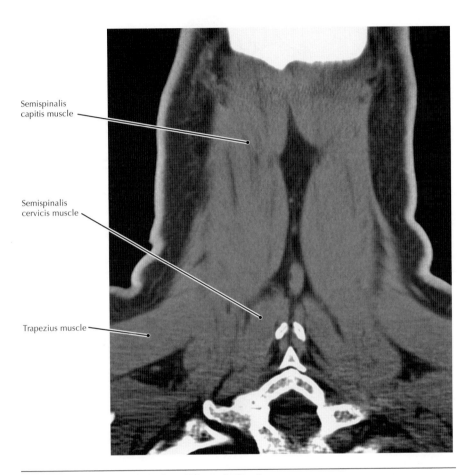

Semispinalis
capitis muscle

Semispinalis
cervicis muscle

Trapezius muscle

Curved coronal reconstruction, CT cervical spine

- The semispinalis capitis muscle forms the bulk of the muscle mass on either side of the nuchal furrow.
- The semispinalis capitis muscle extends and laterally flexes the neck.

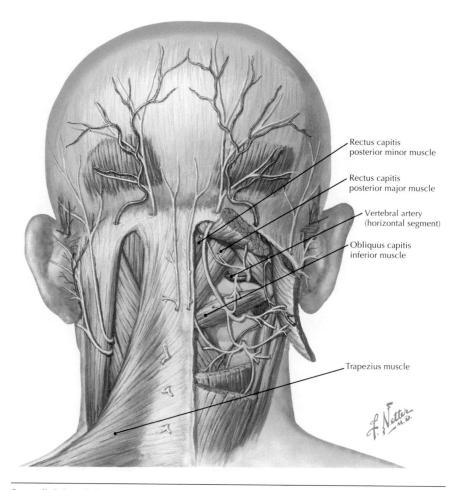

Rectus capitis
posterior minor muscle

Rectus capitis
posterior major muscle

Vertebral artery
(horizontal segment)

Obliquus capitis
inferior muscle

Trapezius muscle

Superficial and deep muscles of the posterior neck *(Atlas of Human Anatomy, 6th edition, Plate 175)*

Clinical Note The rectus posterior muscles may play a role in cervicogenic headaches via a dense fascial connection between these muscles and the cervical dura.

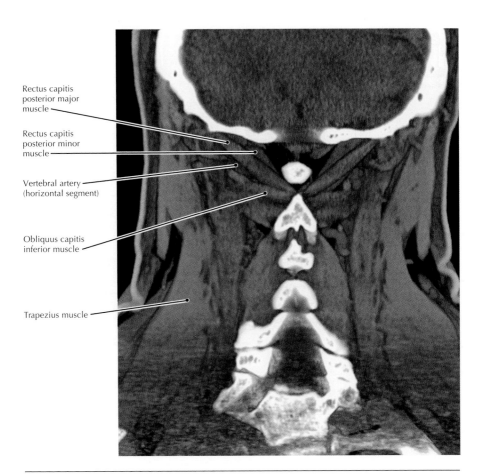

Rectus capitis
posterior major
muscle

Rectus capitis
posterior minor
muscle

Vertebral artery
(horizontal segment)

Obliquus capitis
inferior muscle

Trapezius muscle

Curved 15-mm slab, volume rendered display, cervical spine CT

- The rectus posterior muscles function in lateral rotation and extension of the head.
- All the muscles of the suboccipital triangle are innervated by the suboccipital nerve (dorsal ramus of C1).

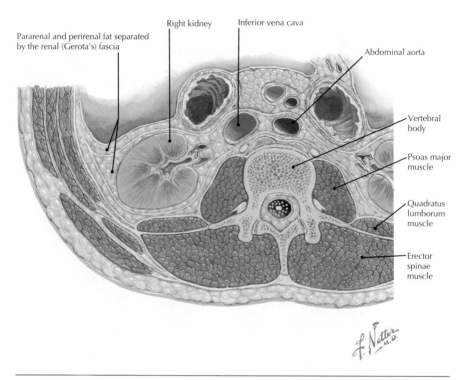

Right kidney

Inferior vena cava

Pararenal and perirenal fat separated
by the renal (Gerota's) fascia

Abdominal aorta

Vertebral
body

Psoas major
muscle

Quadratus
lumborum
muscle

Erector
spinae
muscle

Cross section of back and posterior abdominal wall at L2 *(Atlas of Human Anatomy, 6th edition, Plate 176)*

Clinical Note Back pain may be caused by retroperitoneal disease. Occasionally, a lumbar spine MR image requested to evaluate back pain will reveal, for example, an abdominal aortic aneurysm or retroperitoneal adenopathy.

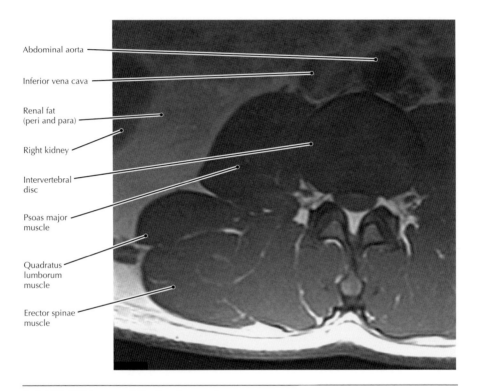

Abdominal aorta

Inferior vena cava

Renal fat
(peri and para)

Right kidney

Intervertebral
disc

Psoas major
muscle

Quadratus
lumborum
muscle

Erector spinae
muscle

Axial T1 MR image of the lumbar region

- Imbalanced patterns of erector spinae muscle activity and reduced trunk extension strength are associated with low back pain.
- Perirenal and pararenal fat is thought to act as a cushion that protects the kidney from injury.
- The diaphragm, psoas, quadratus lumborum, and transversus abdominis comprise the posterior relations of the kidney.

Section 3   **Thorax**

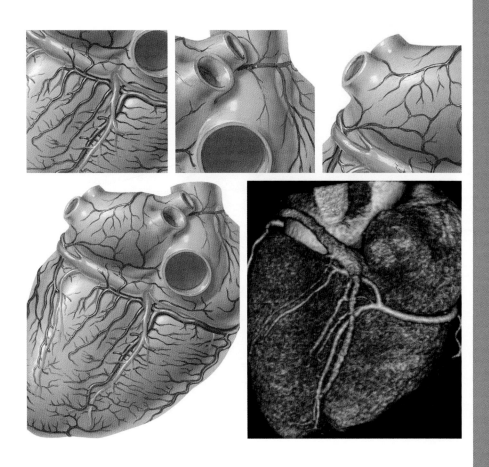

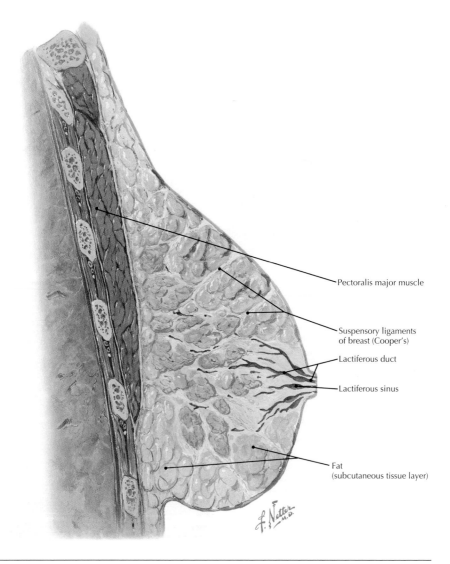

Pectoralis major muscle

Suspensory ligaments
of breast (Cooper's)

Lactiferous duct

Lactiferous sinus

Fat
(subcutaneous tissue layer)

Sagittal section of breast and chest wall *(Atlas of Human Anatomy, 6th edition, Plate 179)*

Clinical Note Dimpling of the skin of the breast over a carcinoma is caused by involvement and retraction of the suspensory ligaments (of Cooper), and obstruction of lymphatic drainage by carcinoma may cause edematous skin changes known as *peau d'orange*.

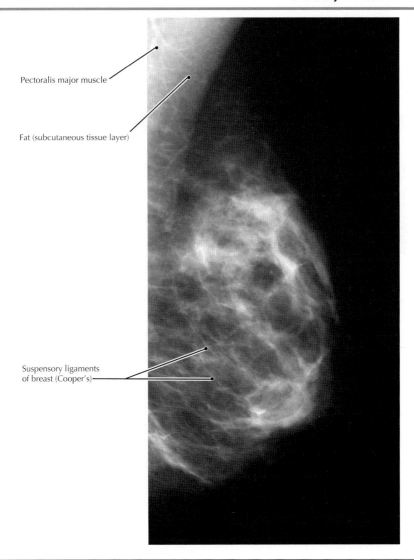

Pectoralis major muscle

Fat (subcutaneous tissue layer)

Suspensory ligaments
of breast (Cooper's)

Mammogram, mediolateral oblique (MLO) view

- Standard projections for screening mammography are the MLO view shown above and a craniocaudal (CC) projection.

- When clinical breast examination reveals a suspicious finding, diagnostic mammography should be requested. Sometimes, routine screening MLO and CC views are not adequate for visualization of a mass, so additional mammographic views such as spot compression, magnification, and 90-degree mediolateral ones are performed and are often followed by ultrasonography.

- Cooper's ligaments appear in mammograms as very thin white lines.

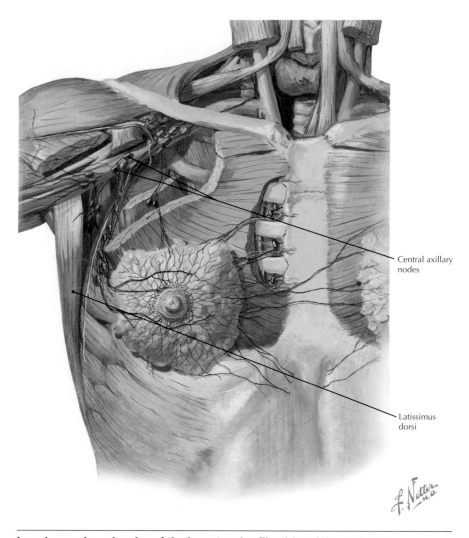

Central axillary nodes

Latissimus dorsi

Lymph vessels and nodes of the breast and axilla *(Atlas of Human Anatomy, 6th edition, Plate 181)*

Clinical Note When operating on a tumor of the breast, the surgeon will often harvest some axillary lymph nodes for histologic examination. Presence or absence of cancerous cells in the nodes is important for staging of the cancer.

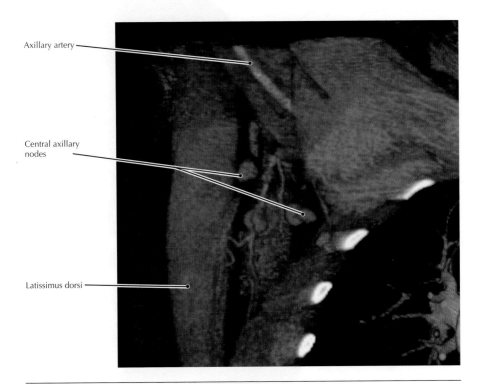

Axillary artery

Central axillary nodes

Latissimus dorsi

Volume rendered display, CE CT of the chest

- The arm is elevated in this patient.
- In subclavian venous puncture for central line placement the vein initially punctured is technically the axillary vein, which becomes the subclavian at the first rib. Thus, it is clinically important that the axillary vein lies anterior and inferior (i.e., superficial) to the axillary artery and the cords of the brachial plexus.

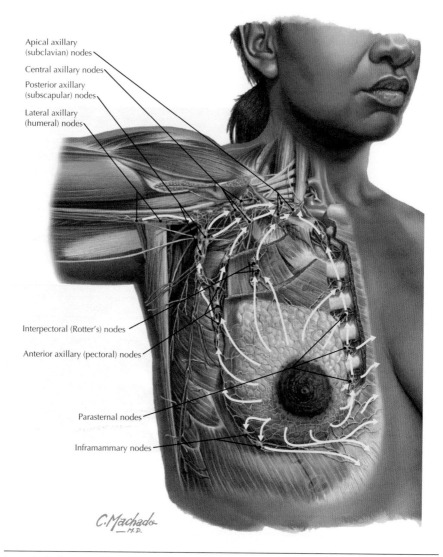

Apical axillary
(subclavian) nodes

Central axillary nodes

Posterior axillary
(subscapular) nodes

Lateral axillary
(humeral) nodes

Interpectoral (Rotter's) nodes

Anterior axillary (pectoral) nodes

Parasternal nodes

Inframammary nodes

C. Machado
M.D.

Lymph drainage of the breast *(Atlas of Human Anatomy, 6th edition, Plate 182)*

Clinical Note   The axillary lymph nodes drain most of the breast as well as the upper limb and thus are of paramount importance in the staging of breast cancer. These nodes are classically divided into five groups, with the pectoral group being the first of the chain to receive lymph from the breast. Extensive axillary node dissection can result in lymphedema of the upper limb.

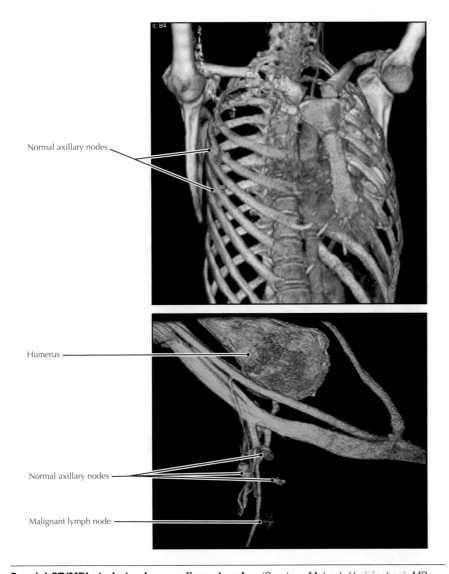

Normal axillary nodes

Humerus

Normal axillary nodes

Malignant lymph node

Special CT/MRI study to show malignant nodes *(Courtesy Mukesh Harisinghani, MD, Harvard Medical School, Cambridge, Mass)*

- These MR lymph node images are superimposed on CT data (showing bones and vessels) from the same patient. The brown tubular structures in lower image are blood vessels.
- The red nodes indicate malignancy, determined by MR signal characteristics.

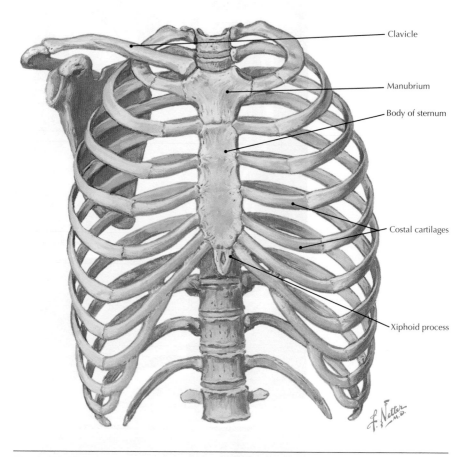

Clavicle

Manubrium

Body of sternum

Costal cartilages

Xiphoid process

Thoracic cage *(Atlas of Human Anatomy, 6th edition, Plate 183)*

> **Clinical Note** The middle ribs are fractured more frequently than the superior or inferior ribs because they are more prominent and/or less protected by other structures. The fractured ends of ribs can injure thoracic or abdominal organs (e.g., lungs, spleen). Rib fractures are very painful because the ribs move during inspiration and expiration.

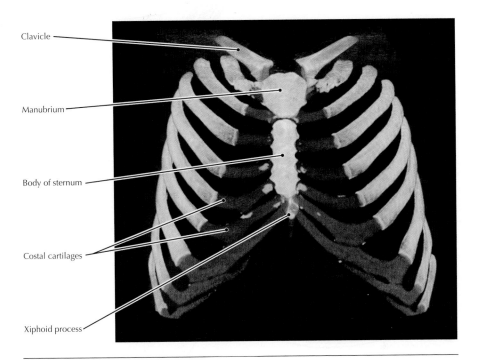

Clavicle

Manubrium

Body of sternum

Costal cartilages

Xiphoid process

Volume rendered display, CT of the chest

- Portions within the costal cartilages have calcified in this CT image. The calcification of costal cartilages is highly variable in the adult.

- The xiphoid process has also ossified in this CT image; it is typically cartilaginous in persons under 40.

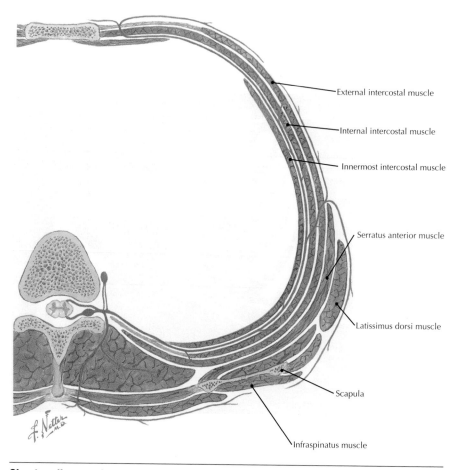

External intercostal muscle

Internal intercostal muscle

Innermost intercostal muscle

Serratus anterior muscle

Latissimus dorsi muscle

Scapula

Infraspinatus muscle

Chest wall musculature and intercostal nerve *(Atlas of Human Anatomy, 6th edition, Plate 177)*

Clinical Note Serratus anterior free flaps are often used for reconstruction of anatomic structures such as parts of the face, limbs, or diaphragm. The serratus anterior flap is very versatile because variable sizes of flap and pedicle lengths can be taken. Furthermore, using these flaps does not typically produce major functional or aesthetic sequelae.

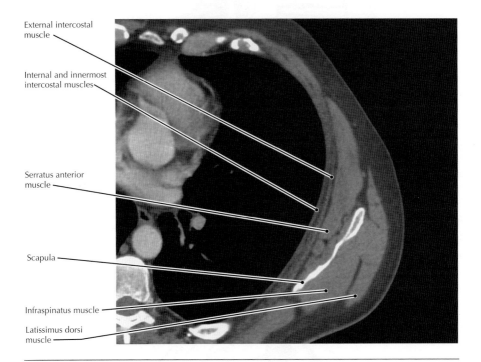

External intercostal muscle

Internal and innermost intercostal muscles

Serratus anterior muscle

Scapula

Infraspinatus muscle

Latissimus dorsi muscle

Oblique axial CT (parallel to ribs at level of intercostal space)

- The internal and innermost intercostal muscles are not easily differentiated in radiographic images because they are typically not well separated by a fatty layer.

- During quiet respiration, the actions of the intercostal muscles contribute only marginally to inhalation and expiration.

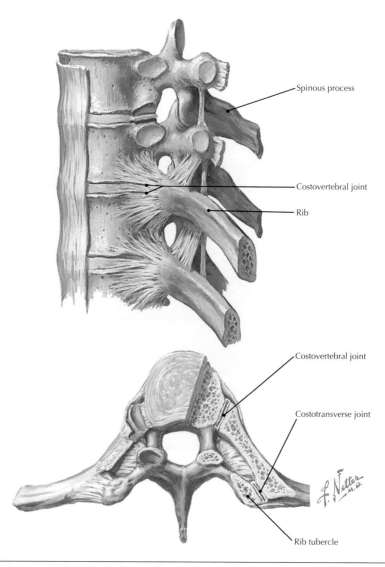

Spinous process

Costovertebral joint

Rib

Costovertebral joint

Costotransverse joint

Rib tubercle

Lateral and superior views of the joints between the ribs and vertebrae *(Atlas of Human Anatomy, 6th edition, Plate 184)*

Clinical Note Injury and dysfunction of the costovertebral joint complex (costotransverse and costovertebral joints) may be associated with direct blows, forceful rib cage compression, and excessive trunk flexion.

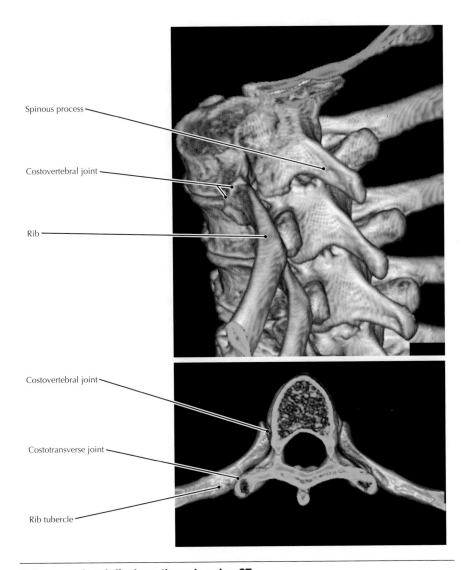

Spinous process

Costovertebral joint

Rib

Costovertebral joint

Costotransverse joint

Rib tubercle

Volume rendered displays, thoracic spine CT

- Most of the ribs have two demifacets on their heads to articulate with the same numbered vertebra and the one superior to it.
- Both the costovertebral and costotransverse joints are synovial and accordingly may become arthritic, causing pain.

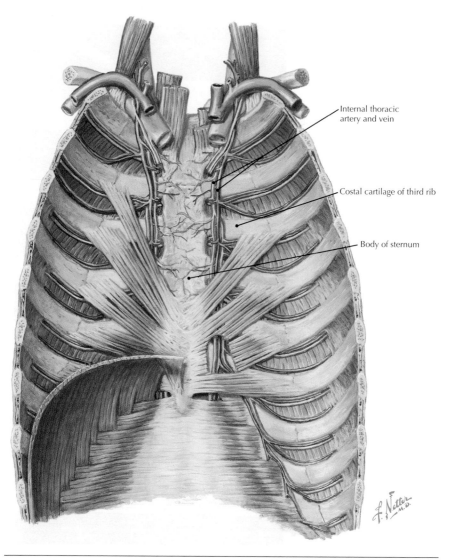

Internal view of anterior chest wall *(Atlas of Human Anatomy, 6th edition, Plate 187)*

Internal thoracic artery and vein

Costal cartilage of third rib

Body of sternum

Clinical Note Parasternal lymph nodes and channels parallel the internal thoracic (mammary) artery and vein. These channels receive lymphatic drainage from the breast and therefore may be a pathway for lymphatic spread of breast cancer.

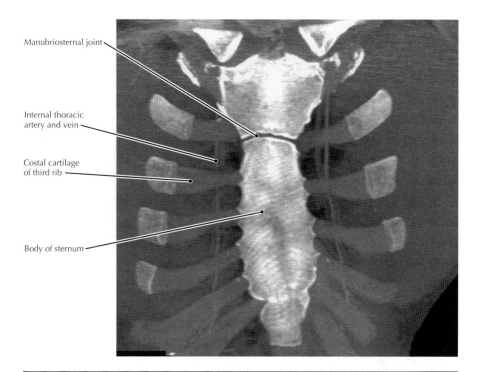

Manubriosternal joint

Internal thoracic
artery and vein

Costal cartilage
of third rib

Body of sternum

Curved coronal MIP from CTA of the chest

- The internal thoracic (mammary) artery and vein give rise to the anterior intercostal vessels, which anastomose with the posterior intercostal vessels, which are branches of the thoracic aorta.

- The joints between the costal cartilages and the ribs are classified as primary cartilaginous joints (synchondroses), whereas the joint between the manubrium and the sternum is a secondary cartilaginous joint (symphysis).

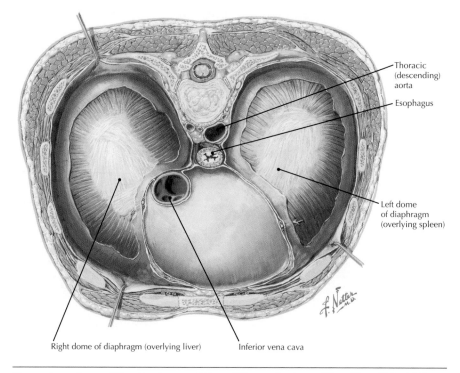

Thoracic
(descending)
aorta

Esophagus

Left dome
of diaphragm
(overlying spleen)

Right dome of diaphragm (overlying liver)

Inferior vena cava

Thoracic surface of the diaphragm *(Atlas of Human Anatomy, 6th edition, Plate 191)*

Clinical Note Hiccups result from spasmodic contractions of the diaphragm and, if protracted, can have serious consequences (e.g., cardiac dysrhythmias). The medical term for hiccups is *singultus*.

Left dome of diaphragm
(overlying spleen)

Thoracic
(descending) aorta

Esophagus

Inferior vena cava

Right dome of
diaphragm
(overlying liver)

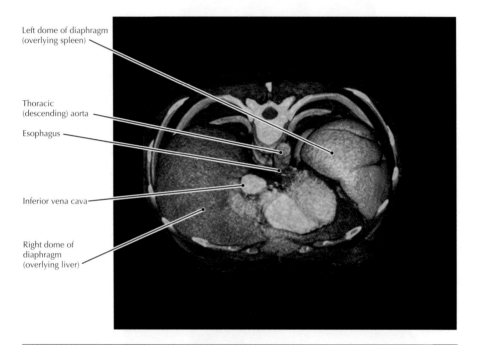

Volume rendered display, CE CT of the chest

- The diaphragm is innervated by the phrenic nerve, which is typically composed of segments from the ventral rami of the C3, C4, and C5 spinal nerves.
- Because the supraclavicular nerves also receive innervation from C3 and C4, pain from much of the diaphragm is referred to the shoulder region.
- The liver and spleen are partially protected from injury from the lower part of the rib cage as seen in this CT image.

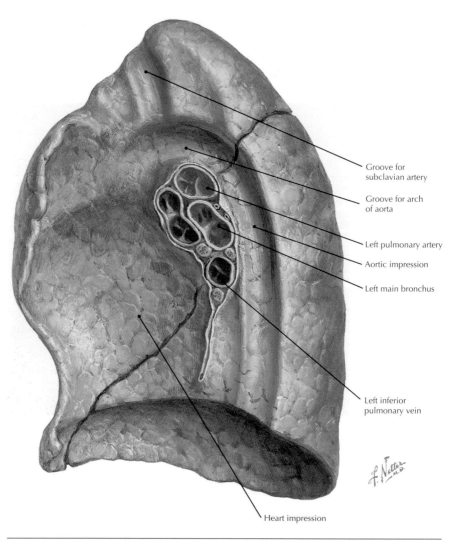

Groove for
subclavian artery

Groove for arch
of aorta

Left pulmonary artery

Aortic impression

Left main bronchus

Left inferior
pulmonary vein

Heart impression

Medial view of the left lung showing hilar structures *(Atlas of Human Anatomy, 6th edition, Plate 196, presented as a mirror image of the original Netter drawing to match the standard radiologic orientation of the CT scan.)*

Clinical Note   Bronchogenic carcinoma, the vast majority of which is caused by cigarette smoking, typically metastasizes early to the bronchopulmonary lymph nodes at the hilum of the lung.

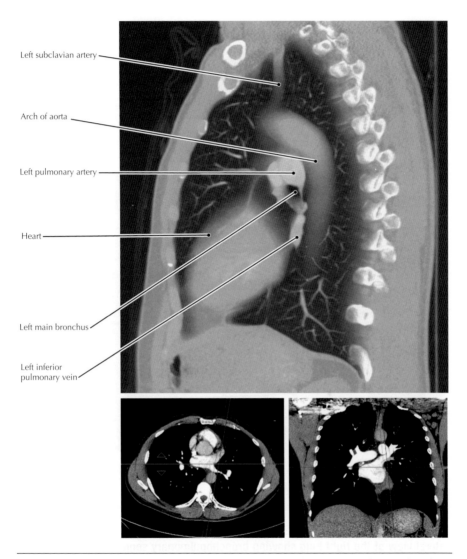

Left subclavian artery

Arch of aorta

Left pulmonary artery

Heart

Left main bronchus

Left inferior
pulmonary vein

2-cm thick MIP, CE CT showing major lung hilar structures (*red* and *blue lines* in the reference images indicate the position and orientation of the main image)

- Typically, sagittal radiologic images are viewed from the patient's left as shown in this CT image.
- Note the very low CT density (indicated by blackness) of air in the lungs and airways, which results because air does not stop or scatter many photons.

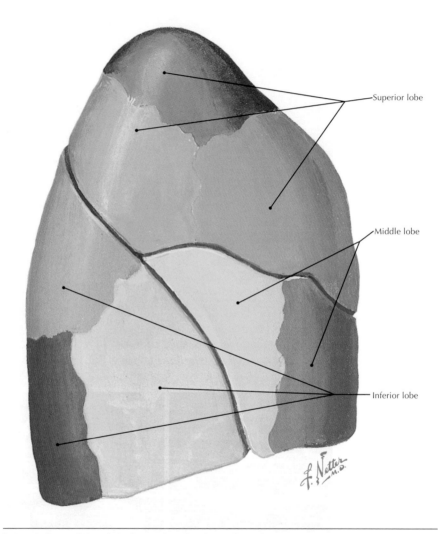

Superior lobe

Middle lobe

Inferior lobe

Lateral view of the right lung showing bronchopulmonary segments *(Atlas of Human Anatomy, 6th edition, Plate 198)*

Clinical Note There are 18 to 20 bronchopulmonary segments, 10 in the right and 8 to 10 in the left, depending on the branching pattern of the bronchi. These segments are separated from adjacent segments by connective tissue and are surgically resectable.

Superior lobe

Middle lobe

Inferior lobe

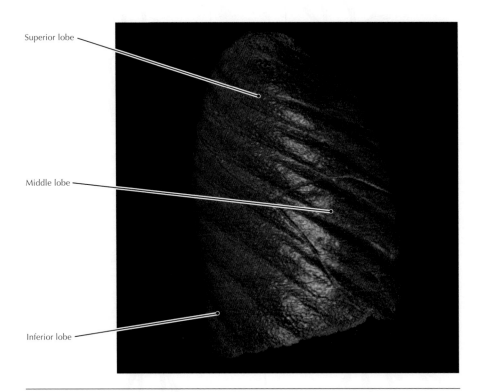

CE CT shaded surface display of the right lung from scan of the thorax

- The left lung is composed of two lobes (superior and inferior) separated by an oblique (major) fissure.
- The right lung is composed of three lobes (superior, middle, and inferior) separated by horizontal (minor) and oblique (major) fissures.

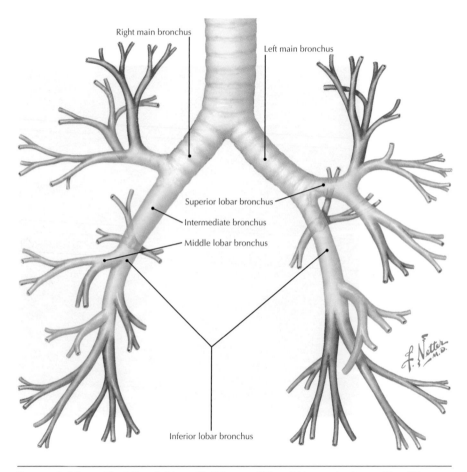

Segmental bronchi of the right and left lungs *(Atlas of Human Anatomy, 6th edition, Plate 200)*

Clinical Note Bronchiectasis is characterized by chronic bronchial dilation associated with loss of muscular and supporting tissues within the bronchi. Patients typically have chronic cough and purulent sputum production.

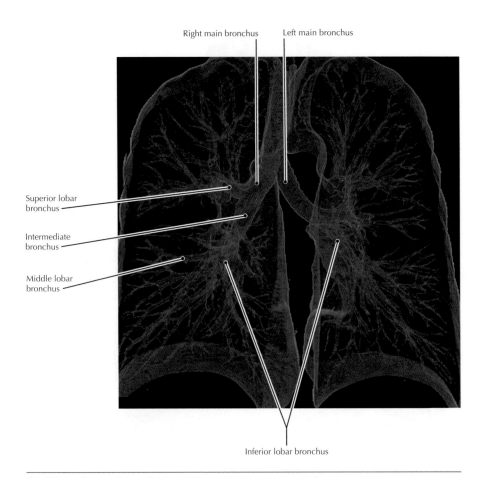

Right main bronchus   Left main bronchus

Superior lobar bronchus

Intermediate bronchus

Middle lobar bronchus

Inferior lobar bronchus

CE CT shaded surface display of bronchi from scan of the thorax

- Standard procedures for evaluating airway disease include pulmonary function testing, which quantifies the volume and rate of flow of air movement into and out of the lungs, fiberoptic bronchoscopy, and high resolution pulmonary CT scanning.
- Volume rendered images such as this are not usually fundamental for initial diagnosis, but can be useful for showing whether a tumor is resectable.

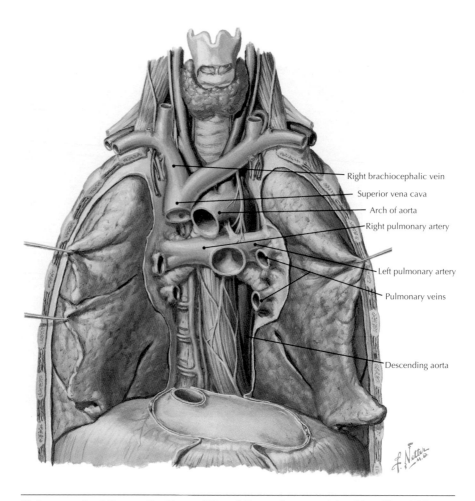

Right brachiocephalic vein

Superior vena cava

Arch of aorta

Right pulmonary artery

Left pulmonary artery

Pulmonary veins

Descending aorta

Major vessels of the mediastinum *(Atlas of Human Anatomy, 6th edition, Plate 203)*

Clinical Note Occlusion of a pulmonary artery by an embolus (blood clot) causes a mismatch between ventilation and perfusion of affected lung segments. The resulting hypoxemia (decreased partial pressure of oxygen in the blood) may be fatal.

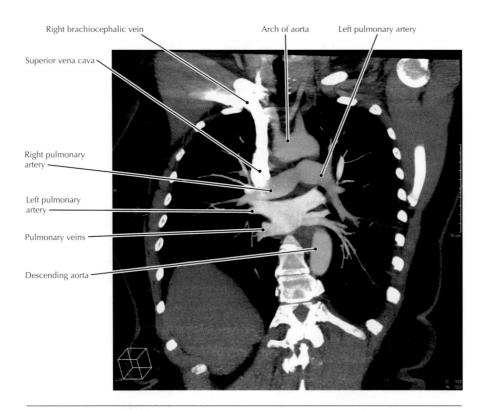

Right brachiocephalic vein
Arch of aorta
Left pulmonary artery
Superior vena cava
Right pulmonary artery
Left pulmonary artery
Pulmonary veins
Descending aorta

Coronal CE CT of the chest

- Intravenous (IV) contrast material was injected rapidly into a right arm vein, resulting in intense enhancement of the right brachiocephalic vein and superior vena cava (SVC).
- The intensity of enhancement of various vascular structures is critically dependent on the timing and rate of the IV contrast injection and the start of the CT scan.

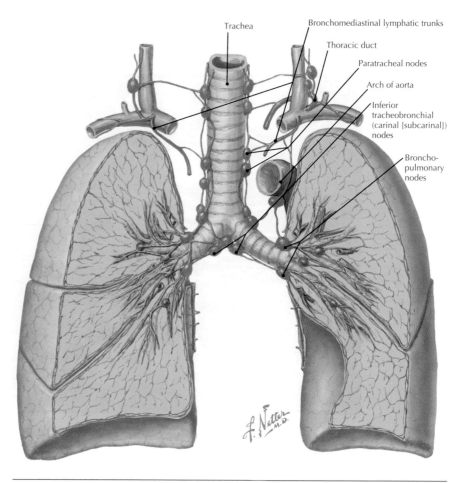

Trachea

Bronchomediastinal lymphatic trunks

Thoracic duct

Paratracheal nodes

Arch of aorta

Inferior tracheobronchial (carinal [subcarinal]) nodes

Broncho-pulmonary nodes

Lymph nodes and vessels of the lung *(Atlas of Human Anatomy, 6th edition, Plate 205)*

Clinical Note The staging of lung cancer is based, in part, on whether or not cancer has metastasized to hilar and mediastinal lymph nodes or more distant sites. Accurate tumor staging provides prognosis and guides optimal therapy.

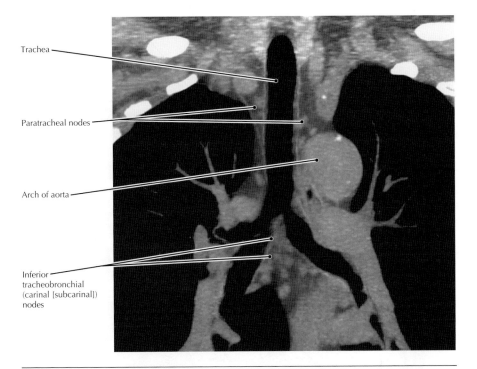

Trachea

Paratracheal nodes

Arch of aorta

Inferior tracheobronchial (carinal [subcarinal]) nodes

Coronal reconstruction, CT of the chest

- Lymph from the lung flows to a superficial subpleural plexus and a deep plexus that accompanies the pulmonary vessels and bronchi.

- Because lymph nodes are located near the main bronchi, metastases to these nodes may also involve the bronchi, complicating surgical removal of the cancerous tissues.

- Before the clinical use of positron emission tomography (PET) scanning, imaging criteria for pathology of lymph nodes was based solely on size. However, the sensitivity and specificity of PET scans for detection of lymph node metastases allows for more accurate staging.

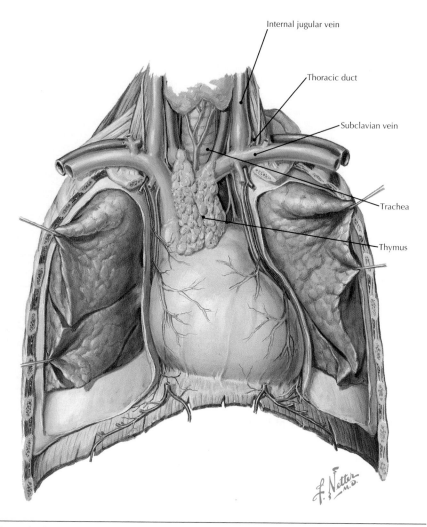

Internal jugular vein

Thoracic duct

Subclavian vein

Trachea

Thymus

Thoracic duct, trachea, and thymus *(Atlas of Human Anatomy, 6th edition, Plate 208)*

> **Clinical Note**   Although the thoracic duct usually terminates as a single channel into the junction of the left internal jugular and subclavian veins, bifid and trifid terminations are not rare. Iatrogenic transection of one of these terminations during radical neck surgery can result in a chylous fistula.

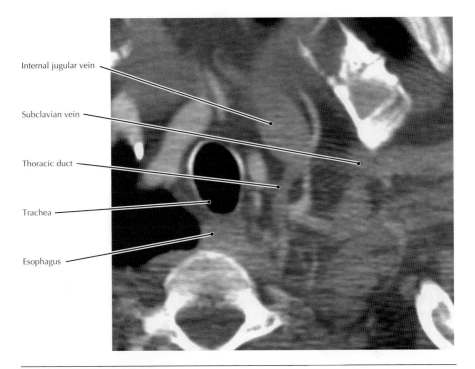

Internal jugular vein

Subclavian vein

Thoracic duct

Trachea

Esophagus

Oblique axial CE CT at the thoracic inlet

- The thoracic duct conducts lymph to the venous system from all of the body except the right side of the head, thorax, and upper limb.
- When the esophagus is empty, its walls are apposed and no lumen is apparent on imaging.
- The trachea, which is approximately circular in axial section, appears ovoid in this CT image because the image is oblique to its axis.

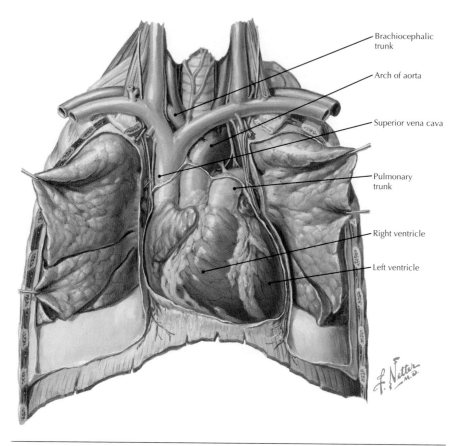

Brachiocephalic trunk

Arch of aorta

Superior vena cava

Pulmonary trunk

Right ventricle

Left ventricle

Anterior exposure of the heart *(Atlas of Human Anatomy, 6th edition, Plate 209)*

Clinical Note Aortic valve stenosis necessitates higher systolic pressure to maintain cardiac output. This leads to left ventricular hypertrophy.

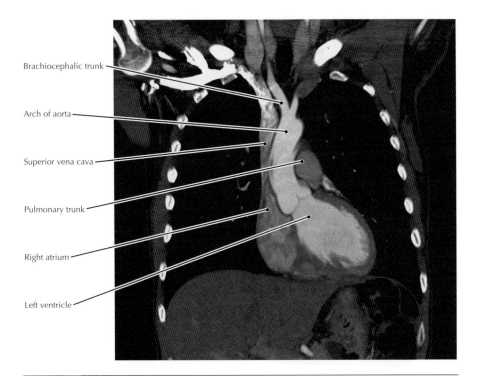

Brachiocephalic trunk

Arch of aorta

Superior vena cava

Pulmonary trunk

Right atrium

Left ventricle

Coronal reconstruction, CE CT of the chest

- This coronal section is approximately halfway through the anterior-posterior (AP) dimension of the heart, so it is posterior to the right ventricle, which forms most of the anterior surface of the heart. It illustrates the components of the right and left cardiac borders that appear in a posterior-anterior (PA) chest radiograph.

- The high-pitched sounds generated by a stenotic aortic valve are projected into the aorta and are best heard at the right second intercostal space.

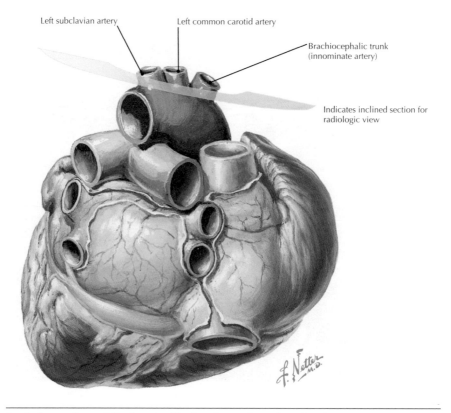

Left subclavian artery

Left common carotid artery

Brachiocephalic trunk (innominate artery)

Indicates inclined section for radiologic view

Posterior surface of the heart with the plane of section showing the radiographic reconstruction through the branches of the arch of the aorta *(Atlas of Human Anatomy, 6th edition, Plate 211)*

Clinical Note Variations in the arch of the aorta are not rare and may have clinical implications. For example, an aberrant origin of the right subclavian artery may pass posterior to the esophagus, compressing it and causing dysphagia.

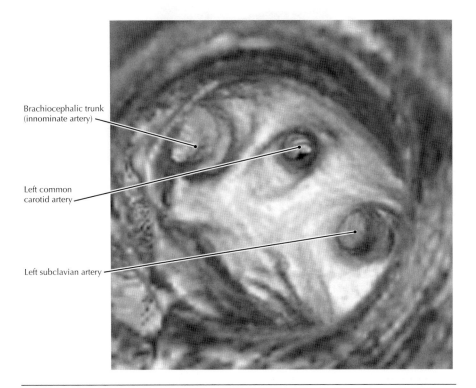

Brachiocephalic trunk
(innominate artery)

Left common
carotid artery

Left subclavian artery

Endoluminal 3-D reconstruction, CT of the arch of the aorta (inferior perspective)
(From Ravenel JG, McAdams HP: Multiplanar and three-dimensional imaging of the thorax. Radiol Clin North Am 41(3):475-489, 2003)

- Atherosclerotic disease of the arch of the aorta may narrow the ostia of the major arch branches.
- After giving off the left subclavian artery, the arch of the aorta becomes the descending or thoracic aorta. The ascending aorta is that portion before the origin of the brachiocephalic trunk.

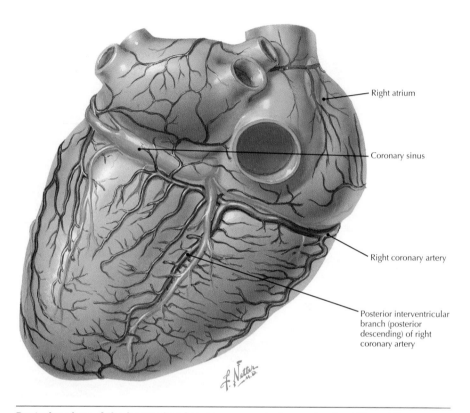

Right atrium

Coronary sinus

Right coronary artery

Posterior interventricular branch (posterior descending) of right coronary artery

Posterior view of the heart showing coronary arteries and veins *(Atlas of Human Anatomy, 6th edition, Plate 215)*

Clinical Note   In the 70% to 80% of individuals who have a right dominant coronary circulation, the right coronary artery (RCA) gives rise to the posterolateral artery (PLA) and continues as the posterior descending artery (PDA), which runs in the posterior interventricular groove. If these arteries arise from the left circumflex (LCX), there is a left dominant circulation. If the PLA arises from the LCX and the PDA is a continuation of the RCA, the coronary circulation is "balanced" or "codominant."

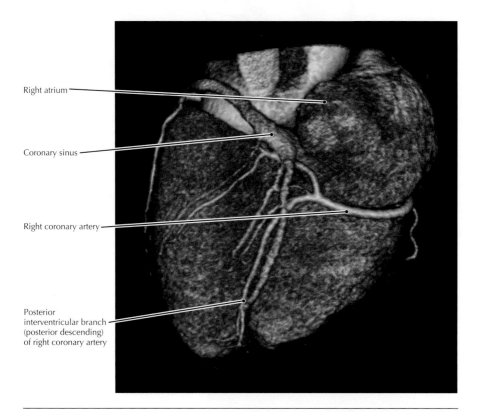

Right atrium

Coronary sinus

Right coronary artery

Posterior
interventricular branch
(posterior descending)
of right coronary artery

3-D reconstruction, coronary CTA

- The coronary sinus drains into the right atrium.
- The right coronary artery traverses the right atrioventricular groove.
- The posterior descending (interventricular) artery arises from the right coronary artery in this individual.

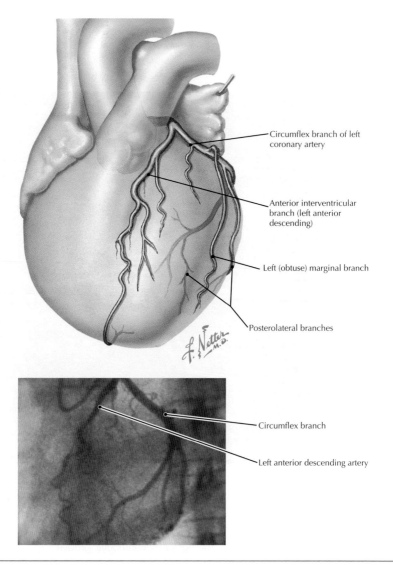

Illustrative and angiographic views of the branches of the left coronary artery *(Atlas of Human Anatomy, 6th edition, Plate 216)*

Clinical Note   If a coronary artery is occluded, the myocardium supplied by that artery becomes infarcted and undergoes necrosis.

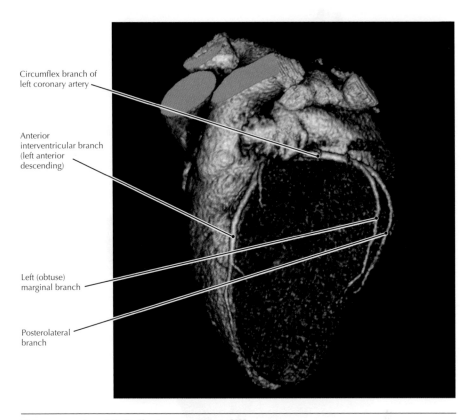

Circumflex branch of
left coronary artery

Anterior
interventricular branch
(left anterior
descending)

Left (obtuse)
marginal branch

Posterolateral
branch

Volume rendered 3-D display, coronary CTA

- Common sites of occlusion for coronary artery disease include the following:
  - Left anterior descending (anterior interventricular; 40% to 50%)
  - Right coronary artery (30% to 40%)
  - Circumflex branch (15% to 20%)
- Coronary artery stenting is performed in conjunction with cardiac catheterization and balloon angioplasty. It requires the insertion of a balloon catheter into the femoral artery in the upper thigh, which is threaded into the blocked coronary artery. When this catheter is positioned at the location of the blockage, it is slowly inflated to widen that artery and then removed. Next, the stent is threaded into the artery and placed around a deflated balloon. This balloon is then inflated, expanding the stent against the walls of the coronary artery. The balloon catheter is finally removed, leaving the stent in place to maintain the patency of the vessel.

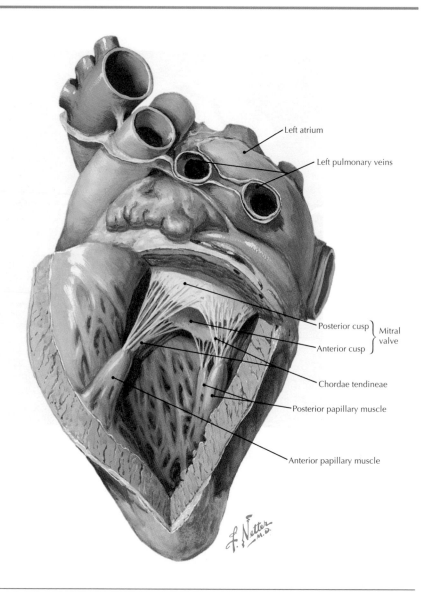

Left atrium

Left pulmonary veins

Posterior cusp ⎫ Mitral
Anterior cusp ⎬ valve

Chordae tendineae

Posterior papillary muscle

Anterior papillary muscle

Flap opened in posterolateral wall of the left ventricle *(Atlas of Human Anatomy, 6th edition, Plate 218)*

Clinical Note Ruptured chordae tendineae in the left ventricle result in an incompetent mitral valve, allowing blood to regurgitate back into the left atrium during systole.

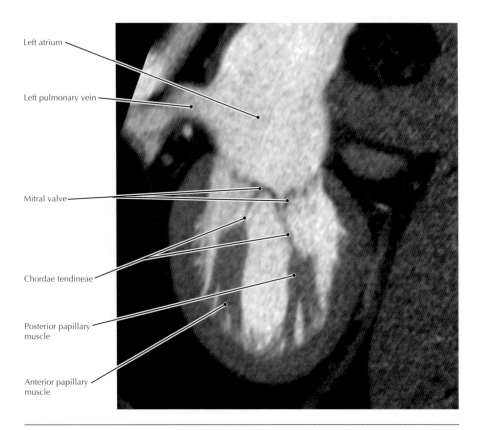

Left atrium

Left pulmonary vein

Mitral valve

Chordae tendineae

Posterior papillary
muscle

Anterior papillary
muscle

Oblique reconstruction, coronary CTA

- In this patient, after beginning a rapid infusion of IV contrast material, a precisely timed CT scan is acquired during optimal enhancement of the left cardiac chambers and coronary arteries.
- Internal cardiac structures are silhouetted against the contrast-enhanced blood.
- Contraction of the papillary muscles maintains the position of the valve cusps during systole, thus preventing blood from regurgitating into the atrium.

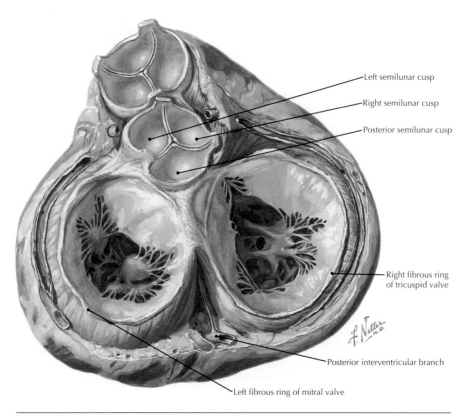

Left semilunar cusp

Right semilunar cusp

Posterior semilunar cusp

Right fibrous ring
of tricuspid valve

Posterior interventricular branch

Left fibrous ring of mitral valve

Aortic valve in diastole (superior perspective) *(Atlas of Human Anatomy, 6th edition, Plate 219)*

Clinical Note The first sound (S1) associated with a heartbeat is produced by the closing of the mitral and tricuspid valves; the closing of the aortic and pulmonary valves produces the second sound (S2).

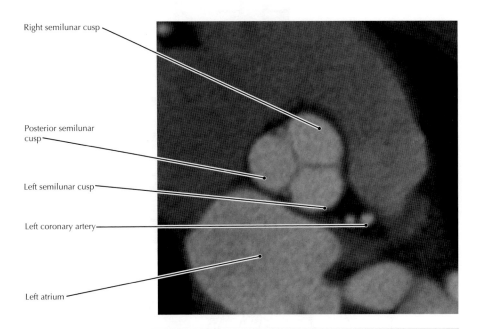

Right semilunar cusp

Posterior semilunar cusp

Left semilunar cusp

Left coronary artery

Left atrium

Oblique axial CE CT of the aortic valve

- The left and right cusps are "coronary" (associated with the left and right coronary arteries), whereas the posterior cusp is "noncoronary."
- Auscultation of valve sounds is best in the region just downstream from the valves because of the turbulent blood flow there.
- Approximately 1% to 2% of the population has a bicuspid aortic valve, which may become calcified and lead to aortic valve stenosis and regurgitation.

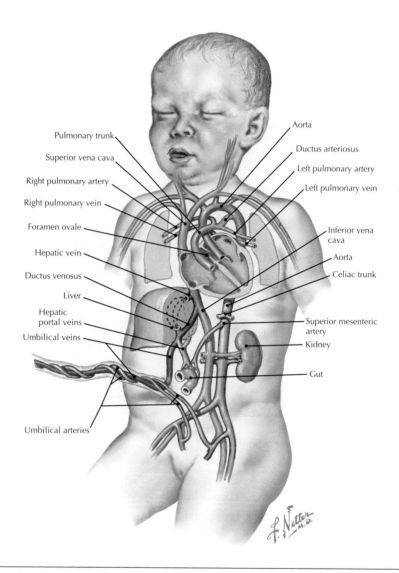

Pulmonary trunk

Superior vena cava

Right pulmonary artery

Right pulmonary vein

Foramen ovale

Hepatic vein

Ductus venosus

Liver

Hepatic portal veins

Umbilical veins

Umbilical arteries

Aorta

Ductus arteriosus

Left pulmonary artery

Left pulmonary vein

Inferior vena cava

Aorta

Celiac trunk

Superior mesenteric artery

Kidney

Gut

Fetus showing umbilical cord *(Atlas of Human Anatomy, 6th edition, Plate 226)*

> **Clinical Note** Umbilical cord blood may be an alternative to bone marrow for treating a variety of leukemias. Cord blood contains stem cells that have the potential to develop into any of the body's blood cell types.

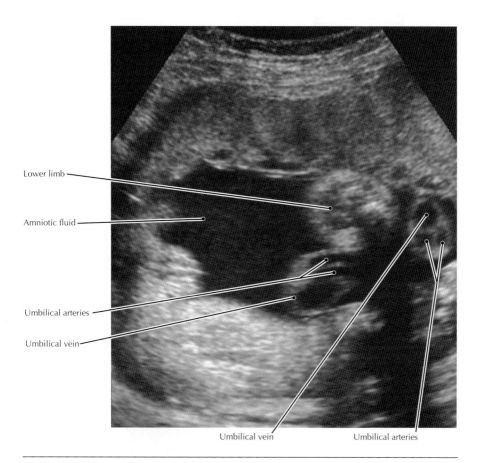

Lower limb

Amniotic fluid

Umbilical arteries

Umbilical vein

Umbilical vein

Umbilical arteries

Obstetric ultrasound

- Image contains two sections of a loop of umbilical cord, each showing two arteries and one large vein within the cord.
- The umbilical arteries carry deoxygenated blood from the fetus to the placenta, and the umbilical vein carries oxygenated blood back to the fetus.
- The umbilical arteries are branches of the internal iliac arteries and in the adult remain partially patent, supplying the superior vesical arteries.

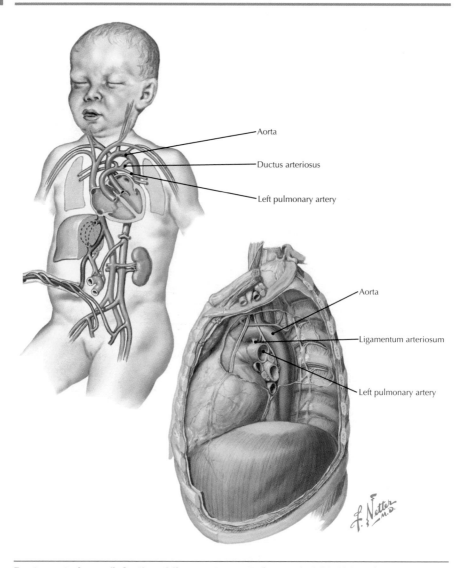

Ductus arteriosus (infant) and ligamentum arteriosum (adult) *(Atlas of Human Anatomy, 6th edition, Plates 226 and 228)*

Clinical Note If the ductus arteriosus fails to close, blood flows from the aorta to the lungs via the pulmonary trunk (termed a *left-to-right shunt*) and may lead to congestive heart failure. Children with a large ductus arteriosus can show difficulty in breathing on moderate physical exercise and fail to gain weight, clinically referred to as a *failure to thrive*.

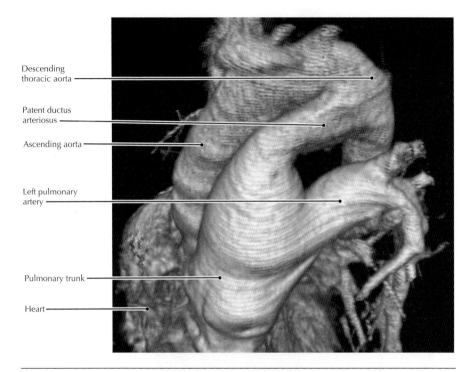

Descending thoracic aorta

Patent ductus arteriosus

Ascending aorta

Left pulmonary artery

Pulmonary trunk

Heart

Volume rendered image, CTA of a patent ductus arteriosus (PDA) *(From Ravenel JG, McAdams HP: Multiplanar and three-dimensional imaging of the thorax. Radiol Clin North Am 41(3):475-489, 2003)*

- The patent ductus arteriosus connects the left pulmonary artery to the descending thoracic aorta.

- The ductus arteriosus normally closes shortly after birth and eventually becomes ligamentous.

- Calcification within the ligamentum arteriosum occurs in a small percentage of children and should not be confused with a pathologic process producing mediastinal calcifications.

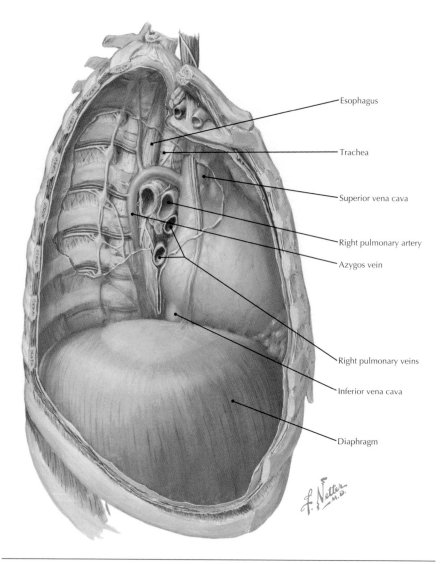

Esophagus

Trachea

Superior vena cava

Right pulmonary artery

Azygos vein

Right pulmonary veins

Inferior vena cava

Diaphragm

Right lateral view of mediastinum *(Atlas of Human Anatomy, 6th edition, Plate 227)*

Clinical Note Posterior mediastinal tumors include esophageal tumors, enlarged lymph nodes, or neural tumors from the sympathetic chain or thoracic nerves. Posterior mediastinal tumors are more common in children than in adults and are typically benign.

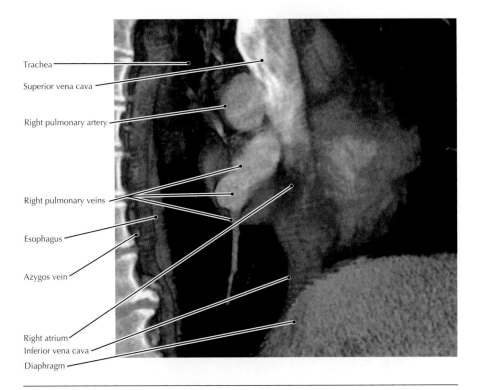

Trachea
Superior vena cava
Right pulmonary artery
Right pulmonary veins
Esophagus
Azygos vein
Right atrium
Inferior vena cava
Diaphragm

Sagittal 30-mm slab, volume rendered display, CE CT of the chest

- The shape of the supradiaphragmatic portion of the inferior vena cava (IVC) is clinically significant. In most individuals the posterior margin of the IVC is concave; a convex margin is a possible marker for elevated right atrial and IVC pressure.
- The CT image shows enhanced blood from the SVC mixing with unenhanced blood from the IVC in the right atrium. The enhancement resulted from an injection of contrast into an upper limb vein.

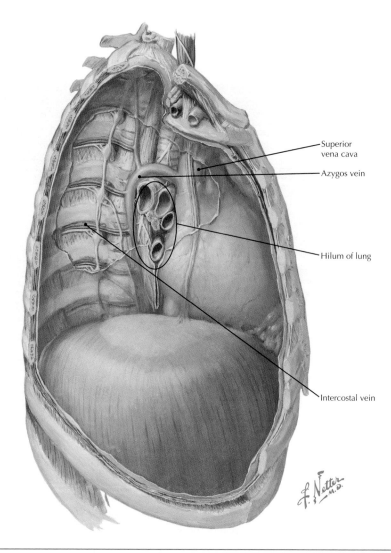

Superior
vena cava

Azygos vein

Hilum of lung

Intercostal vein

Right lateral view of mediastinum *(Atlas of Human Anatomy, 6th edition, Plate 227)*

Clinical Note   If the IVC is obstructed (e.g., by cancer) superior to the abdominal tributaries of the azygos vein, this vein provides an alternative route for blood from the lower body to return to the heart.

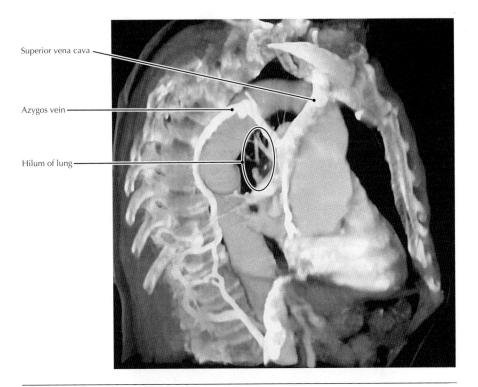

Superior vena cava

Azygos vein

Hilum of lung

Oblique MIP, CE CT of the thorax *(From Lawler LP, Fishman EK: Thoracic venous anatomy: Multidetector row CT evaluation. Radiol Clin North Am 41(3):545-560, 2003)*

- Contrast enhancement of the azygos veins is highly variable during routine CT scanning; with congenital interruption or acquired obstruction of the superior vena cava, collateral venous flow through the azygos system may result in intense opacification of these veins after upper extremity IV injection of contrast material.

- Intercostal veins in the thorax drain both to the azygos system and also to the internal thoracic (mammary) vein, which in turns drains into the brachiocephalic vein.

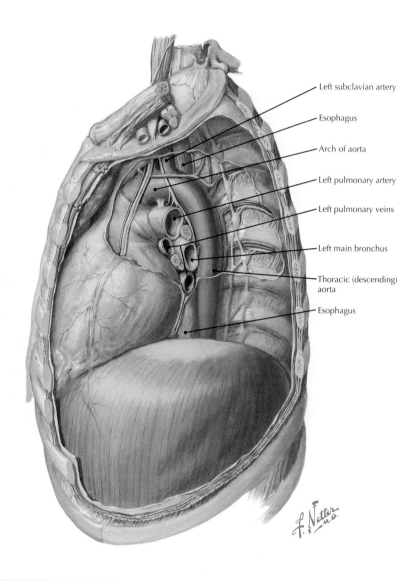

- Left subclavian artery
- Esophagus
- Arch of aorta
- Left pulmonary artery
- Left pulmonary veins
- Left main bronchus
- Thoracic (descending) aorta
- Esophagus

Left lateral view of mediastinum *(Atlas of Human Anatomy, 6th edition, Plate 228)*

Clinical Note An aortic aneurysm is a localized dilation of the aorta that results in a diameter that is 50% greater than normal. A pseudoaneurysm is a perforation of an artery that is contained by adjacent tissue and/or a thrombus.

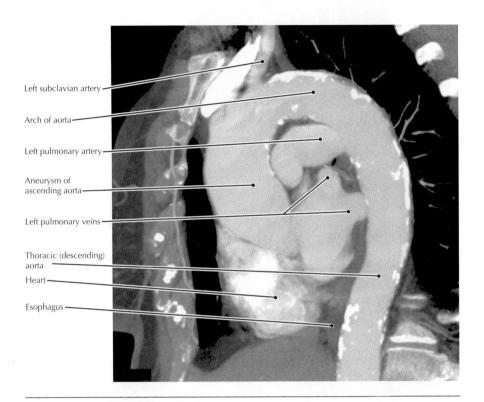

Left subclavian artery

Arch of aorta

Left pulmonary artery

Aneurysm of ascending aorta

Left pulmonary veins

Thoracic (descending) aorta

Heart

Esophagus

Sagittal CE CT of the left mediastinum

- A large ascending aortic aneurysm may compress the SVC, resulting in distended neck veins. Compression of the trachea or bronchus by an aortic aneurysm may result in dyspnea. Occasionally the esophagus may be compressed and the patient will have dysphagia.

- Aortic aneurysms may be asymptomatic, cause pain, or may cause secondary signs by compressing adjacent structures.

- Aneurysms of the arch of the aorta may stretch the left recurrent laryngeal nerve and cause hoarseness.

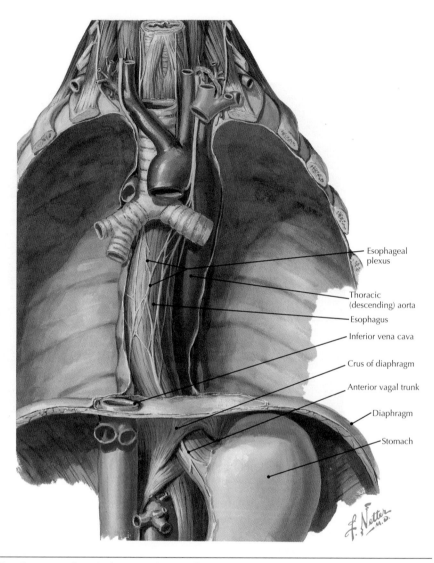

- Esophageal plexus
- Thoracic (descending) aorta
- Esophagus
- Inferior vena cava
- Crus of diaphragm
- Anterior vagal trunk
- Diaphragm
- Stomach

Esophagus and aorta in posterior mediastinum *(Atlas of Human Anatomy, 6th edition, Plate 229)*

Clinical Note Vagotomy (resection of the nerve along the distal esophagus) was once a common treatment for ulcer disease. Laparoscopic vagotomy, by interfering with gastric function, is emerging as a new surgical treatment for morbid obesity.

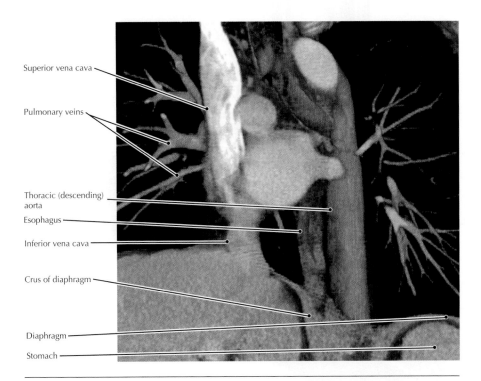

Superior vena cava

Pulmonary veins

Thoracic (descending) aorta

Esophagus

Inferior vena cava

Crus of diaphragm

Diaphragm

Stomach

Oblique sagittal 30-mm slab, volume rendered display, CE CT of the chest

- The three major structures traversing the diaphragm are the IVC at T8, the esophagus at T10, and the aorta at T12.
- The left and right vagus nerves form a plexus on the esophagus (left mainly anterior, right mainly posterior) that follows the esophagus into the abdomen to provide parasympathetic innervation to almost all of the abdominal viscera.

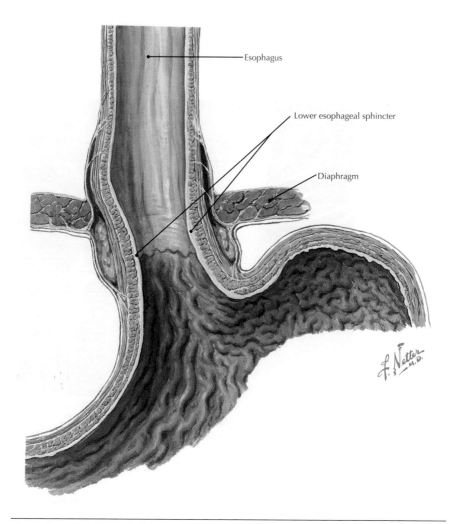

Esophagus

Lower esophageal sphincter

Diaphragm

Coronal section through the esophagogastric junction *(Atlas of Human Anatomy, 6th edition, Plate 232)*

Clinical Note The lower esophageal "sphincter" is sometimes ineffective, allowing gastric contents to enter the lower esophagus. This results in gastroesophageal reflux disease (GERD), which can cause deleterious changes in the epithelium of the esophagus.

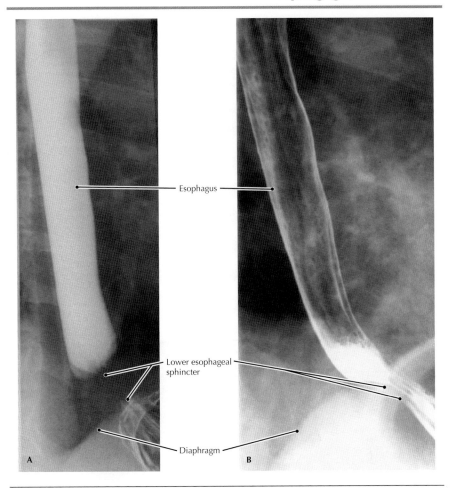

Barium esophagogram radiographic projections of the same patient in the prone (A) and upright (B) positions

- The lower esophageal sphincter is a "physiologic" sphincter rather than an anatomic structure. The right crus of the diaphragm, the phrenicoesophageal ligament, and some smooth muscle in the distal esophagus all probably contribute to this "sphincter."
- Barrett's esophagus is a precancerous condition in which the lining of the esophagus changes from its normal lining to a type that is usually found in the intestines. This change is believed to result from chronic regurgitation (reflux) of damaging stomach contents into the esophagus. In the healing process, intestinal metaplasia replaces the normal squamous-type cells that line the esophagus. Patients with Barrett's esophagus have a 30-fold to 125-fold higher risk of developing cancer of the esophagus than the general population.

Azygos and Hemiazygos Veins

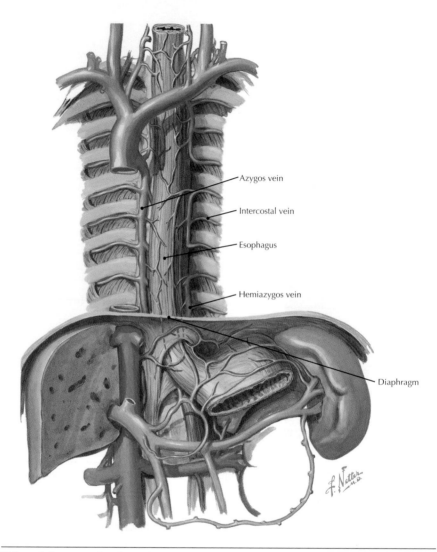

Azygos vein

Intercostal vein

Esophagus

Hemiazygos vein

Diaphragm

Veins of the posterior thoracic wall and esophagus *(Atlas of Human Anatomy, 6th edition, Plate 234)*

Clinical Note Injury to the azygos veins is most commonly the result of penetrating trauma; severe hemorrhage occurs that may lead to death if not treated quickly.

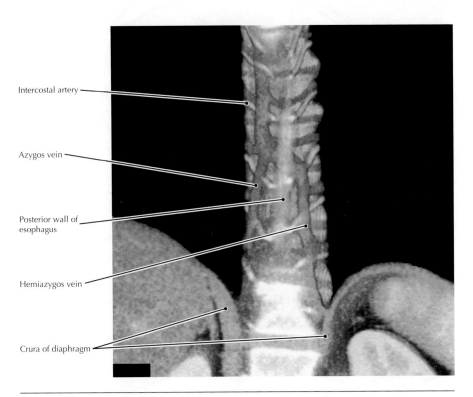

Intercostal artery

Azygos vein

Posterior wall of esophagus

Hemiazygos vein

Crura of diaphragm

Oblique coronal 30-mm slab, volume rendered display, CE CT of the chest

- The azygos system of veins primarily returns blood from both sides of thoracic wall structures to the heart via the intercostal veins.

- The components of the azygos system of veins (i.e., azygos, hemiazygos, and accessory hemiazygos veins) are extremely variable in their arrangement.

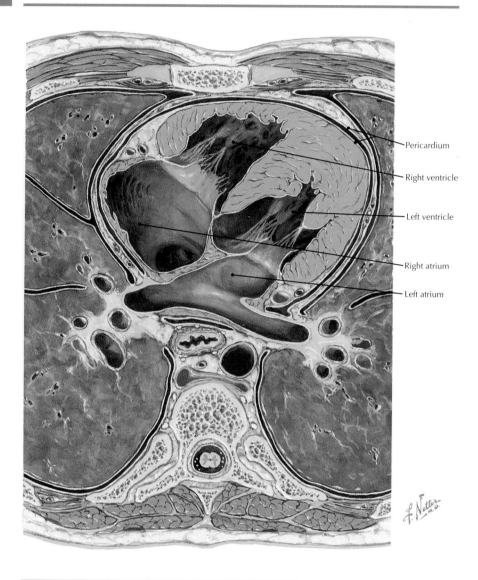

Cross section of heart showing pericardium *(Atlas of Human Anatomy, 6th edition, Plate 213)*

Clinical Note Pericardial effusion, an accumulation of excess fluid in the pericardial cavity, is associated with pericarditis and can mimic symptoms of a myocardial infarction. Pericardial effusion can be treated by pericardiocentesis.

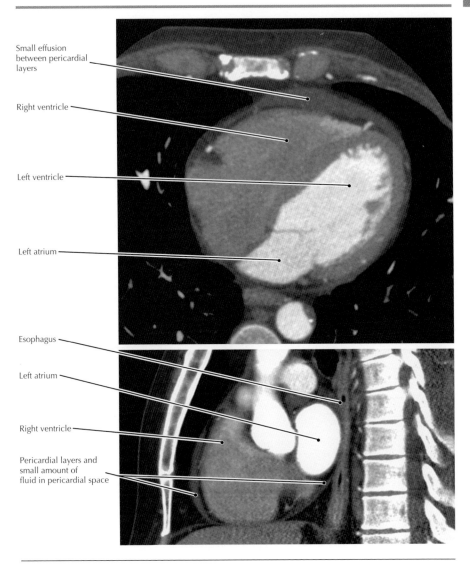

Small effusion between pericardial layers

Right ventricle

Left ventricle

Left atrium

Esophagus

Left atrium

Right ventricle

Pericardial layers and small amount of fluid in pericardial space

Axial and sagittal reconstructions, coronary artery CT arteriogram

- The thick curved line around the heart in this CT image consists of the two pericardial layers (each extremely thin and not individually resolved) and a small amount of pericardial fluid.

- Cardiac tamponade results from excessive fluid in the pericardiac sac, which prevents cardiac filling.

- Pain from the pericardium may be referred to the shoulder via the sensory branches accompanying the phrenic nerve.

Section 4 **Abdomen**

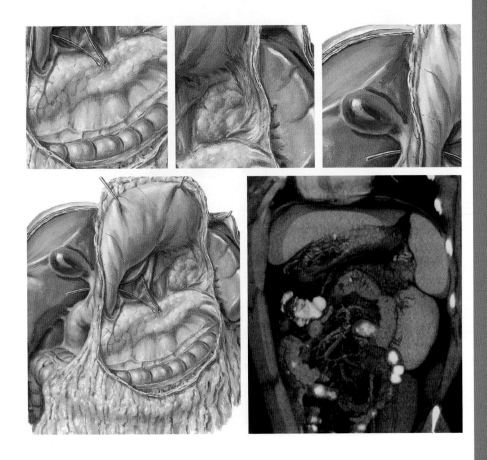

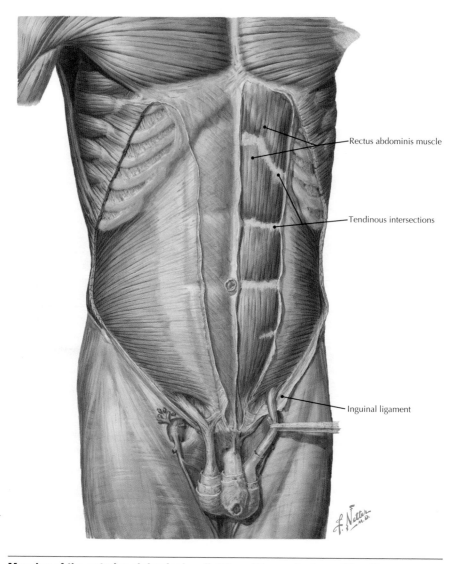

Rectus abdominis muscle

Tendinous intersections

Inguinal ligament

Muscles of the anterior abdominal wall *(Atlas of Human Anatomy, 6th edition, Plate 246)*

Clinical Note Surgical incisions through the rectus abdominis can be made transversely because the abdominal nerves run in that direction and the healed scar appears very similar to one of the many tendinous intersections within the muscle.

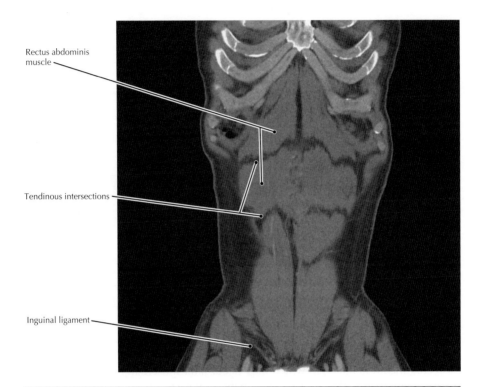

Rectus abdominis
muscle

Tendinous intersections

Inguinal ligament

Curved coronal reconstruction, abdominal CT

- The rectus sheath is composed of the aponeuroses of the abdominal muscles.
- The inguinal ligament (Poupart's) is the thickened inferior border of the external oblique aponeurosis.

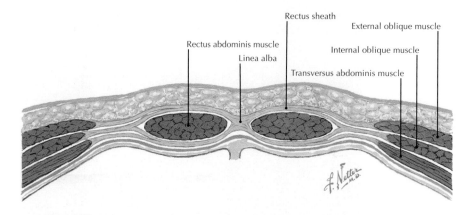

Rectus sheath

External oblique muscle

Rectus abdominis muscle

Internal oblique muscle

Linea alba

Transversus abdominis muscle

Cross section of the muscles of the anterior abdominal wall *(Atlas of Human Anatomy, 6th edition, Plate 248)*

Clinical Note Because of the dense fascia investing the rectus muscles, a rectus sheath hematoma, which may occur after muscle injury in a patient with coagulopathy, develops within a tight, nonelastic space and can become remarkably firm.

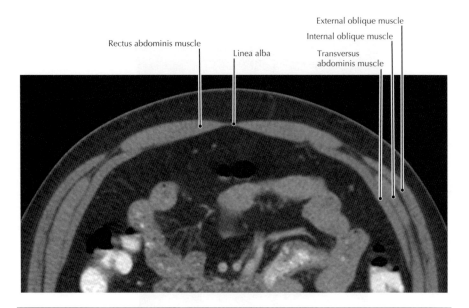

Rectus abdominis muscle

Linea alba

External oblique muscle

Internal oblique muscle

Transversus abdominis muscle

Axial section, abdominal CT

- The linea alba is composed of the interweaving fibers of the aponeuroses of the abdominal muscles and is important surgically because longitudinal incisions in it are relatively bloodless.
- The composition of the anterior and posterior layers of the rectus sheath changes superior and inferior to the arcuate line (of Douglas), which is where the inferior epigastric artery enters the sheath.

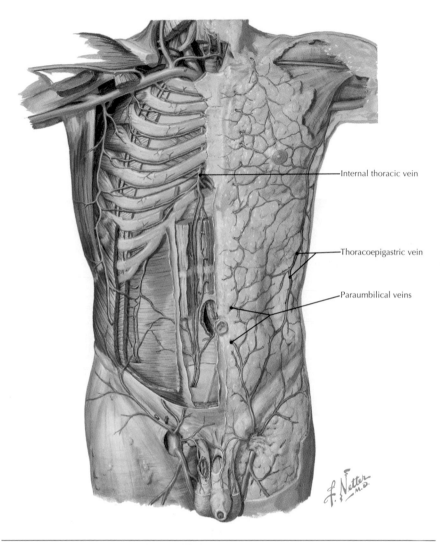

Internal thoracic vein

Thoracoepigastric vein

Paraumbilical veins

Veins of the anterior abdominal wall *(Atlas of Human Anatomy, 6th edition, Plate 252)*

Clinical Note	Varicosity of the paraumbilical veins is associated with portal hypertension (often caused by cirrhosis) and is termed *caput medusa*. Varicosity of the thoracoepigastric vein is similarly associated with portal hypertension and also with increased pressure or obstruction in the IVC because blood from the lower body then uses this vein to return blood to the heart via the SVC.

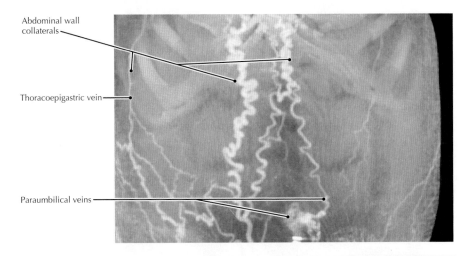

Abdominal wall collaterals

Thoracoepigastric vein

Paraumbilical veins

Coronal volume rendered, CE CT of the superficial abdominal wall veins *(From Lawler LP, Fishman EK: Thoracic venous anatomy: Multidetector row CT evaluation. Radiol Clin North Am 41(3):545-560, 2003)*

- Abdominal wall collaterals join the internal thoracic (mammary) and lateral thoracic veins to return venous blood to the vena cava.

- The paraumbilical veins communicate with the portal vein via the vein in the ligamentum teres hepatis (round ligament of the liver).

- When pathology obstructs normal flow, collateral vessels may dilate and become tortuous as shown in this CT.

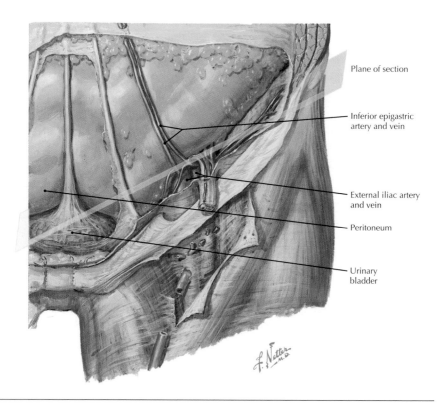

Plane of section

Inferior epigastric artery and vein

External iliac artery and vein

Peritoneum

Urinary bladder

Anterior view of the inguinal region (Atlas of Human Anatomy, 6th edition, Plate 257)

> **Clinical Note** When the bladder fills, it expands in the extraperitoneal space between the peritoneum and the abdominal wall. Thus, the bladder may be penetrated (suprapubic cystotomy) for removal of urinary calculi, foreign bodies, or small tumors without entering the peritoneal cavity.

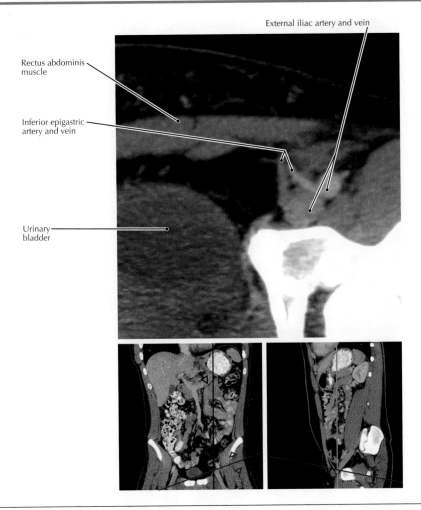

External iliac artery and vein

Rectus abdominis muscle

Inferior epigastric artery and vein

Urinary bladder

Oblique axial 6-mm thick MIP, CE CT of the abdomen and pelvis (*red lines* in the reference images indicate the position and orientation of the main image)

- The inferior epigastric vessels are an important landmark for differentiating between indirect and direct inguinal hernias. Pulsations from the artery can be felt medial to the neck of an indirect hernia and lateral to the neck of a direct hernia.

- The inferior epigastric vessels enter the rectus sheath approximately at the arcuate line, which is where the formation of the sheath changes. Inferior to the line the aponeuroses of all of the abdominal muscles pass anterior to the rectus abdominis muscle whereas superior to the line, half of the aponeurosis of the internal oblique muscle and all of the aponeurosis of the transversus abdominis pass posterior to the rectus muscle.

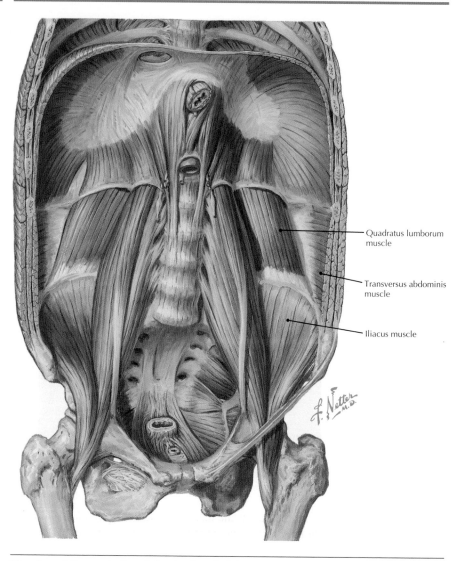

Quadratus lumborum
muscle

Transversus abdominis
muscle

Iliacus muscle

Muscles of the posterior abdominal wall *(Atlas of Human Anatomy, 6th edition, Plate 258)*

Clinical Note Grey-Turner's sign, ecchymosis in the flank resulting from retroperitoneal hemorrhage (most often from hemorrhagic pancreatitis), occurs as the blood spreads from the anterior pararenal space to between the two leaves of the posterior renal fascia and subsequently to the lateral edge of the quadratus lumborum muscle.

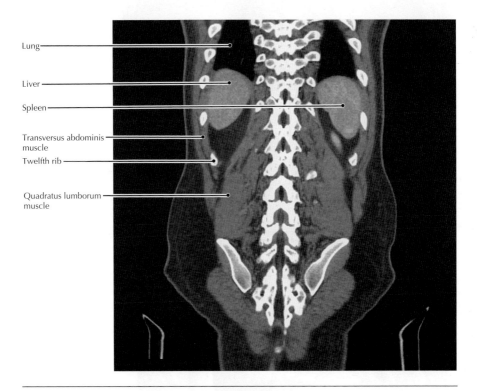

Lung
Liver
Spleen
Transversus abdominis muscle
Twelfth rib
Quadratus lumborum muscle

Curved coronal reconstruction, thoracolumbar CT

- The quadratus lumborum muscle primarily laterally flexes the trunk when acting unilaterally.
- The quadratus lumborum muscle attaches to the 12th rib and thereby can act as an accessory respiratory muscle by allowing the diaphragm to exert greater downward force by preventing upward movement of the 12th rib.

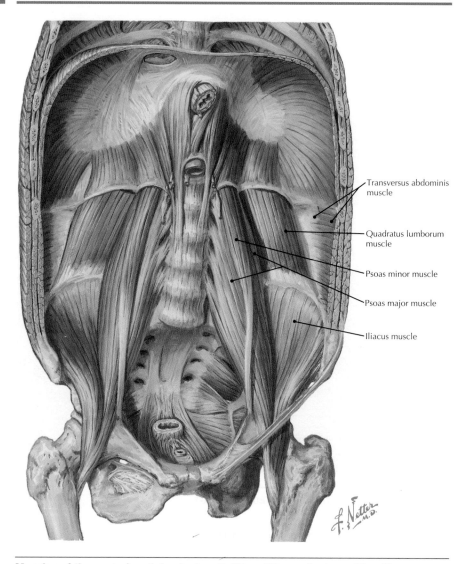

Transversus abdominis
muscle

Quadratus lumborum
muscle

Psoas minor muscle

Psoas major muscle

Iliacus muscle

Muscles of the posterior abdominal wall *(Atlas of Human Anatomy, 6th edition, Plate 258)*

Clinical Note A psoas abscess usually results from disease of the lumbar vertebrae, with the pus descending into the muscle sheath; it may cause swelling in the proximal thigh that refers pain to the hip, thigh, or knee. The infection is most commonly tuberculous or staphylococcal. Before the discovery of antibiotics, these infections were life threatening.

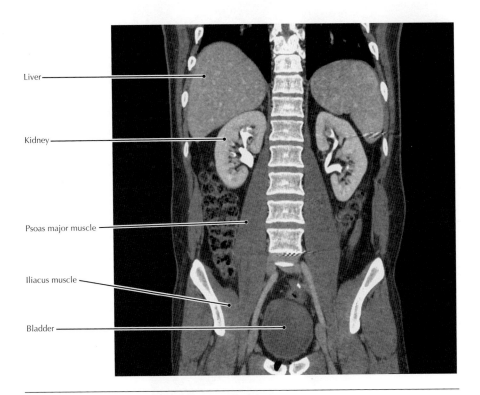

Liver

Kidney

Psoas major muscle

Iliacus muscle

Bladder

Curved coronal reconstruction, abdominal CT

- The psoas major muscle is a primary flexor of the trunk.
- The psoas minor is an inconstant muscle that inserts onto the pubis; the major inserts onto the lesser trochanter.

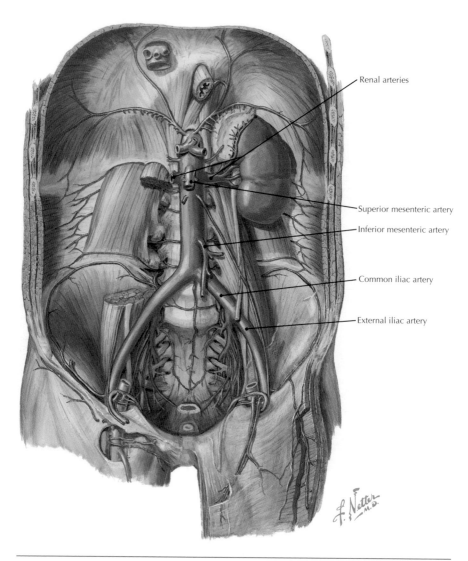

Renal arteries

Superior mesenteric artery

Inferior mesenteric artery

Common iliac artery

External iliac artery

Arteries of the posterior abdominal wall *(Atlas of Human Anatomy, 6th edition, Plate 259)*

Clinical Note A transplanted kidney is typically placed in the pelvis and its associated artery is attached to the external iliac artery, although it may also be attached to the common iliac artery as shown in the MR image.

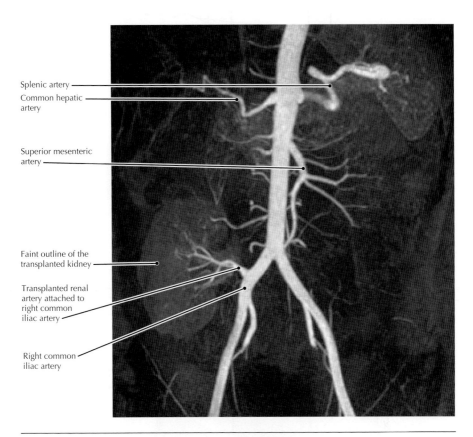

Splenic artery
Common hepatic artery
Superior mesenteric artery
Faint outline of the transplanted kidney
Transplanted renal artery attached to right common iliac artery
Right common iliac artery

Coronal MIP, CE MRA of renal transplant surveillance *(From McGuigan EA, Sears ST, Corse WR, Ho VB: MR angiography of the abdominal aorta. Magn Reson Imaging Clin N Am 13(1):65-89, 2005)*

- Patency of the anastomosis (connection) of the iliac artery to the transplanted renal artery is demonstrated.
- The indication for kidney transplantation is end-stage renal disease (ESRD). Diabetes is the most common cause of ESRD, followed by glomerulonephritis.
- Potential recipients of kidney transplants undergo an extensive immunologic evaluation to minimize transplants that are at risk for antibody-mediated hyperacute rejection.
- The left kidney is the one preferred for transplant because of its longer vein compared to the right.

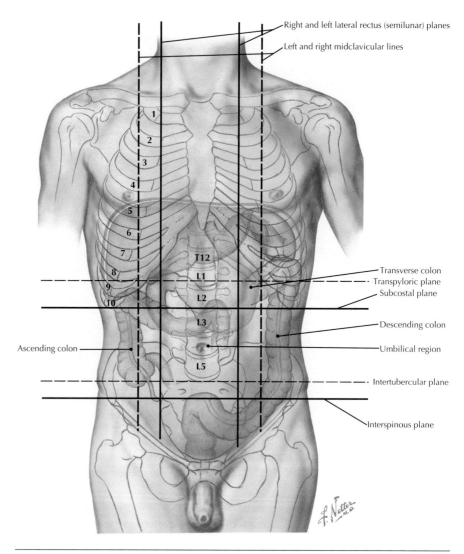

Right and left lateral rectus (semilunar) planes
Left and right midclavicular lines

1
2
3
4
5
6
7
T12
L1
L2
L3
L5
8
9
10

Transverse colon
Transpyloric plane
Subcostal plane

Descending colon

Ascending colon

Umbilical region

Intertubercular plane

Interspinous plane

Relationships of the abdominal viscera to the abdominal regions *(Atlas of Human Anatomy, 6th edition, Plate 244)*

Clinical Note   The umbilical region remains a region of abdominal muscle weakness after birth, and umbilical or paraumbilical hernias can develop at any age.

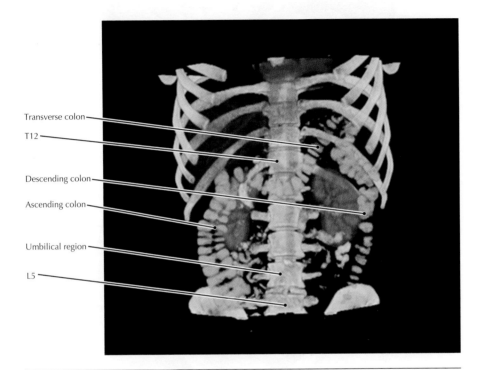

Transverse colon

T12

Descending colon

Ascending colon

Umbilical region

L5

Volume rendered display, abdominal CT

- Classically, the abdomen is divided into four quadrants defined by vertical and horizontal planes through the umbilicus. More recently, it has been divided into nine regions based on subcostal, transtubercular, and right and left lateral rectus (semilunar) planes.

- Note the greater height of the left colic (splenic) flexure compared to the hepatic flexure on the right.

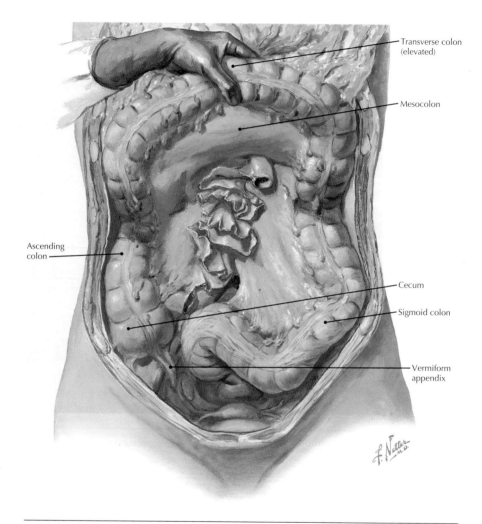

Transverse colon (elevated)

Mesocolon

Ascending colon

Cecum

Sigmoid colon

Vermiform appendix

Appendix, large bowel, mesocolon *(Atlas of Human Anatomy, 6th edition, Plate 265)*

> **Clinical Note**   Appendicitis is a common cause of acute abdominal pain, which usually begins in the periumbilical region and migrates to the right lower quadrant because of associated peritoneal irritation.

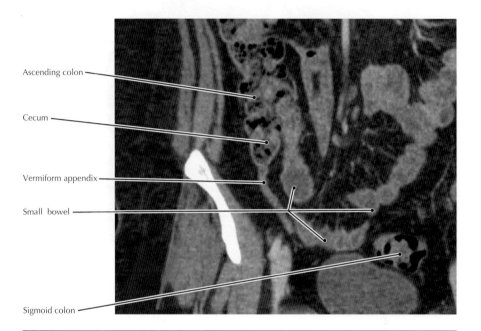

Ascending colon

Cecum

Vermiform appendix

Small bowel

Sigmoid colon

Oblique coronal reconstruction, abdominal CT

- Inspissated bowel contents may lead to development of an appendolith, which is a calcified concretion that may obstruct the proximal lumen of the appendix; stasis, bacterial overgrowth, infection, and swelling (i.e., appendicitis) may follow, as can eventual rupture.
- The appendix is highly variable in its location, including occasionally being posterior to the cecum (retrocecal).

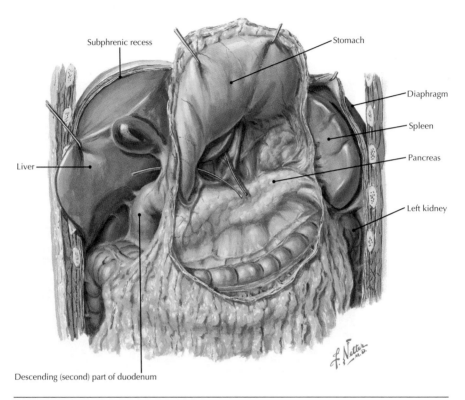

Subphrenic recess

Stomach

Diaphragm

Spleen

Pancreas

Liver

Left kidney

Descending (second) part of duodenum

Upper abdominal viscera with stomach reflected thus revealing the omental bursa
(Atlas of Human Anatomy, 6th edition, Plate 266)

Clinical Note A collection of pus between the diaphragm and the liver is known as a subphrenic abscess and may be secondary to the following: (1) peritonitis following a perforated peptic ulcer, appendicitis, pelvic inflammatory disease, or infection subsequent to cesarean section; (2) trauma that ruptures a hollow viscus and contaminates the peritoneal cavity; (3) a laparotomy during which the peritoneal cavity is contaminated; and (4) a ruptured liver abscess. Treatment is placement of a drainage tube until the abscess heals.

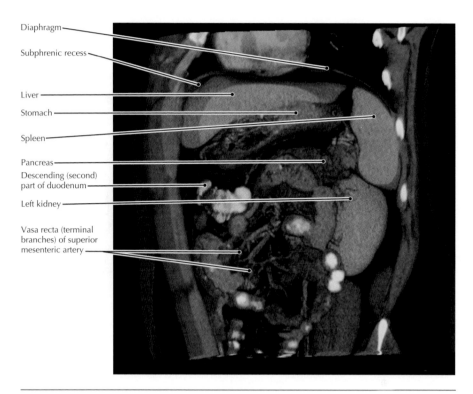

Diaphragm
Subphrenic recess
Liver
Stomach
Spleen
Pancreas
Descending (second) part of duodenum
Left kidney
Vasa recta (terminal branches) of superior mesenteric artery

Oblique coronal slab, volume rendered display, abdominal CT

- The right kidney is not apparent in this image because of the obliquity of the image (the plane of the "coronal" image is angled so that it passes anterior to the right kidney but through the left kidney).

- The vasa recta (terminal branches) of the superior mesenteric artery (SMA) supply loops of small bowel.

- The terminal or fourth segment of the duodenum is attached to the diaphragm by a variable band of smooth muscle known as the suspensory ligament of the duodenum (ligament of Treitz). It is not recognizable on CT images.

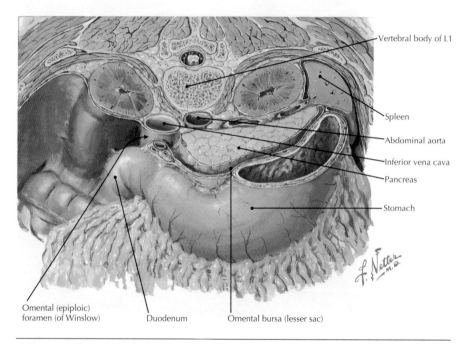

Vertebral body of L1

Spleen

Abdominal aorta

Inferior vena cava

Pancreas

Stomach

Omental (epiploic) foramen (of Winslow)

Duodenum

Omental bursa (lesser sac)

Oblique section at the level of the first lumbar vertebra *(Atlas of Human Anatomy, 6th edition, Plate 267)*

> **Clinical Note**   Ascites is an accumulation of excess fluid in the peritoneal cavity. The finding of a disproportionate amount of ascites in the bursa may help narrow the differential diagnosis to organs bordering the lesser sac.

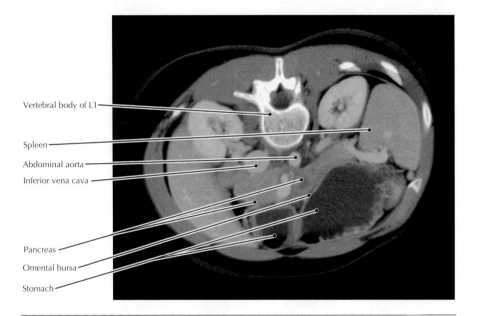

Vertebral body of L1

Spleen

Abdominal aorta

Inferior vena cava

Pancreas

Omental bursa

Stomach

Volume rendered display, CE CT of the abdomen

- The omental bursa, also known as the lesser sac, is the portion of the peritoneal cavity that is directly posterior to the stomach.
- The only natural connection between the omental bursa and the remainder of the peritoneal cavity (greater sac) is the epiploic foramen (of Winslow).

Abdomen   **243**

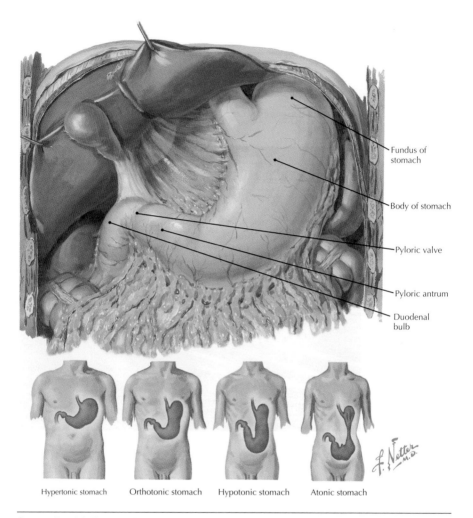

Fundus of stomach

Body of stomach

Pyloric valve

Pyloric antrum

Duodenal bulb

Hypertonic stomach   Orthotonic stomach   Hypotonic stomach   Atonic stomach

Stomach with liver and gallbladder elevated *(top);* **variations in positions of the stomach** *(bottom)* *(Atlas of Human Anatomy, 6th edition, Plate 269)*

Clinical Note Adjustable gastric banding, or lap band surgery, is a form of restrictive weight loss surgery (bariatric surgery) for morbidly obese patients with a body mass index (BMI) of 40 or more. The gastric band is an inflatable silicone prosthetic device that is laparoscopically placed around the fundus of the stomach to reduce the amount of food that can be ingested at any one time.

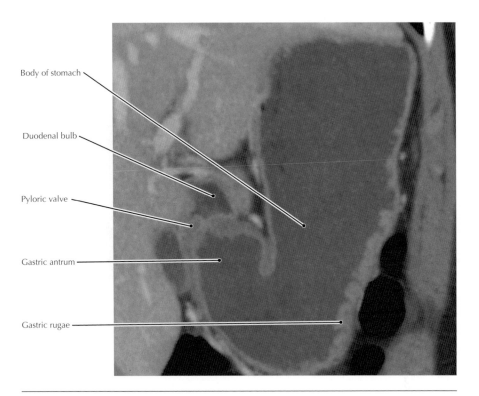

Body of stomach

Duodenal bulb

Pyloric valve

Gastric antrum

Gastric rugae

Oblique curved CE CT of the abdomen

- The stomach is filled with whole milk in this patient, the fat content of which decreases the CT density of the stomach fluid in order to enhance contrast differences with other tissues, such as the stomach wall. Note that the pyloric valve is closed, as it is most of the time.
- The position of the stomach is variable in relation to the body habitus. This patient has an "orthotonic" stomach.
- The term *gastric antrum* is a clinical term referring to the distal part of the stomach immediately proximal to the pyloric valve (pylorus). Anatomically, this part of the stomach would be referred to as the gastric antrum.

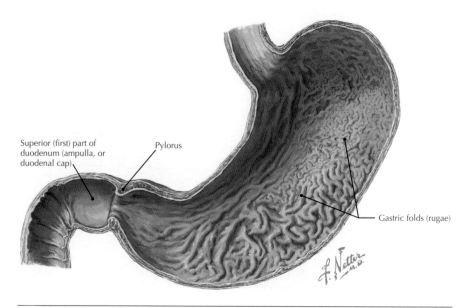

Superior (first) part of
duodenum (ampulla, or
duodenal cap)

Pylorus

Gastric folds (rugae)

Longitudinal section of the stomach and proximal duodenum *(Atlas of Human Anatomy, 6th edition, Plate 270)*

Clinical Note Gastric ulcers are lesions in the mucosa of the stomach that are typically associated with an infection by *Helicobacter pylori* bacteria.

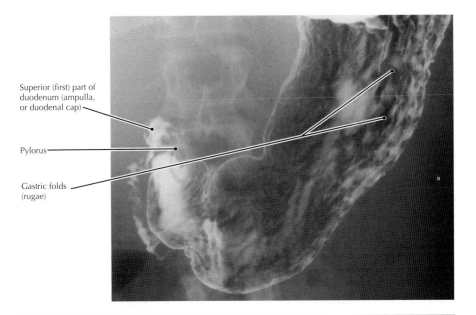

Superior (first) part of
duodenum (ampulla,
or duodenal cap)

Pylorus

Gastric folds
(rugae)

Air contrast upper gastrointestinal (GI) examination

- In the air contrast upper GI examination, the mucosa is coated with a thin layer of orally administered barium and the stomach is distended by CO_2 given off by effervescent granules swallowed by the patient.
- Mucosal malignancies can be ruled out with a very low false-negative rate by a radiographic upper GI examination.
- Herniation of the stomach through the diaphragm is referred to as a hiatal hernia.

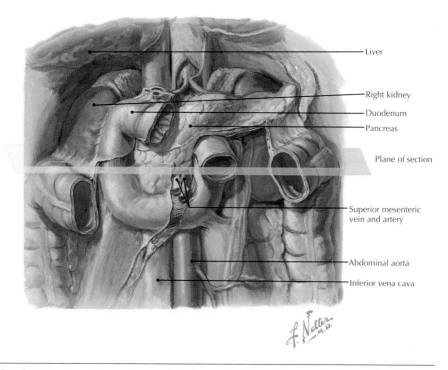

Liver

Right kidney

Duodenum

Pancreas

Plane of section

Superior mesenteric vein and artery

Abdominal aorta

Inferior vena cava

Duodenum, pancreas, and associated vessels *(Atlas of Human Anatomy, 6th edition, Plate 271)*

Clinical Note Obstruction of the common bile duct by a pancreatic malignancy frequently leads to jaundice as a presenting sign of that malignancy.

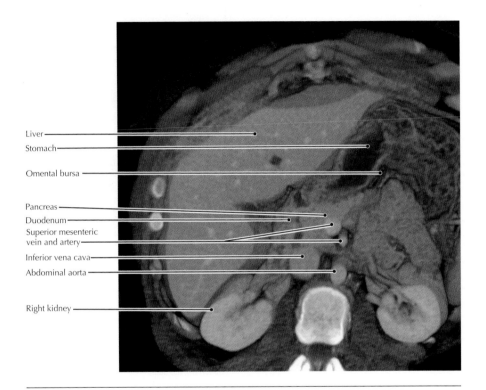

Liver
Stomach
Omental bursa
Pancreas
Duodenum
Superior mesenteric
vein and artery
Inferior vena cava
Abdominal aorta
Right kidney

Volume rendered display, CE CT of the abdomen

- The portion of the pancreas that lies posterior to the SMA and superior mesenteric vein (SMV) is the uncinate process.
- The omental bursa is shown to be collapsed in this image because in a healthy patient it is a potential space. Distention of the bursa is a sign of disease.

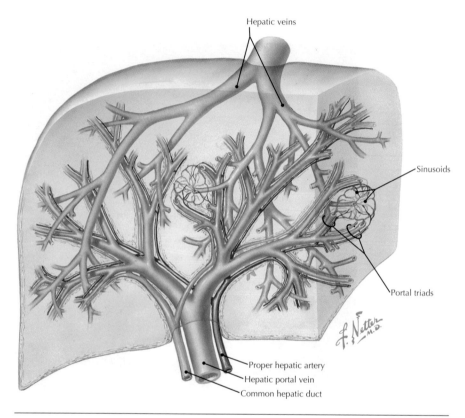

Hepatic veins

Sinusoids

Portal triads

Proper hepatic artery
Hepatic portal vein
Common hepatic duct

Intrahepatic vascular and duct system *(Atlas of Human Anatomy, 6th edition, Plate 278)*

Clinical Note In liver cirrhosis, bridging fibrous septae link portal tracts with one another and with terminal hepatic veins. This interferes with liver function and results in the liver's surface becoming rough instead of smooth. Alcoholism and hepatitis C are the primary causes of liver cirrhosis in the United States.

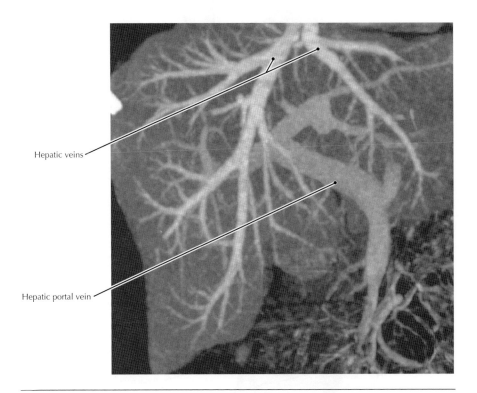

Hepatic veins

Hepatic portal vein

Coronal MIP, CE CT of hepatic/portal circulation within the liver *(From Kamel IR, Liapi E, Fishman E: Liver and biliary system: Evaluation by multidetector CT. Radiol Clin North Am 43(6):977-997, 2005)*

- A portal system is one in which the blood passes through two vascular beds before returning to the heart.
- In the liver, the blood passes through the capillary beds in the digestive tract and the spleen, and then the liver sinusoids.
- All hepatic veins lead to the IVC.

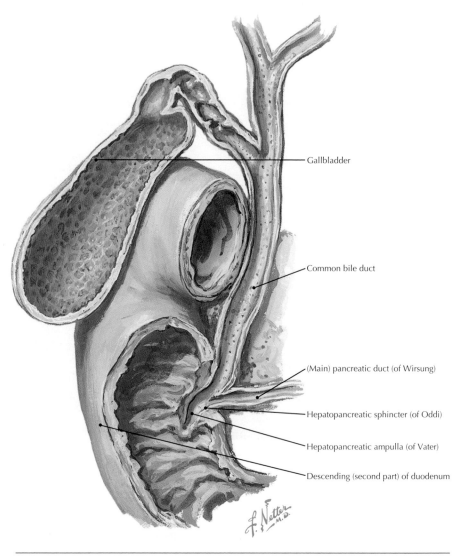

Gallbladder

Common bile duct

(Main) pancreatic duct (of Wirsung)

Hepatopancreatic sphincter (of Oddi)

Hepatopancreatic ampulla (of Vater)

Descending (second part) of duodenum

Union of common bile and (main) pancreatic ducts as they enter the duodenum
(Atlas of Human Anatomy, 6th edition, Plate 280)

Clinical Note Obstruction of the common bile and pancreatic ducts will cause obstructive jaundice and may lead to pancreatitis. Possible causes of obstructions can be a small gallstone at the hepatopancreatic sphincter (of Oddi) or a tumor at the hepatopancreatic ampulla (of Vater).

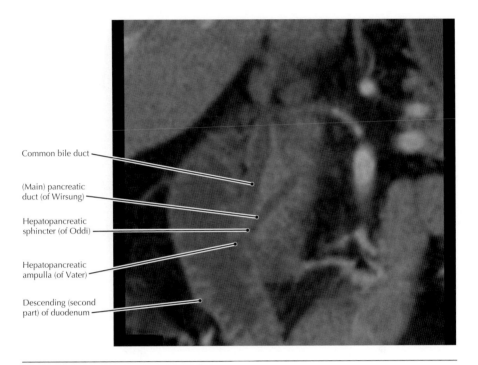

Common bile duct

(Main) pancreatic
duct (of Wirsung)

Hepatopancreatic
sphincter (of Oddi)

Hepatopancreatic
ampulla (of Vater)

Descending (second
part) of duodenum

Oblique coronal reconstruction, CE CT of the abdomen

- The "negative opacification" of the duodenal lumen is achieved by the patient ingesting whole milk before the scan.
- Often there is an accessory pancreatic duct (of Santorini) that can provide an alternative route for pancreatic enzymes to enter the duodenum.
- There is substantial variation in the manner in which the common bile and pancreatic ducts join.

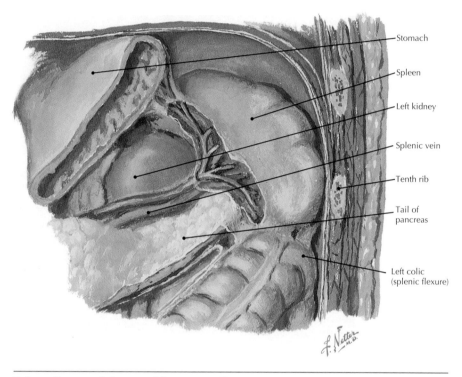

Stomach

Spleen

Left kidney

Splenic vein

Tenth rib

Tail of pancreas

Left colic (splenic flexure)

Spleen, its vasculature, and its surrounding structures *(Atlas of Human Anatomy, 6th edition, Plate 282)*

> **Clinical Note** The spleen is the most commonly injured abdominal organ because it is friable and can be easily pierced by rib fragments or damaged by blunt trauma. If ruptured, it is usually removed to prevent severe hemorrhage.

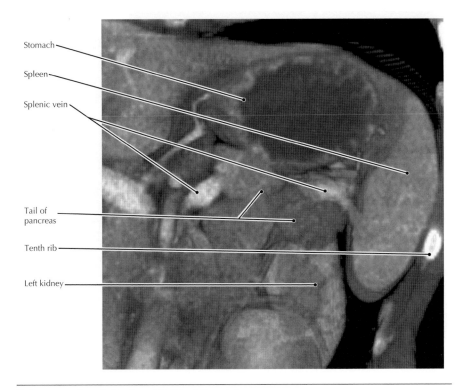

Stomach

Spleen

Splenic vein

Tail of pancreas

Tenth rib

Left kidney

Volume rendered display, CE CT of the abdomen

- Accessory spleens are common and are often located in the tail of the pancreas.
- The spleen is supported by a "shelf" of peritoneum, the phrenicocolic ligament.
- The splenic vessels run a tortuous course from the celiac trunk to the spleen, so they may be seen more than once in a single plane of a cross-sectional image.

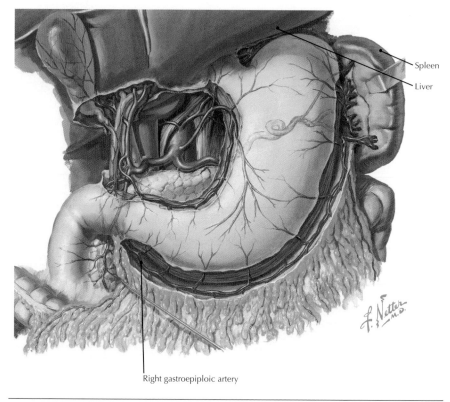

Spleen

Liver

Right gastroepiploic artery

Arterial supply of the stomach, liver, spleen, and greater omentum *(Atlas of Human Anatomy, 6th edition, Plate 283)*

Clinical Note The right gastroepiploic artery is sometimes used for coronary artery bypass grafts in cases of coronary artery disease.

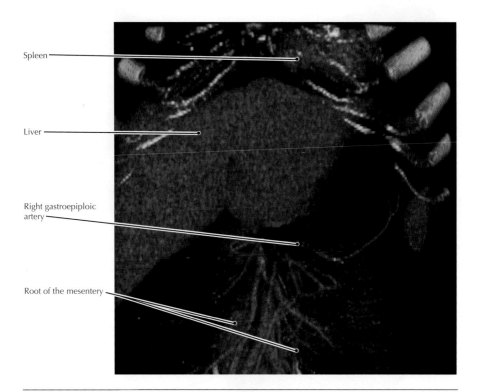

Spleen

Liver

Right gastroepiploic artery

Root of the mesentery

Volume rendered display, abdominal CT arteriogram

- Because the CT arteriogram shown displays only tissues above a threshold value of CT density, the stomach itself is not visualized.

- The epiploic arteries provide redundant collateral arterial supply to the stomach.

- The right gastroepiploic artery arises from the gastroduodenal artery, and the left gastroepiploic artery is from the splenic artery. Because the greater curvature of the stomach is supplied from both sides, the right gastroepiploic artery can be harvested for use as a bypass graft.

Porta Hepatis

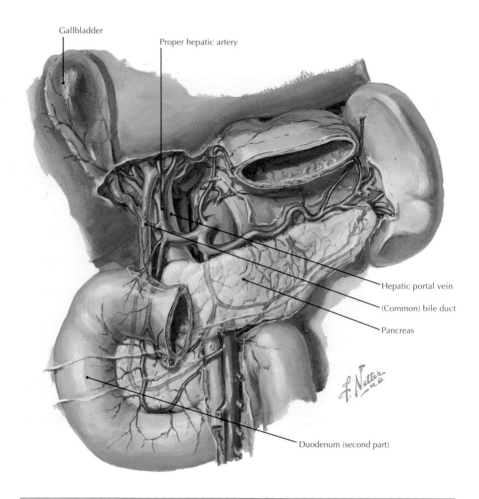

Gallbladder

Proper hepatic artery

Hepatic portal vein

(Common) bile duct

Pancreas

Duodenum (second part)

Anterior view of structures entering and exiting the liver *(Atlas of Human Anatomy, 6th edition, Plate 284)*

Clinical Note In surgical emergencies, such as a laceration of the liver due to blunt trauma, all blood flow to the liver can be stopped by the surgeon passing an index finger into the epiploic foramen (of Winslow) posterior to the portal vein and compressing the hepatoduodenal ligament with the thumb (Pringle maneuver).

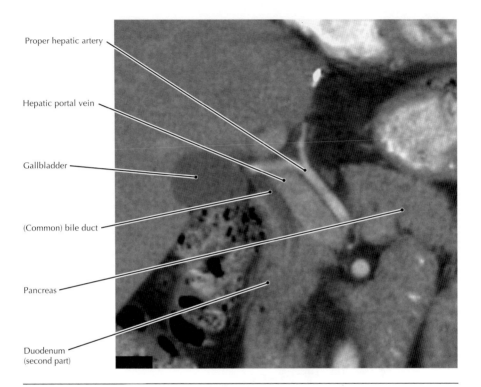

Proper hepatic artery

Hepatic portal vein

Gallbladder

(Common) bile duct

Pancreas

Duodenum
(second part)

Oblique coronal reconstruction, CE CT of the abdomen

- The hepatic portal vein, proper hepatic artery, and (common) bile duct (the hepatic triad) and their branches and tributaries are found together, even at the microscopic level within the liver.

- The hepatic triad is in the hepatoduodenal ligament in a relatively constant relationship to each other; the portal vein is posterior, the artery is anterior, and the duct is to the right (mnemonic: the portal is posterior, the artery is anterior, and the duct is dexter).

Celiac Trunk, Normal and Variant

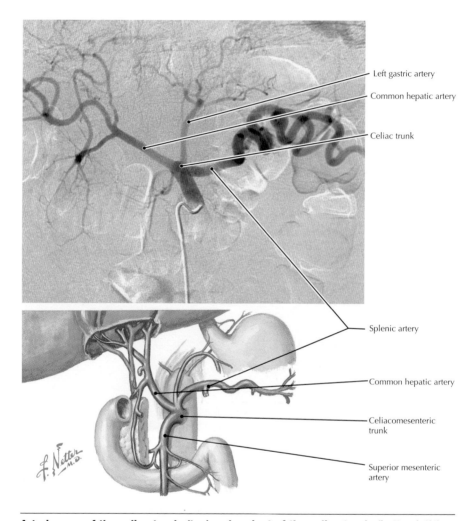

Left gastric artery

Common hepatic artery

Celiac trunk

Splenic artery

Common hepatic artery

Celiacomesenteric trunk

Superior mesenteric artery

Arteriogram of the celiac trunk *(top)* and variant of the celiac trunk *(bottom)* (*Atlas of Human Anatomy, 6th edition, Plate 285*)

Clinical Note A standard arteriogram is an invasive procedure in that a catheter is introduced into an artery, whereas CT arteriography requires only an IV injection. Hepatic and splenic arterial bleeding can be demonstrated with either technique. Variations in the celiac trunk are common and are clinically significant in any surgical approach to the region.

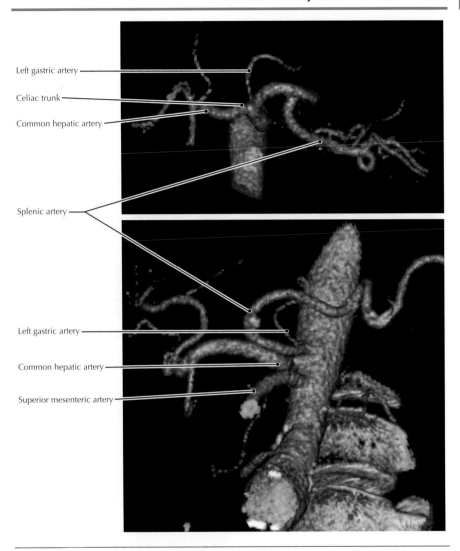

Left gastric artery

Celiac trunk

Common hepatic artery

Splenic artery

Left gastric artery

Common hepatic artery

Superior mesenteric artery

Volume rendered displays, abdominal CTAs

- The lower volume rendered display and the drawing of the celiac trunk variant show very similar anatomy, with a common origin for the celiac trunk and superior mesenteric artery.

- The splenic artery has a tortuous path along the superior border of the pancreas, supplying many branches to this organ including the dorsal and greater pancreatic arteries.

- The left gastric artery supplies the left side of the lesser curvature of the stomach and also has branches that supply the lower portion of the esophagus.

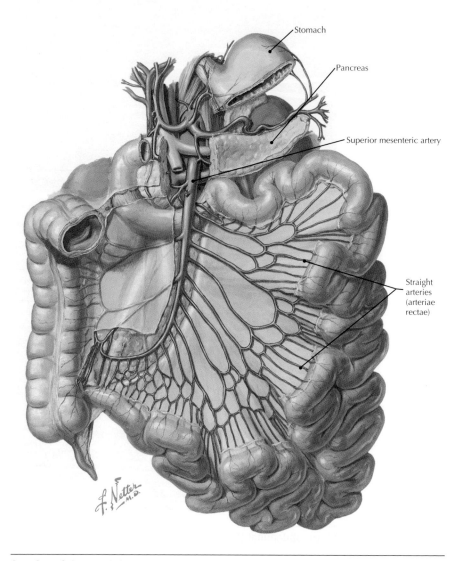

Stomach

Pancreas

Superior mesenteric artery

Straight arteries (arteriae rectae)

f. Netter.
M.D.

Arteries of the small intestines *(Atlas of Human Anatomy, 6th edition, Plate 287)*

Clinical Note If the lumen of the superior mesenteric artery (SMA) becomes obstructed and if there is insufficient collateral blood supplied by branches of the celiac and inferior mesenteric arteries, then postprandial (after eating) abdominal pain may result from intestinal ischemia. This is referred to as mesenteric angina. Accordingly, patients tend not to eat and to lose weight rapidly.

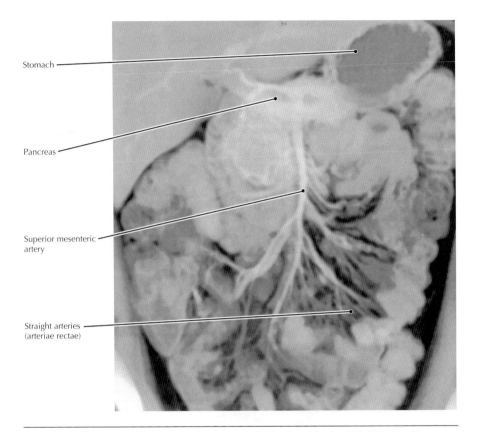

Stomach

Pancreas

Superior mesenteric
artery

Straight arteries
(arteriae rectae)

Coronal MIP, CE CTA of the branches of the SMA *(From Horton KM, Fishman EK: The current status of multidetector row CT and three-dimensional imaging of the small bowel. Radiol Clin North Am 41(2):199-212, 2003)*

- The SMA passes posterior to the body of the pancreas but anterior to the third part of the duodenum.
- The vasa rectae are "straight arteries" that run from the arterial arcades to the walls of the small intestines.

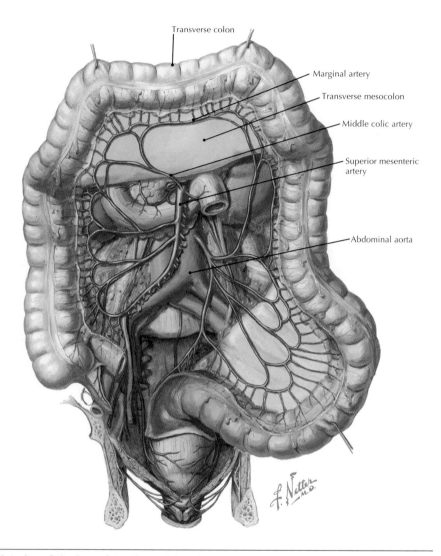

Transverse colon

Marginal artery

Transverse mesocolon

Middle colic artery

Superior mesenteric artery

Abdominal aorta

Arteries of the large intestines *(Atlas of Human Anatomy, 6th edition, Plate 288)*

Clinical Note The marginal artery (of Drummond) parallels the mesenteric border of the colon and receives blood from both the SMA and inferior mesenteric artery (IMA). Because of this dual arterial supply, occlusion of one does not usually lead to vascular compromise.

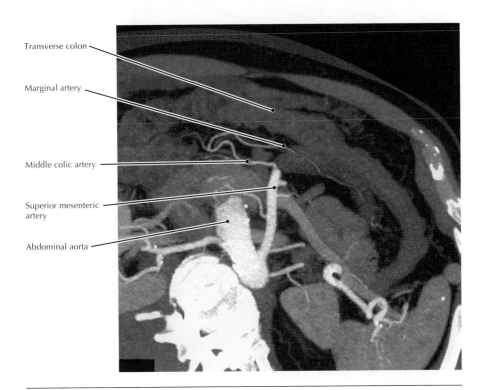

Transverse colon

Marginal artery

Middle colic artery

Superior mesenteric artery

Abdominal aorta

Oblique axial MIP, CE CT of the abdomen

- The middle colic artery is the first branch of the SMA. It runs in the transverse mesocolon to reach the transverse colon.

- Haustra are the sacculations of the colon caused by the longitudinal muscle of the colon, the taenia coli.

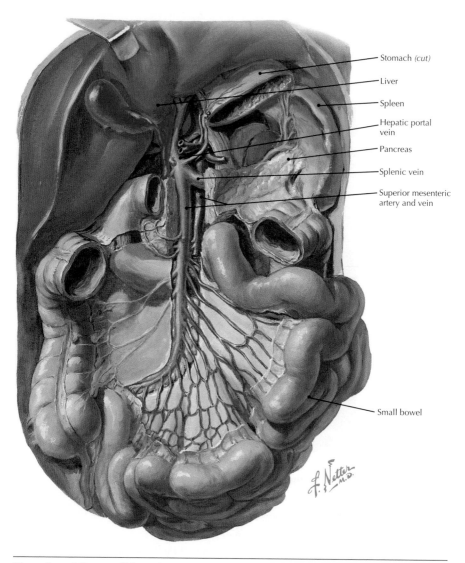

Stomach *(cut)*

Liver

Spleen

Hepatic portal
vein

Pancreas

Splenic vein

Superior mesenteric
artery and vein

Small bowel

The veins of the small bowel *(Atlas of Human Anatomy, 6th edition, Plate 290)*

Clinical Note The SMV joins with the splenic vein posterior to the neck of
the pancreas to form the portal vein. Pancreatic cancer may invade and
obstruct the SMV and splenic vein.

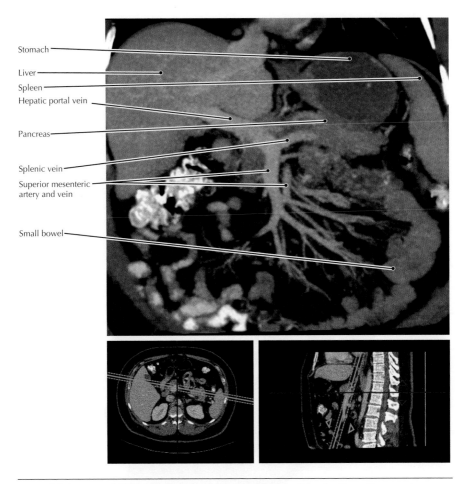

Stomach
Liver
Spleen
Hepatic portal vein
Pancreas
Splenic vein
Superior mesenteric artery and vein
Small bowel

3-cm thick coronal MIP, CE CT of the abdomen (*green lines* in the reference images indicate the position and orientation of the main image)

- In typical clinical imaging, bowel segments may not be uniformly opacified. If suspected pathology is in the upper abdomen, CT scanning may be done before oral contrast material has reached the distal gastrointestinal tract.

- This CT scan was done during the "portal venous phase" of hepatic enhancement, approximately 65 seconds after starting an IV infusion of iodinated contrast material.

- High-density oral contrast material (barium) is seen in some small bowel loops and in the colon to the level of the splenic flexure; low-density oral contrast material (ingested tap water) is seen in the gastric lumen.

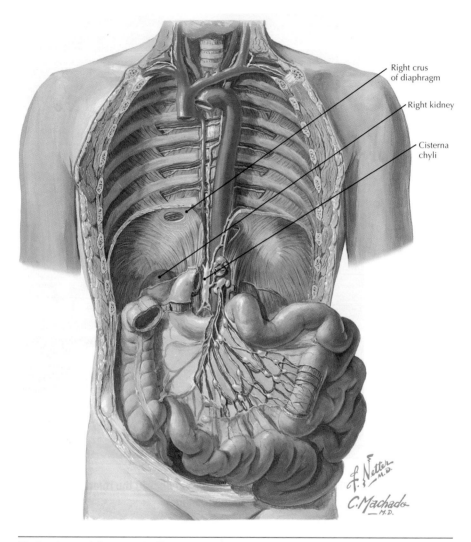

Right crus
of diaphragm

Right kidney

Cisterna
chyli

Chyle cistern (cisterna chyli), and lymph vessels and nodes of the small intestines
(Atlas of Human Anatomy, 6th edition, Plate 295)

Clinical Note   The thoracic duct along with the chyle cistern is a major lymphatic pathway near the anterior thoracolumbar spine. Although the lymphatic system is very delicate, chylorrhea and chylothorax are very rare complications of spinal surgery.

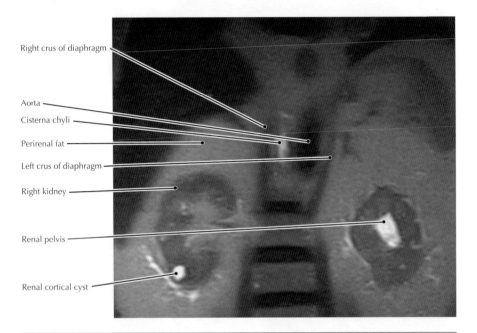

Right crus of diaphragm

Aorta
Cisterna chyli
Perirenal fat
Left crus of diaphragm
Right kidney

Renal pelvis

Renal cortical cyst

Coronal T2 single shot FSE MR image, abdomen

- The four main abdominal lymph channels all converge to form an abdominal confluence of lymph trunks. The shape of this convergence is variable; it may be singular, duplicated, triplicated, or plexiform. A singular (fusiform) structure is only occasionally found but is the form most associated with the term *cisterna chyli*.

- Most typically the lymphatic confluence is located at the inferior border of T12 or at the thoracolumbar intervertebral disc.

- The high signal from the renal pelvis on the left results because the image passes through more of the collecting system on that side, which contains fluid (urine).

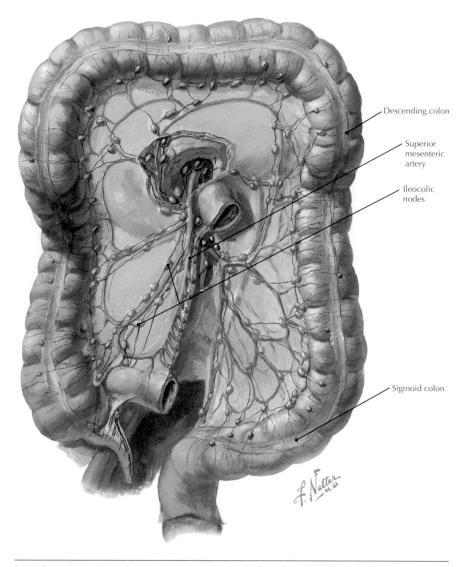

Lymph nodes and vessels of the large bowel *(Atlas of Human Anatomy, 6th edition, Plate 296)*

Descending colon

Superior mesenteric artery

Ileocolic nodes

Sigmoid colon

Clinical Note During bowel resection for malignancy, the surgeon attempts to mobilize the associated mesentery and remove as many infiltrated lymph nodes as possible.

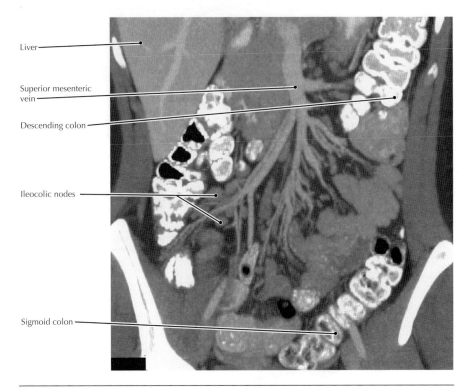

Liver

Superior mesenteric vein

Descending colon

Ileocolic nodes

Sigmoid colon

2-cm thick coronal MIP, CE CT of the abdomen

- This image is from a young adult woman with mild adenopathy. Unless enlarged by disease as in this case, mesenteric lymph nodes are difficult to discern in axial images.

- In axial images of normal patients, lymph nodes appear as round or ovoid structures similar in size to some mesenteric vessels, thus making differentiation problematic. However, coronal reconstructions enable clearer discrimination between lymph nodes and vessels.

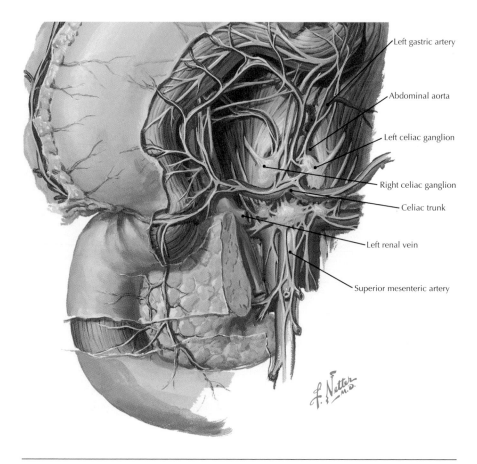

Left gastric artery

Abdominal aorta

Left celiac ganglion

Right celiac ganglion

Celiac trunk

Left renal vein

Superior mesenteric artery

Anterior view of the upper abdominal autonomic plexuses and nerves (Atlas of Human Anatomy, 6th edition, Plate 299)

Clinical Note The celiac ganglia provide autonomic (predominantly sympathetic) innervation to the upper abdominal viscera. The ganglia receive preganglionic fibers from approximately T5-T10 spinal nerves. Visceral afferent fibers accompany both the preganglionic and postganglionic fibers that are associated with the ganglia, transmitting the poorly localized (or referred) pain impulses that occur with disorders of the abdominal viscera.

Inferior vena cava
Left gastric artery
Abdominal aorta
Celiac trunk
Right celiac ganglion
Left celiac ganglion
Superior mesenteric artery
Left renal vein
Left suprarenal (adrenal) gland and vein

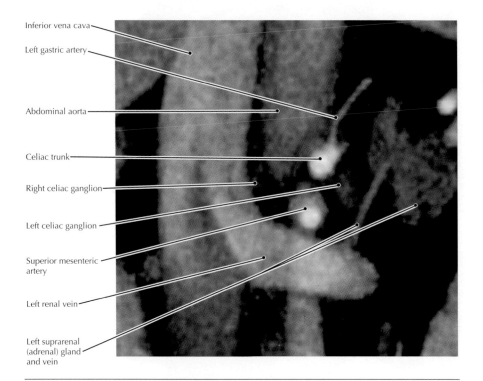

Volume rendered display, CE CT of the abdomen

- The fibers uniting the right and left celiac ganglia around the celiac trunk with the ganglia comprise the celiac (solar) plexus.
- Intractable pancreatic pain associated with pancreatic cancer is sometimes treated by ablation of the celiac ganglia.

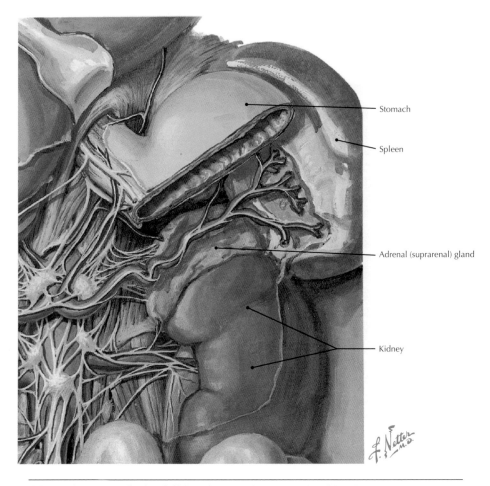

Adrenal (suprarenal) gland *(Atlas of Human Anatomy, 6th edition, Plate 301)*

> **Clinical Note**   On MRI and CT, the normal adrenal (suprarenal) glands show two or three slender limbs, depending on the imaging plane. This appearance often varies because of tumor. The most common adrenal tumor is a benign adenoma, which is usually not a hormone-secreting tumor and therefore of no clinical significance.

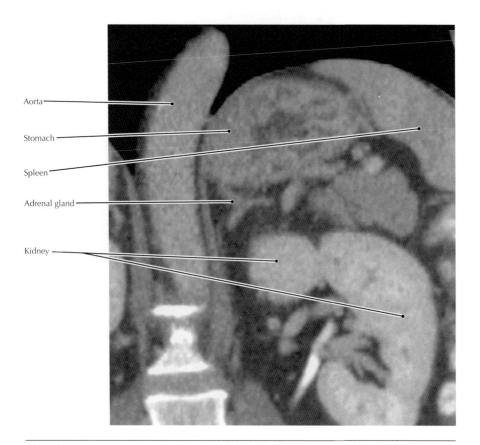

Aorta

Stomach

Spleen

Adrenal gland

Kidney

Coronal CT

- The fatty retroperitoneal tissue in which the adrenal gland is embedded may account for the difference in appearance between the adrenal gland seen in vivo by diagnostic imaging and its classic depiction in anatomy illustrations.

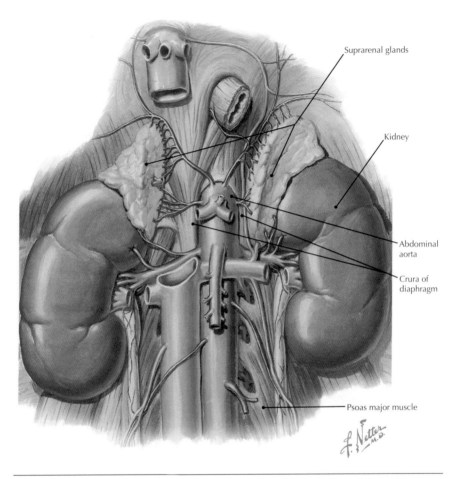

Kidneys, suprarenal (adrenal) glands, and associated vasculature *(Atlas of Human Anatomy, 6th edition, Plate 310)*

Clinical Note Cortisol is a corticosteroid hormone that is produced by the suprarenal gland. Disorders of the glands can result in insufficient cortisol production (Addison's disease) or overproduction (Cushing's disease).

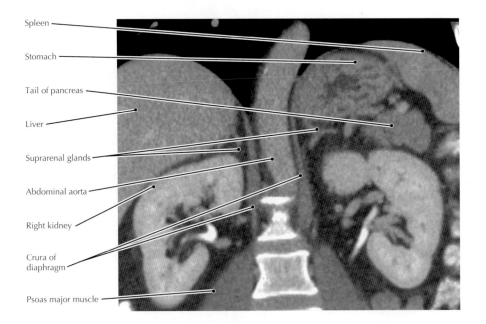

Spleen

Stomach

Tail of pancreas

Liver

Suprarenal glands

Abdominal aorta

Right kidney

Crura of diaphragm

Psoas major muscle

Coronal reconstruction, CE CT of the abdomen

- The crura of the diaphragm are those parts of the diaphragm that arise from the bodies of the lumbar vertebrae.
- The suprarenal gland tends to appear as a three-armed star in coronal section.

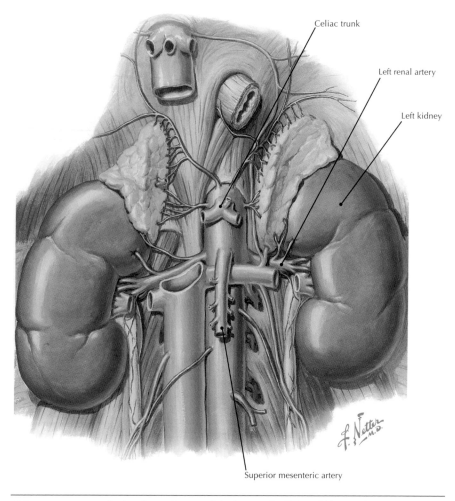

Celiac trunk

Left renal artery

Left kidney

Superior mesenteric artery

Kidneys, suprarenal glands, and associated vessels *(Atlas of Human Anatomy, 6th edition, Plate 310)*

Clinical Note   The abdominal aorta is a common site for aneurysms, which may be associated with abdominal or back pain, nausea, and rapid satiety, and can lead to fatal rupture, especially when greater than 5 cm.

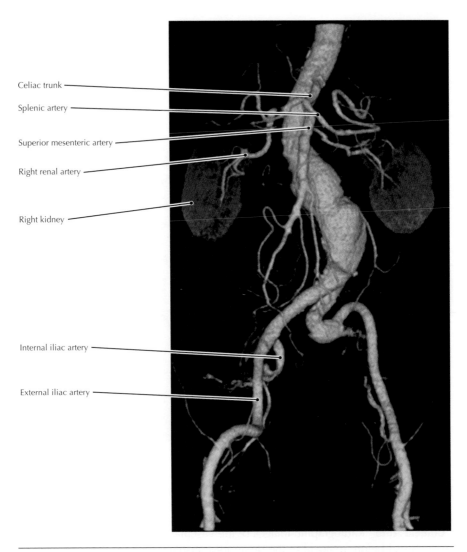

Celiac trunk

Splenic artery

Superior mesenteric artery

Right renal artery

Right kidney

Internal iliac artery

External iliac artery

3-D display, CE CTA of the entire abdominal aorta and its major branches *(From Kundra V, Silverman PM: Impact of multislice CT on imaging of acute abdominal disease. Radiol Clin North Am 41(6):1083-1093, 2003)*

- Mild aneurysms of the lumbar aorta and the left common iliac arteries are visible in this image.
- The three branches of the celiac trunk are the common hepatic, splenic, and left gastric arteries.

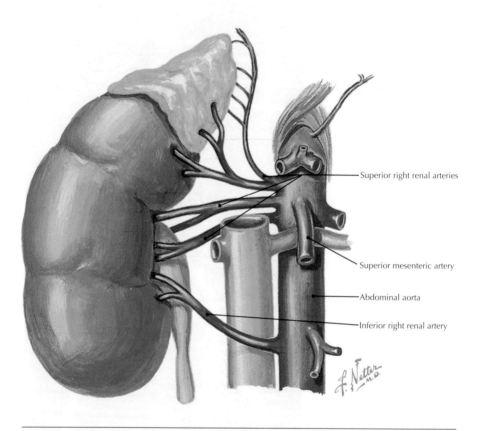

Superior right renal arteries

Superior mesenteric artery

Abdominal aorta

Inferior right renal artery

Multiple renal arteries with inferior artery passing anterior to IVC

Clinical Note Radiographic images of the vasculature supply of the kidney are critical before removal of the organ for transplant because the transplant surgeon needs to know the number of renal arteries present on each side. Although the left kidney is typically preferred for transplant because of its longer vein, if the left has more than one renal artery and the right has only one, the right will be used.

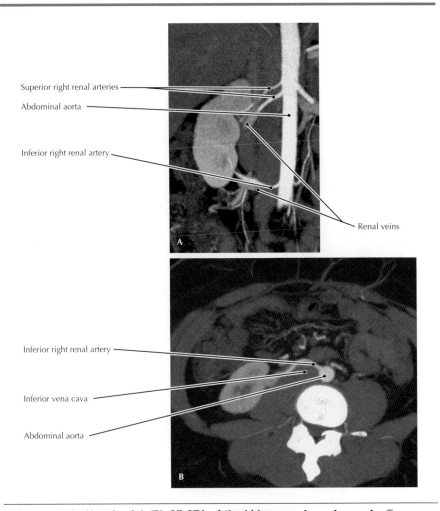

Superior right renal arteries

Abdominal aorta

Inferior right renal artery

Renal veins

A

Inferior right renal artery

Inferior vena cava

Abdominal aorta

B

MIPs, coronal (A) and axial (B), CE CTA of the kidneys and renal vessels *(From Kang PS, Spain JW: Multidetector CT angiography of the abdomen. Radiol Clin North Am 43(6):963-976, 2005)*

- The left kidney is not visible in B because its lower pole is superior to the level of the image.

- The presence of supernumerary renal arteries arising from the abdominal aorta is common (about 28% of cases). Such vessels are more common on the left and more common superior to the main vessel than inferior to it.

- The renal arteries may also give rise to vessels that normally do not arise from them, such as the inferior phrenic, hepatic and middle suprarenals, gonadal, pancreatic, some of the colic arteries, and one or more of the lumbar arteries.

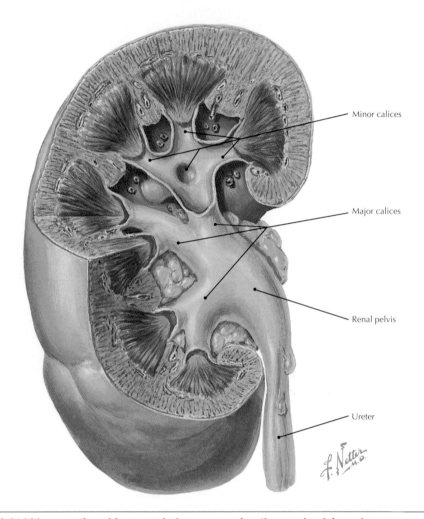

Minor calices

Major calices

Renal pelvis

Ureter

Right kidney sectioned in several planes, exposing the renal pelvis and parenchyma *(Atlas of Human Anatomy, 6th edition, Plate 311)*

Clinical Note   The severe pain of renal colic, resulting from a ureter obstructed by a calculus (stone), seems disproportionate relative to the size of a calculus, and the poorly localized pain does not identify the location of the impacted calculus.

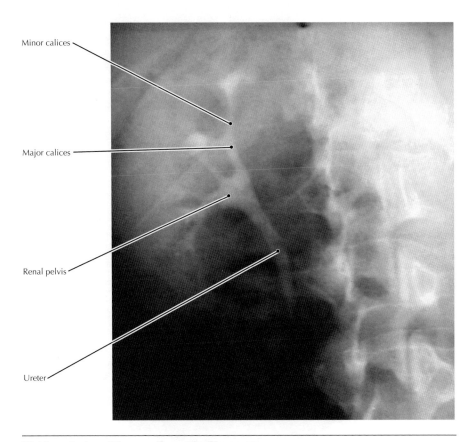

Minor calices

Major calices

Renal pelvis

Ureter

Right posterior oblique radiograph, IV urogram

- The complex embryologic development of the urinary system may result in duplication of the collecting system and ureter. Similarly, renal agenesis can occur unilaterally or bilaterally, isolated or combined with other abnormalities (bilateral agenesis is not compatible with life).

- Urine formed in the kidney passes through a papilla at the apex of the pyramid into a minor calyx and then into major calyx (infundibulum) before passing through the renal pelvis into the ureter.

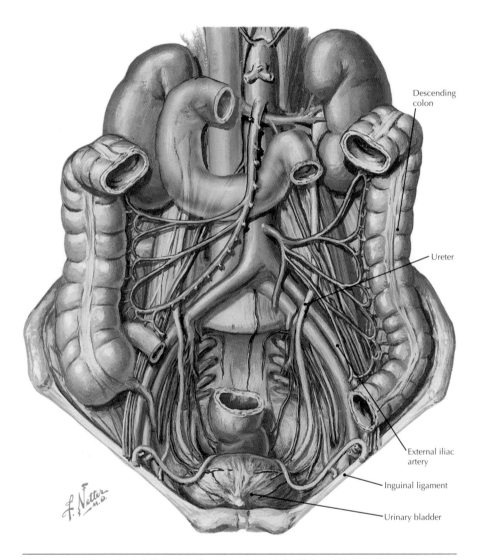

Descending colon

Ureter

External iliac artery

Inguinal ligament

Urinary bladder

Ureter crossing external iliac arteries to enter pelvis *(Atlas of Human Anatomy, 6th edition, Plate 313)*

Clinical Note   Pelvic surgery is the most common cause of iatrogenic injury to the ureter. If this occurs, patients typically have flank pain, tenderness in the costovertebral region, ileus, fever, and a small rise in serum creatinine.

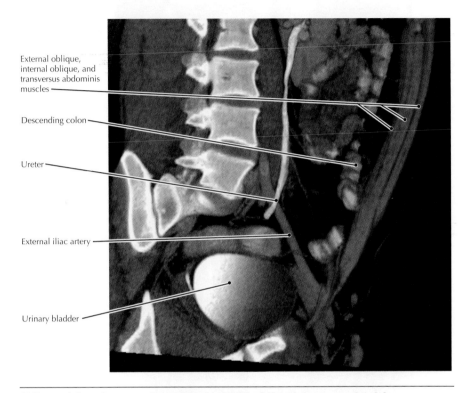

External oblique, internal oblique, and transversus abdominis muscles

Descending colon

Ureter

External iliac artery

Urinary bladder

Oblique slab, volume rendered image, CE CT of the abdomen and pelvis

- The ureter is not seen to enter the bladder in this image because it passes posterior to the plane of the image reconstruction.
- The three layers of the abdominal wall musculature are visible in the CT image.
- The left and right external iliac arteries branch from the common iliac arteries at the level of the lumbosacral intervertebral disc and become the femoral arteries as they pass deep to the inguinal ligaments.

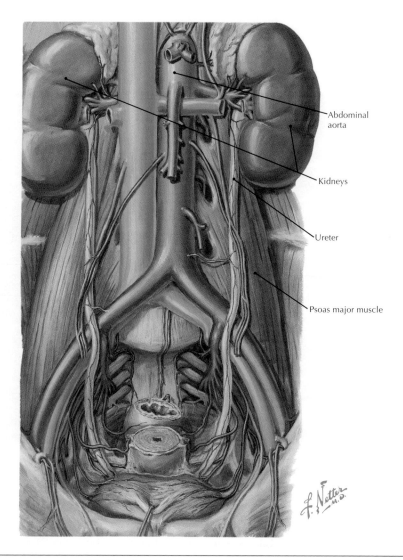

Abdominal aorta

Kidneys

Ureter

Psoas major muscle

Kidneys, ureter, and bladder *in situ* (Atlas of Human Anatomy, 6th edition, Plate 314)

Clinical Note Renal calculi (kidney stones) form within the drainage system of either kidney, but tend to lodge and cause excruciating pain in one of three places: the pelvoureteric junction, where the ureter crosses the pelvic brim, and where the ureter enters the bladder (ureterovesical junction).

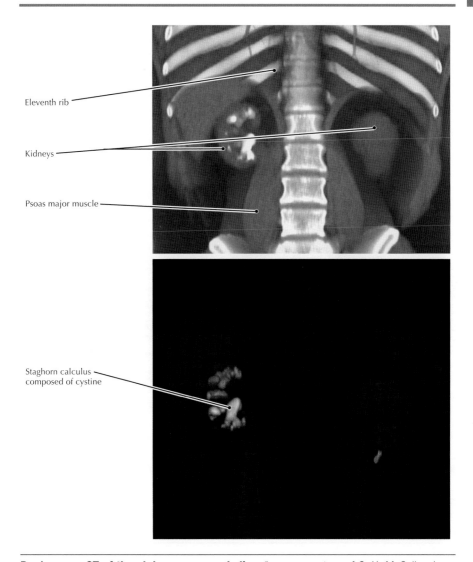

Eleventh rib

Kidneys

Psoas major muscle

Staghorn calculus
composed of cystine

Dual energy CT of the abdomen, coronal slice *(Images courtesy of C. H. McCollough, PhD, Mayo Clinic College of Medicine)*

- Semitransparent 3-D rendering of the kidneys shows a staghorn calculus filling the intrarenal collecting system of the right kidney and a small stone in the lower pole of the left kidney.

- Data acquired using a dual energy CT technique, which can use the energy dependence of CT values to determine stone composition. The calculi in this patient were shown to be cystine stones.

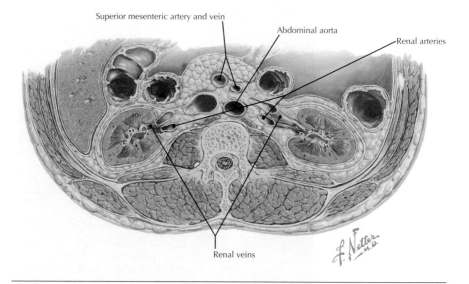

Superior mesenteric artery and vein

Abdominal aorta

Renal arteries

Renal veins

Kidneys and associated vessels *(Atlas of Human Anatomy, 6th edition, Plate 315)*

Clinical Note The SMA passes anterior to the left renal vein, which can be compressed between it and the aorta, producing the "nutcracker syndrome."

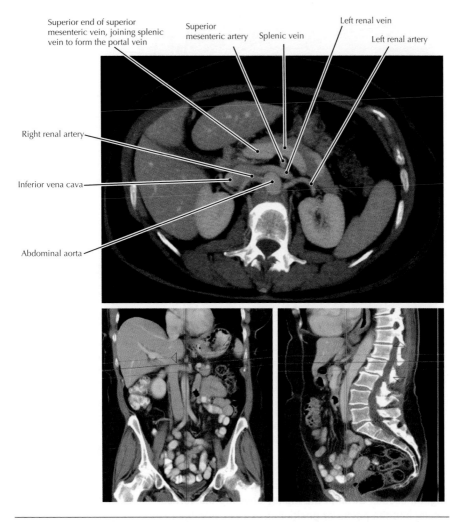

3-cm thick MIP, CE CT of the abdomen (*red lines* in the reference images indicate the position and orientation of the main image, and the thickness of the MIP slab)

- The thick slab MIP allows for better visualization of the vessels than a routine thin axial CT or MR image.
- The close relationships of the renal vessels to each other and the SMA provide an important and easily recognizable landmark during abdominal ultrasonography.

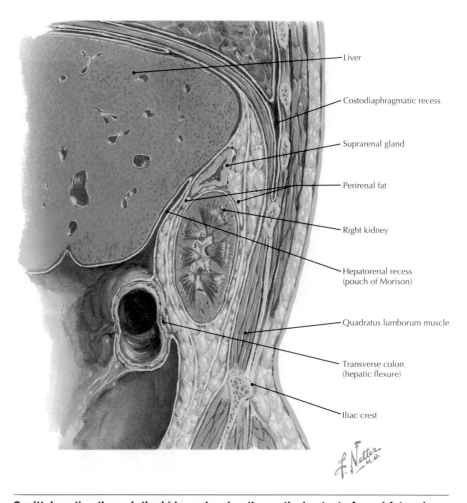

Liver

Costodiaphragmatic recess

Suprarenal gland

Perirenal fat

Right kidney

Hepatorenal recess
(pouch of Morison)

Quadratus lumborum muscle

Transverse colon
(hepatic flexure)

Iliac crest

Sagittal section through the kidney showing the vertical extent of renal fat and fascia, and the posterior position of the hepatorenal recess *(Atlas of Human Anatomy, 6th edition, Plate 315)*

Clinical Note The hepatorenal recess (Morison's pouch) is a peritoneal space that lies between the liver anteriorly, and the right kidney and suprarenal gland posteriorly. In the supine position it can fill with peritoneal fluid from any intraperitoneal sepsis, for example, from gallbladder disease.

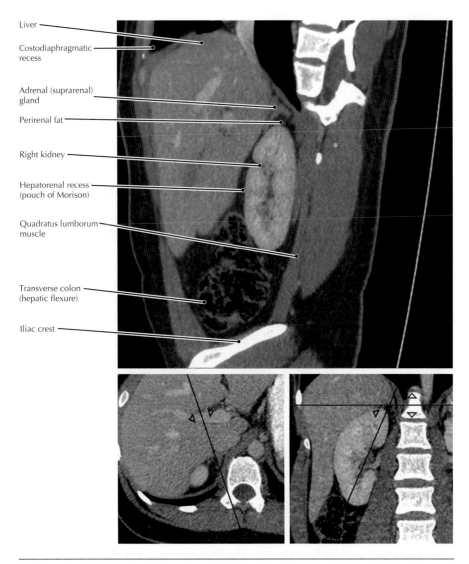

Liver

Costodiaphragmatic recess

Adrenal (suprarenal) gland

Perirenal fat

Right kidney

Hepatorenal recess (pouch of Morison)

Quadratus lumborum muscle

Transverse colon (hepatic flexure)

Iliac crest

Oblique sagittal reconstruction, CE CT of the abdomen (*blue lines* in the reference images indicate the position and orientation of the main image)

- Note that the pleural cavity and lung descend posterior to the liver as indicated by the costodiaphragmatic recess.
- Because of the close relationship of the liver and right kidney, the clinical presentation of pain caused by stretching of the liver capsule by liver disease can initially be confused with right flank pain caused by right kidney disease.

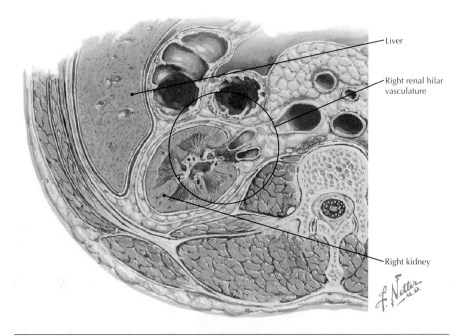

Liver

Right renal hilar vasculature

Right kidney

Renal fasciae *(Atlas of Human Anatomy, 6th edition, Plate 315)*

Clinical Note   Renal ultrasound (US) with Doppler imaging of renal arterial flow for suspected renovascular hypertension can be diagnostic, but the sensitivity and specificity of this examination is variable. Renal US may reveal a renal or adrenal mass that could cause hypertension. US of the kidneys may be done to rule out hydronephrosis. The most common renal mass is a simple cyst (often multiple in same patient) that, depending on the patient's body habitus, may be confidently diagnosed as a simple benign cyst by US.

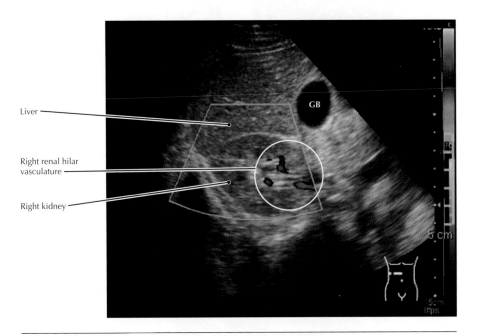

Liver

Right renal hilar
vasculature

Right kidney

GB

Axial US through the right kidney with Doppler color flow imaging

- The vasculature in the right renal hilum is highlighted by colored pixels at locations where there is Doppler signal from flowing blood.
- The homogeneous texture of the liver provides a sonographic "window" that allows good visualization of the right kidney on US studies.

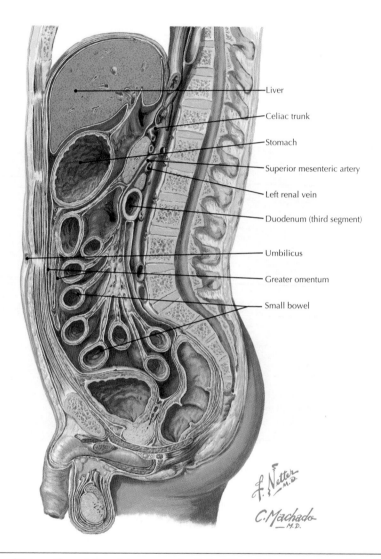

Parasagittal section of the abdomen and pelvis *(Atlas of Human Anatomy, 6th edition, Plate 321)*

Clinical Note In superior mesenteric artery (Wilkie's) syndrome, the organs supplied by the SMA descend, causing the SMA to compress the third portion of the duodenum, resulting in epigastric pain and other symptoms of intestinal obstruction.

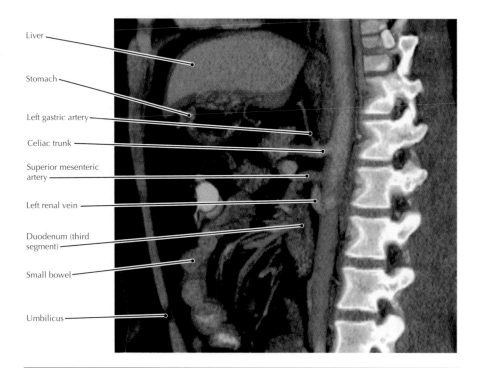

Liver

Stomach

Left gastric artery

Celiac trunk

Superior mesenteric artery

Left renal vein

Duodenum (third segment)

Small bowel

Umbilicus

30-mm sagittal slab, volume rendered display, CE CT of the abdomen

- The left renal vein typically passes anterior to the abdominal aorta to enter the IVC.
- The left gastric artery is the smallest branch of the celiac trunk and supplies the lesser curvature of the stomach and inferior part of the esophagus.

Section 5 **Pelvis and Perineum**

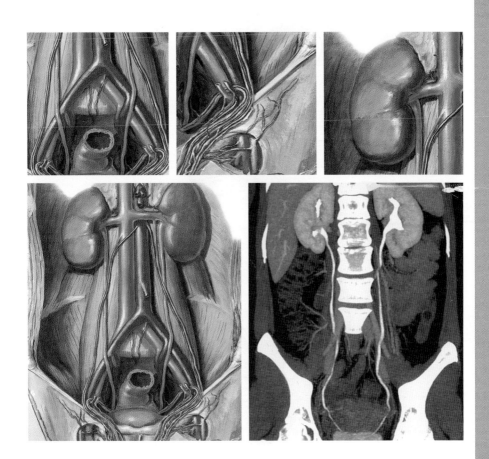

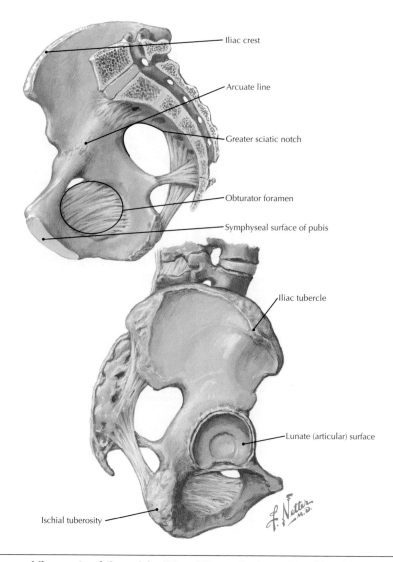

- Iliac crest
- Arcuate line
- Greater sciatic notch
- Obturator foramen
- Symphyseal surface of pubis
- Iliac tubercle
- Lunate (articular) surface
- Ischial tuberosity

Bones and ligaments of the pelvis *(Atlas of Human Anatomy, 6th edition, Plate 334)*

Clinical Note The crest of the ilium is the most common site for the harvesting of red bone marrow for allogenic or autologous transplantation after loss of marrow due to disease, or chemotherapeutic or radiation treatments for cancer. It is also the site for obtaining small samples of marrow for diagnostic purposes.

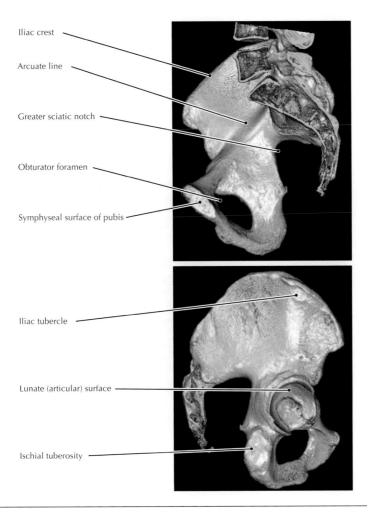

Iliac crest

Arcuate line

Greater sciatic notch

Obturator foramen

Symphyseal surface of pubis

Iliac tubercle

Lunate (articular) surface

Ischial tuberosity

Volume rendered display, CT of the pelvis

- The external surface of the iliac blade is the attachment site for the gluteus medius and minimus muscles. These two muscles are primarily responsible for maintaining pelvic stability when one foot is lifted off the ground (e.g., during the swing phase of walking). They both insert into the greater trochanter of the femur.
- The lunate surface is the articular part of the acetabulum.
- The symphyseal surface of the pubis undergoes predictable changes with aging so that the surface can be used to estimate the age of skeletal material collected forensically or archeologically.

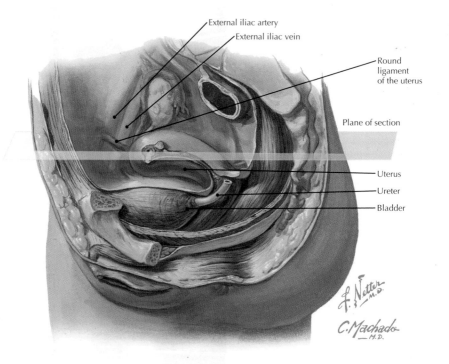

External iliac artery

External iliac vein

Round ligament of the uterus

Plane of section

Uterus

Ureter

Bladder

Parasagittal view of the female pelvic viscera *(Atlas of Human Anatomy, 6th edition, Plate 340)*

Clinical Note Lipomas of the round ligament can mimic signs of hernia. They should be suspected in a woman with groin pain whose physical examination is normal.

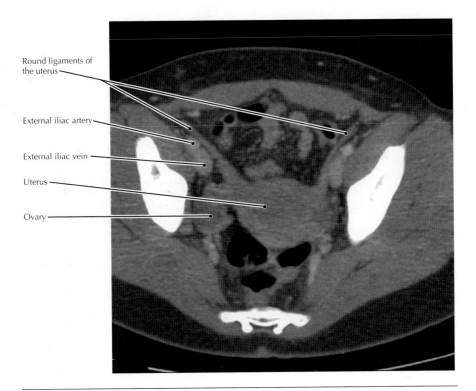

Round ligaments of
the uterus

External iliac artery

External iliac vein

Uterus

Ovary

Axial CE CT of the pelvis

- The round ligament passes through the inguinal canal to reach the labia majus. Lymph vessels travel with the ligament so that some lymph from the uterus drains to the inguinal nodes.
- The position of the ovary can vary within a patient with the amount of bladder and bowel distention and the patient's position.

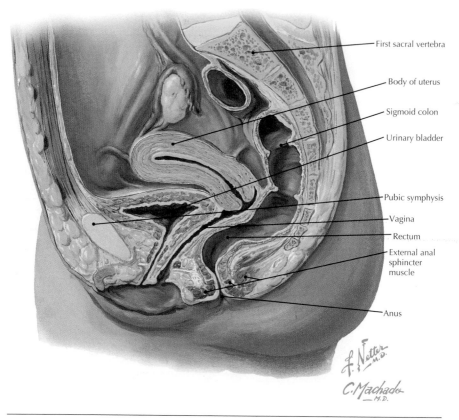

First sacral vertebra

Body of uterus

Sigmoid colon

Urinary bladder

Pubic symphysis

Vagina

Rectum

External anal sphincter muscle

Anus

Midsagittal view of the female pelvis showing viscera (Atlas of Human Anatomy, 6th edition, Plate 340)

Clinical Note A rectocele occurs when the anterior wall of the rectum bulges into the vagina; this occurs because of weaknesses in pelvic support mechanisms (i.e., pelvic ligaments) that sometimes are associated with repeated stretching due to multiple pregnancies.

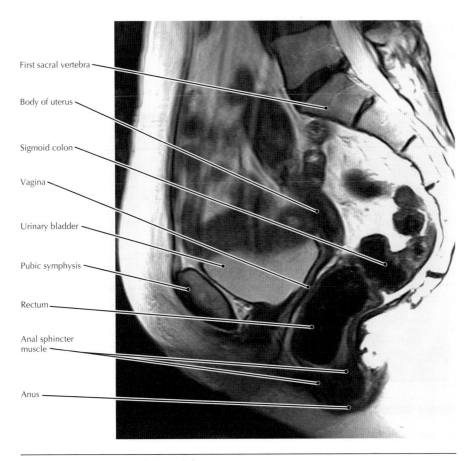

First sacral vertebra

Body of uterus

Sigmoid colon

Vagina

Urinary bladder

Pubic symphysis

Rectum

Anal sphincter
muscle

Anus

Sagittal T2 MR image of the pelvis

- The anal sphincter has both internal (innervated by pelvic splanchnic [parasympathetic] nerves) and external (innervated by the inferior rectal [somatic] nerves) divisions.

- The uterus is not well seen in this patient because much of it extends to one side, out of the plane of this midline sagittal image. Such "tilting" and other variations of the uterus are common and must be kept in mind when viewing cross-sectional images so that erroneous conclusions pertaining to uterine conditions are not made.

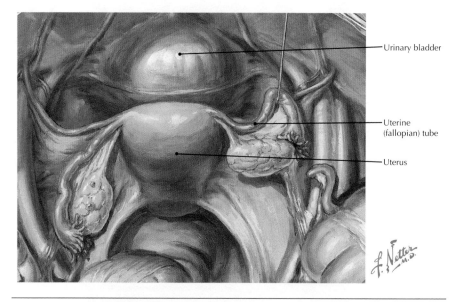

Urinary bladder

Uterine
(fallopian) tube

Uterus

Uterine (fallopian) tubes *(Atlas of Human Anatomy, 6th edition, Plate 341)*

Clinical Note Ligation of the uterine (fallopian) tubes (tubal ligation), once a common surgical procedure for elective sterilization, now is often done with devices inserted into the uterine tubes during hysteroscopy. Hysterosalpingography (HSG) is used to identify tubal occlusion as a cause of infertility and to document tubal occlusion after elective sterilization.

Uterine
(fallopian) tube

HSG catheter

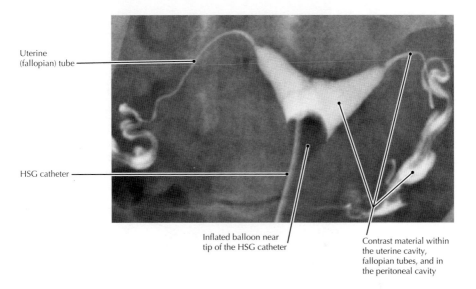

Inflated balloon near
tip of the HSG catheter

Contrast material within
the uterine cavity,
fallopian tubes, and in
the peritoneal cavity

AP radiograph during HSG

- The cornua of the uterine cavity lead to the fallopian tubes.
- The uterine tubes can be very mobile.
- The fimbriated ends of the uterine tubes open to the peritoneal cavity.

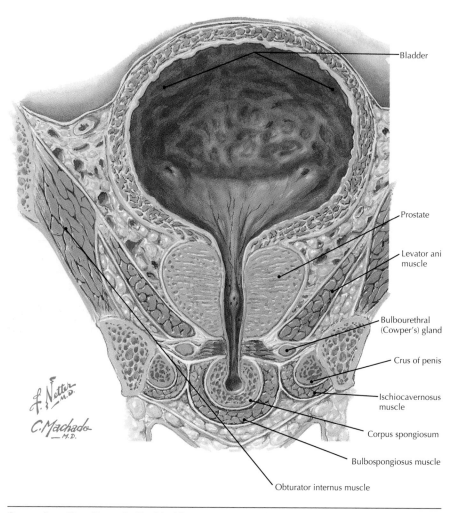

Bladder

Prostate

Levator ani muscle

Bulbourethral (Cowper's) gland

Crus of penis

Ischiocavernosus muscle

Corpus spongiosum

Bulbospongiosus muscle

Obturator internus muscle

Coronal section through the bladder, prostate, and bulb of penis (*Atlas of Human Anatomy, 6th edition, Plate 348*)

Clinical Note A Cowper's cyst or syringocele is a cyst-like swelling of a bulbourethral gland or one of its ducts. This condition is typically found in infant boys or occasionally in older men.

Bladder

Prostate

Levator ani
muscle

Bulbourethral
(Cowper's) gland

Crus of penis

Ischiocavernosus
muscle

Corpus spongiosum

Bulbospongiosus
muscle

Obturator externus
muscle

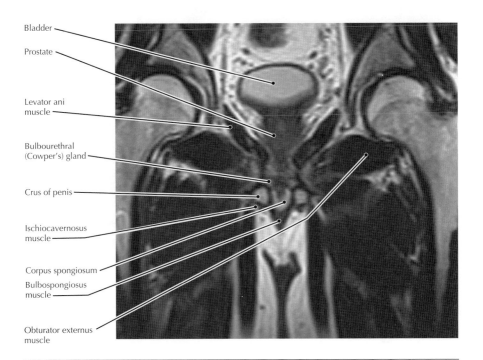

Coronal T2 MR image of the pelvis

- The levator ani muscle comprises most of the pelvic diaphragm and is critical to the maintenance of urinary and fecal continence.
- The bulbospongiosus muscle is a sphincter of the urethra and may play a role in maintaining an erection by forcing blood into the distal penis.
- The ischiocavernous muscles also function in that manner to maintain an erection.

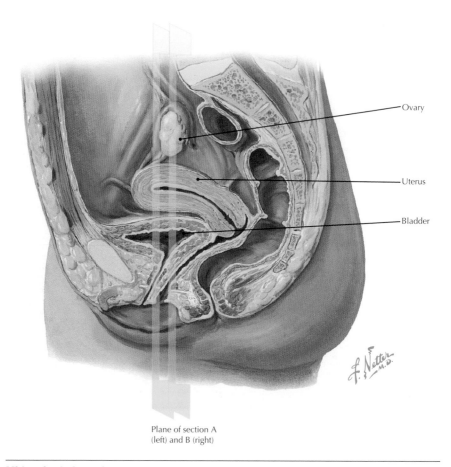

Ovary

Uterus

Bladder

Plane of section A
(left) and B (right)

Midsagittal view of the female pelvis showing viscera *(Atlas of Human Anatomy, 6th edition, Plate 340)*

Clinical Note As shown in the upper image on the opposite page, the intrinsic soft tissue contrast in MRI is clinically useful in examining the uterus. Note the central hyperintense (bright) endometrium surrounded by the hypointense (darker) transitional zone, as well as the intermediate to high signal of the myometrium. Uterine fibroids, adenomyosis, and endometrial hyperplasia and carcinoma are clearly shown in pelvic MRI.

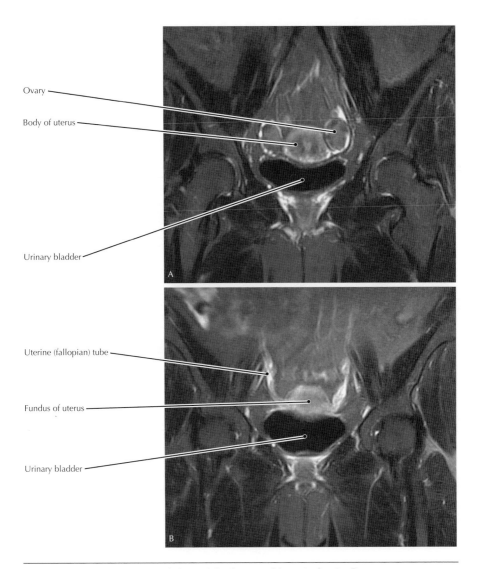

Ovary

Body of uterus

Urinary bladder

A

Uterine (fallopian) tube

Fundus of uterus

Urinary bladder

B

Coronal FS T2 MR images of the pelvis; image *A* is anterior to *B*

- Image is a cross section along short axis of the uterus, which is in its common anteverted position.
- Notice the small, rounded foci of high T2 signal in the periphery of both ovaries, representing small, fluid-filled follicles.

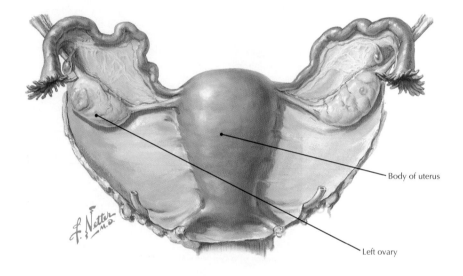

Body of uterus

Left ovary

Posterior view of the uterus and associated structures *(Atlas of Human Anatomy, 6th edition, Plate 352)*

Clinical Note Pelvic pain in female patients can have many causes—for example, ovarian cysts, ectopic pregnancy, endometriosis, and pelvic inflammatory disease (PID). Ultrasound offers a relatively easy (and non-ionizing) procedure that can confirm or rule out many of these conditions.

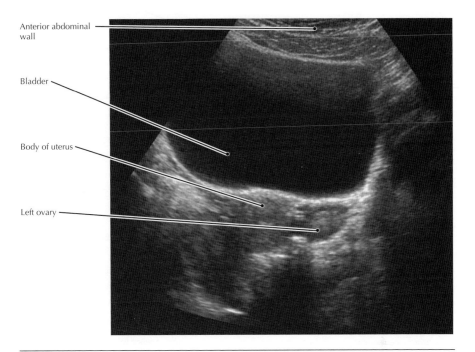

Anterior abdominal wall

Bladder

Body of uterus

Left ovary

Transabdominal sonogram (ultrasound) of the female pelvis, transverse image

- The ultrasound transducer used to generate this image was placed on the anterior abdominal wall and the fluid-filled bladder provided a "window" through which the more posterior structures were imaged.

- The right ovary is obscured by shadowing from a gas-filled bowel loop. Because of the mobility of bowel loops and of the ovaries, as well as varied orientations of the uterus, obtaining ideal ultrasound images of pelvic structures can be challenging with transabdominal scanning. Transvaginal ultrasound scanning is therefore commonly used.

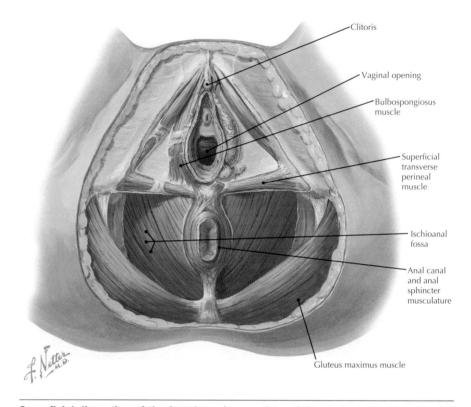

Clitoris

Vaginal opening

Bulbospongiosus muscle

Superficial transverse perineal muscle

Ischioanal fossa

Anal canal and anal sphincter musculature

Gluteus maximus muscle

Superficial dissection of the female perineum *(Atlas of Human Anatomy, 6th edition, Plate 356)*

Clinical Note Congenital obstructing lesions of the vagina—hydrometrocolpos and hematocolpos—present at various ages. Typical presentations in neonates are abdominal mass, neonatal sepsis, and respiratory distress. In adolescents, presentation includes abdominal pain, voiding dysfunction, and backache. Adults may present with infertility or inability to have intercourse (or both).

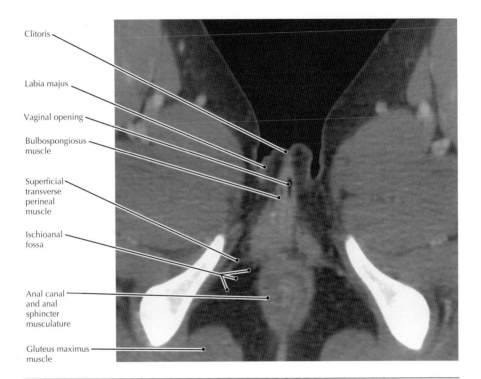

Clitoris

Labia majus

Vaginal opening

Bulbospongiosus
muscle

Superficial
transverse
perineal
muscle

Ischioanal
fossa

Anal canal
and anal
sphincter
musculature

Gluteus maximus
muscle

Oblique axial reconstruction, CE CT of the pelvis

- The clitoris is an erectile body composed only of the corpus cavernosus.
- The superficial transverse perineal muscle attaches to the perineal body and provides support to this region.
- The bulbospongiosus muscle is a sphincter of the vagina.

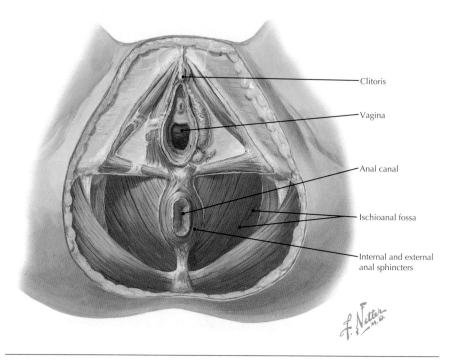

Clitoris

Vagina

Anal canal

Ischioanal fossa

Internal and external
anal sphincters

Female perineum and deep perineum *(Atlas of Human Anatomy, 6th edition, Plate 356)*

Clinical Note Perineal ultrasound is not a common procedure but is sometimes used during parturition to assess fetal progress and in women to evaluate stress incontinence.

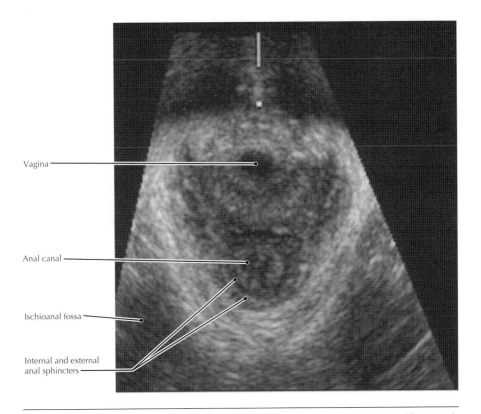

Vagina

Anal canal

Ischioanal fossa

Internal and external
anal sphincters

Perineal US *(From Unger CA, Weinstein MM, Pretorius DH: Pelvic floor imaging. Ultrasound Clin 5:313-330, 2010)*

- Mucosal folds of the anal canal are hyperechoic (bright) and clearly apparent on the image.
- The thin ring of hypoechoic internal anal sphincter surrounds the mucosa. The external anal sphincter is a ring of hyperechoic tissue. The difference in echogenicity of the two muscle layers reflects different internal architecture.

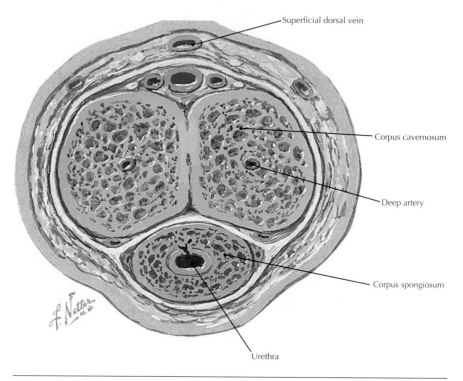

Superficial dorsal vein

Corpus cavernosum

Deep artery

Corpus spongiosum

Urethra

Cross section through the body of the penis *(Atlas of Human Anatomy, 6th edition, Plate 359)*

Clinical Note Hypospadias is the most common congenital abnormality of the penis; in hypospadias the urethra opens on the ventral (underside) of the penis or on the scrotum.

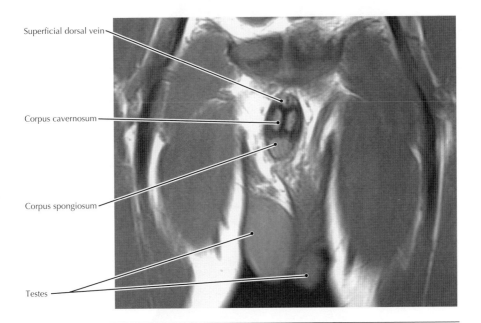

Superficial dorsal vein

Corpus cavernosum

Corpus spongiosum

Testes

Coronal T1 MR image through the penis

- The thin walls of the urethra are normally collapsed and indistinguishable from the surrounding corpus spongiosum on MRI. If an image was taken during urination, the urethra would appear as dark (flow void) in this T1 image.

- Engorgement of the corpora cavernosa with blood is primarily responsible for penile erection. The blood is derived from the internal pudendal artery through the deep and dorsal arteries of the penis.

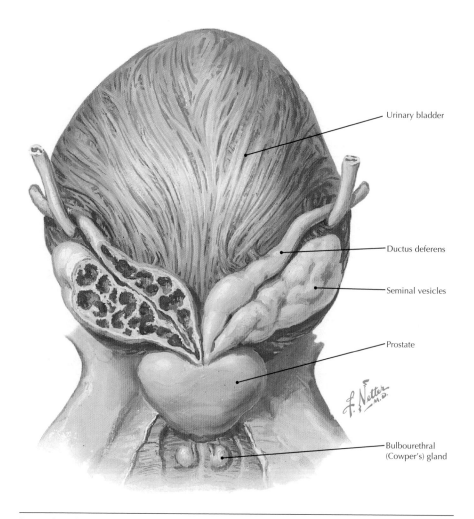

Urinary bladder

Ductus deferens

Seminal vesicles

Prostate

Bulbourethral
(Cowper's) gland

Posterior view of seminal vesicles *(Atlas of Human Anatomy, 6th edition, Plate 362)*

Clinical Note Dilation of the seminal vesicles is associated with ejaculatory duct obstruction and infertility and is visible on a transrectal ultrasound (TRUS) image (see p. 319)

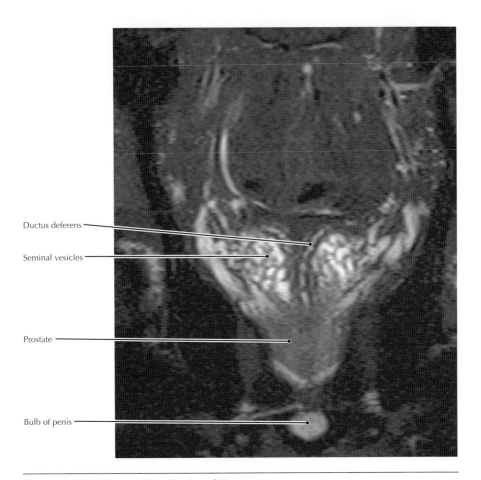

Ductus deferens

Seminal vesicles

Prostate

Bulb of penis

T2 coronal MR image of seminal vesicles

- The bladder is not visible in this scan because it is anterior to this coronal section.
- The ampulla of the ductus deferens and the duct of the seminal vesicle combine to form the ejaculatory duct.

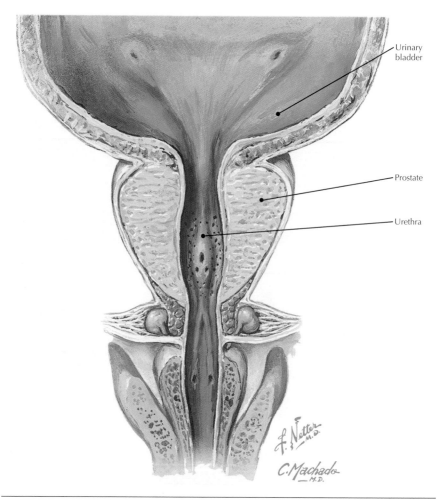

Urinary
bladder

Prostate

Urethra

Coronal section of the bladder, prostate, and bulbous portion of the spongy urethra
(Atlas of Human Anatomy, 6th edition, Plate 362)

Clinical Note Prostate carcinoma (cancer of the prostate) is the most
common visceral cancer in men. In over 70% of cases, cancer arises in the
peripheral zone of the gland, classically in a posterior location, and thus is
palpable via a rectal examination.

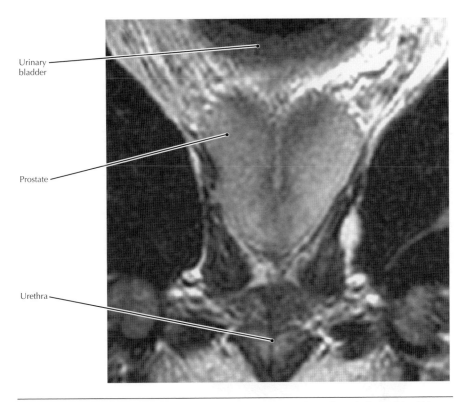

Urinary bladder

Prostate

Urethra

Coronal T2 MR image of the prostate in a young man *(From Rajesh A, Coakley FV: MR imaging and MR spectroscopic imaging of prostate cancer. Magn Reson Imaging Clin N Am 12(3):557-579, 2004)*

- The prostate is small in this patient and zonal differentiation is not appreciable.
- Zonal differentiation becomes more apparent with aging and, in contrast to carcinoma, benign prostatic hypertrophy (BPH) typically arises in the transitional zone.
- Zonal differentiation may be better appreciated in a TRUS image.
- The cavernous nerves (parasympathetic) that stimulate penile erection adhere to the prostate and must be "peeled" off the gland during radical prostatectomy for cancer in order to prevent impotence.

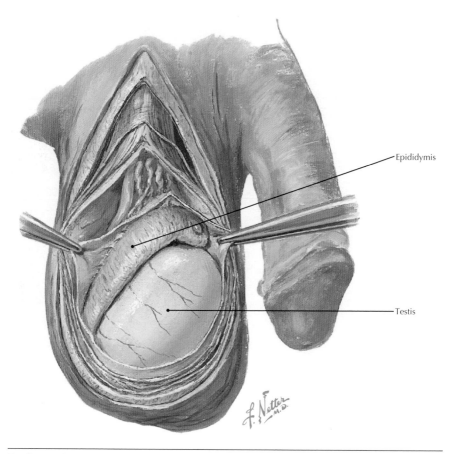

Epididymis

Testis

Penis, testis, and epididymis *(Atlas of Human Anatomy, 6th edition, Plate 365)*

Clinical Note Acute inflammation of the epididymis, epididymitis, results in swelling of the scrotum and pain in the testes. It can be shown on color flow Doppler sonography.

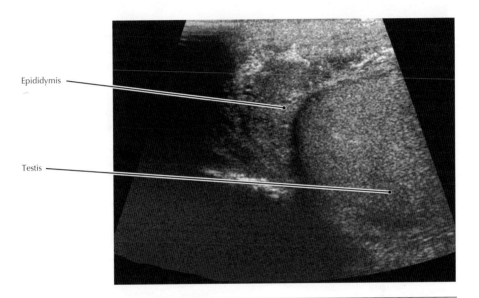

Epididymis

Testis

Ultrasound of the testis and epididymis

- Ultrasound is the procedure of choice for a suspected testicular mass because the echogenicity of testicular masses can clearly differentiate them from normal testicular tissue.
- The epididymis allows for sperm storage and maturation; it is located between the testis and the ductus deferens.

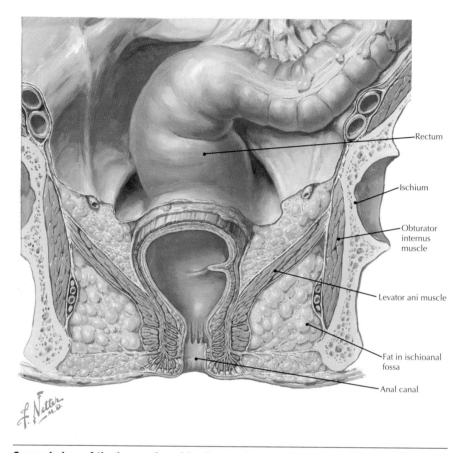

Rectum

Ischium

Obturator internus muscle

Levator ani muscle

Fat in ischioanal fossa

Anal canal

Coronal view of the lower sigmoid colon, rectum, anal canal, and ischioanal fossa
(Atlas of Human Anatomy, 6th edition, Plate 370)

Clinical Note   Whether or not disease processes involve the ischioanal fossa is important for determining the extent of a wide variety of disease processes, including congenital and developmental lesions (e.g., anal fistula); inflammatory, traumatic, and hemorrhagic conditions (e.g., Crohn's disease); and tumors.

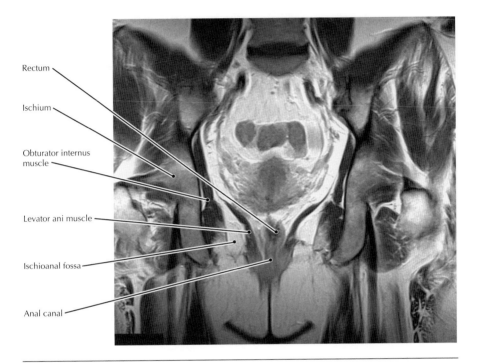

Rectum

Ischium

Obturator internus muscle

Levator ani muscle

Ischioanal fossa

Anal canal

Coronal T1 MR image of the pelvis

- The fat within the ischioanal fossa allows for the distention of the anal canal as feces are expelled.
- The levator ani muscle comprises most of the pelvic diaphragm and is the muscle that is contracted during Kegel exercises, which may be done in women to reduce urinary incontinence.

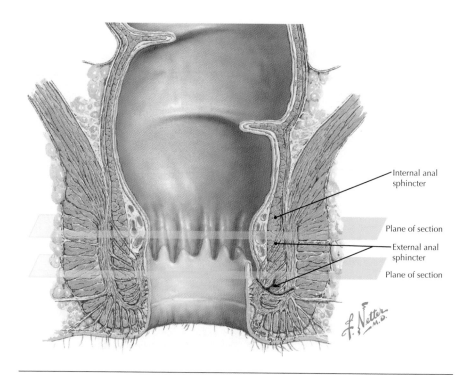

Internal anal sphincter

Plane of section

External anal sphincter

Plane of section

Anal sphincters *(Atlas of Human Anatomy, 6th edition, Plate 371)*

Clinical Note Transrectal ultrasound (TRUS) is used to evaluate patients with fecal incontinence believed to result from structural causes. TRUS is also used for examination of the prostate gland and to guide needle biopsy of the prostate.

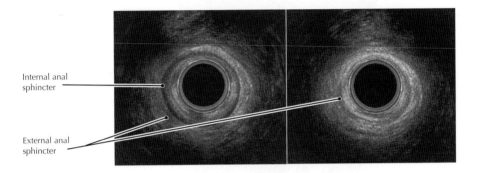

Internal anal
sphincter

External anal
sphincter

Middle and distal TRUS *(From Unger CA, Weinstein MM, Pretorius DH: Pelvic floor imaging. Ultrasound Clin 5:313-330, 2010)*

- The internal anal sphincter is under autonomic (parasympathetic) control, whereas the external anal sphincter is under somatic control.
- The puborectalis muscle, which is part of the levator ani muscle, is instrumental in maintaining continence and is seen in more proximal, endoanal US images than shown here.
- The internal anal sphincter is hypoechoic and does not extend to the distal anal canal, while the external anal sphincter is hyperechoic and does extend distally. This difference in echogenicity correlates with the histologic differences in these muscles (smooth and striated).

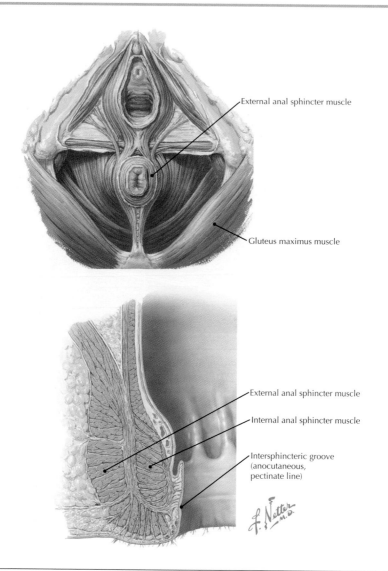

External anal sphincter muscle

Gluteus maximus muscle

External anal sphincter muscle

Internal anal sphincter muscle

Intersphincteric groove (anocutaneous, pectinate line)

f. Netter M.D.

Anal musculature *(Atlas of Human Anatomy, 6th edition, Plates 372 and 373)*

Clinical Note A fistula is an abnormal channel from a hollow body cavity to another surface. An anal fistula opens on the skin near the anus. It may begin with inflammation of the mucous lining of the rectum, perhaps triggered by tuberculosis or Crohn's disease. The area becomes an abscess because it is constantly reinfected by feces; eventually a fistula forms.

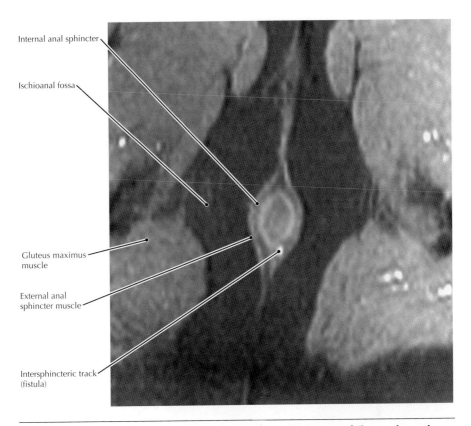

Internal anal sphincter

Ischioanal fossa

Gluteus maximus
muscle

External anal
sphincter muscle

Intersphincteric track
(fistula)

Axial short tau inversion recovery (STIR) sequence MR image of the anal canal
(From Bartram C, Buchanan G: Imaging and fistula. Radiol Clin North Am 41(2):443-457, 2003)

- In this patient, the anal fistula is very limited and does not extend into the ischioanal fossa.

- The external anal sphincter is innervated by the inferior rectal branches of the pudendal (somatic) nerve, and the internal anal sphincter is innervated by pelvic splanchnic nerves (parasympathetic).

- The intersphincteric groove (anocutaneous or pectinate line) marks the junction between the embryologic hindgut (visceral endoderm) and the proctodeum (somatic ectoderm). Thus, whereas inferior to this line the anal canal is sensitive to various somatic sensations (e.g., cutting, temperature), superior to the line the canal is only sensitive to ischemia and stretching.

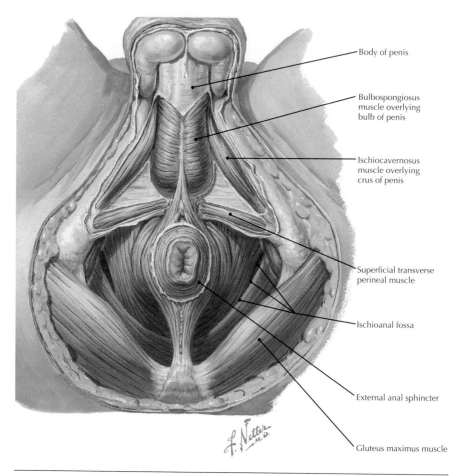

Body of penis

Bulbospongiosus muscle overlying bulb of penis

Ischiocavernosus muscle overlying crus of penis

Superficial transverse perineal muscle

Ischioanal fossa

External anal sphincter

Gluteus maximus muscle

Inferior view of the male perineum *(Atlas of Human Anatomy, 6th edition, Plate 373)*

Clinical Note Peyronie's disease is characterized by the development of hardened tissue (fibrosis) in the penis that causes pain, curvature, and distortion, usually during erection.

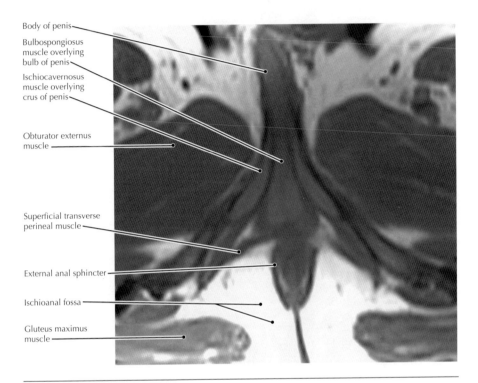

Body of penis

Bulbospongiosus muscle overlying bulb of penis

Ischiocavernosus muscle overlying crus of penis

Obturator externus muscle

Superficial transverse perineal muscle

External anal sphincter

Ischioanal fossa

Gluteus maximus muscle

Axial T1 MR image of the pelvis

- The deep layer of the superficial fascia (Scarpa's) of the abdominal wall attaches laterally to the fascia lata of the thigh and continues into the perineum as its superficial (Colles') fascia, which in turn attaches posteriorly to the perineal membrane. These attachments limit the spread of urine from a ruptured spongy urethra to the perineum and lower abdominal wall.

- The bulbospongiosus muscle in the male assists in the production of an erection by forcing blood into the distal parts of the penis and also acts as a sphincter of the urethra.

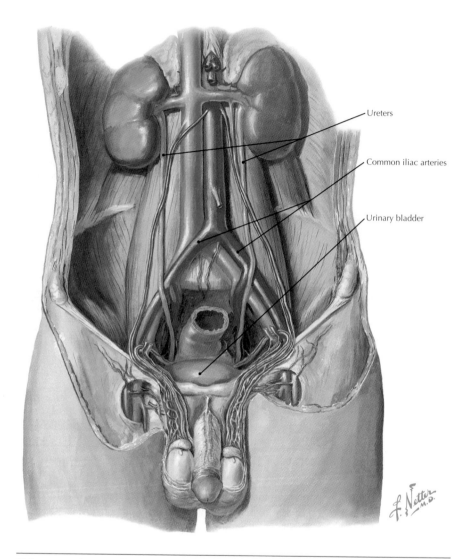

Ureters

Common iliac arteries

Urinary bladder

Kidneys, ureters, and arteries and veins of the testes *(Atlas of Human Anatomy, 6th edition, Plate 379)*

Clinical Note The ureters are highly susceptible to iatrogenic injury during abdominal and pelvic surgery because of their long abdominal and pelvic paths. Such injuries must be corrected as soon as possible to prevent the development of urethral strictures, fistulas, and/or loss of renal function.

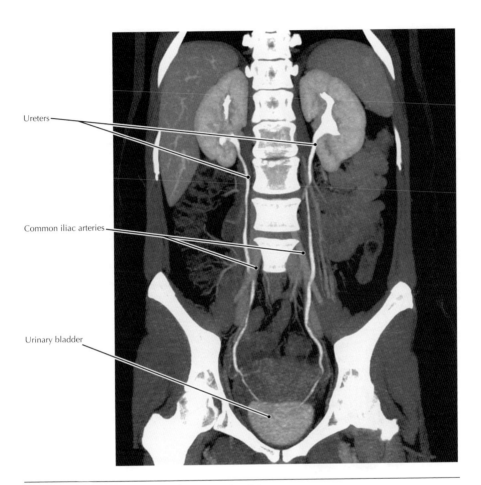

Ureters

Common iliac arteries

Urinary bladder

Coronal MIP, CE CT of the abdomen and pelvis

- The pain from a ureteric calculus (stone) is referred to the cutaneous areas that are associated with the visceral nerves supplying the ureter and changes as the calculus moves. Typically, the pain moves from the "loin to the groin."

- Imaging at any one moment is not likely to show the entire length of both ureters because of peristaltic contractions of these muscular structures that force contrast out of the lumen.

- It is normal for ureters to appear narrow where they cross vessels because their walls can be compressed by mild extrinsic pressure.

Pelvis and Perineum

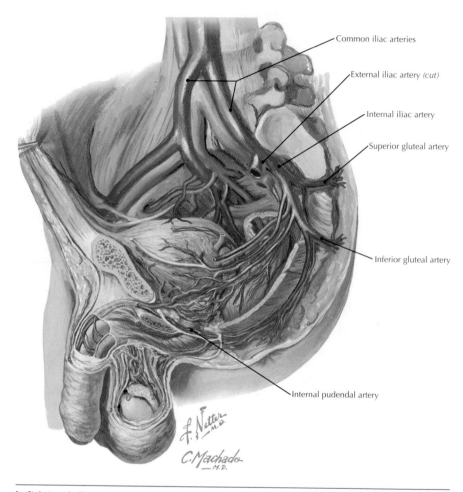

Common iliac arteries

External iliac artery *(cut)*

Internal iliac artery

Superior gluteal artery

Inferior gluteal artery

Internal pudendal artery

Left lateral dissection of the male pelvis *(Atlas of Human Anatomy, 6th edition, Plate 381)*

Clinical Note The superior gluteal artery is at risk of laceration in fractures of the pelvis that involve the greater sciatic notch. An iatrogenic injury can result from procedures in the region of the notch, such as harvesting a bone graft from the ilium.

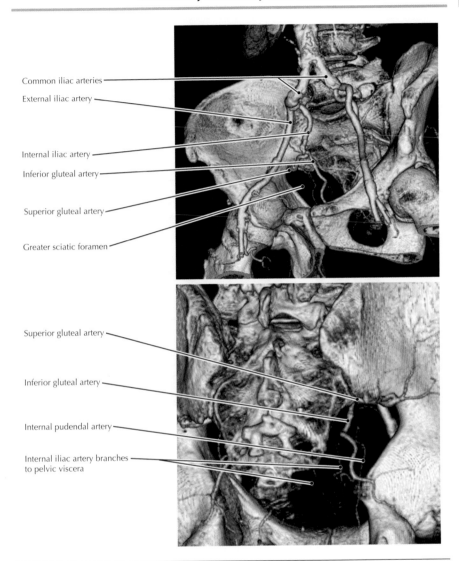

Common iliac arteries

External iliac artery

Internal iliac artery

Inferior gluteal artery

Superior gluteal artery

Greater sciatic foramen

Superior gluteal artery

Inferior gluteal artery

Internal pudendal artery

Internal iliac artery branches
to pelvic viscera

Volume rendered displays, abdominal/pelvic CTA

- Both the superior and inferior gluteal arteries branch from the internal iliac artery within the pelvis and then pass through the greater sciatic foramen to supply the gluteal muscles. They are accompanied by similarly named nerves that innervate the muscles (superior: gluteus medius and minimus; inferior: gluteus maximus).

- The internal pudendal artery is the primary vascular supply of the perineum; in this region the artery has many branches, including the dorsal and deep arteries of the penis or clitoris.

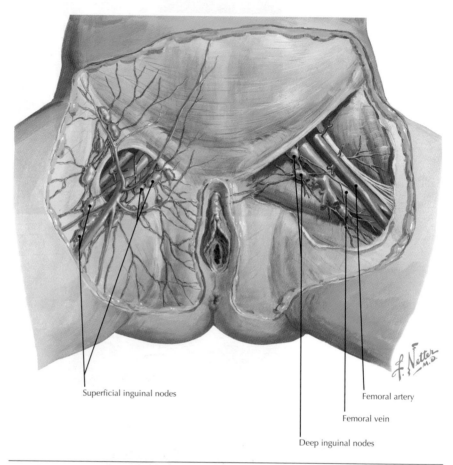

Superficial inguinal nodes

Femoral artery

Femoral vein

Deep inguinal nodes

Superficial and deep inguinal lymph nodes *(Atlas of Human Anatomy, 6th edition, Plate 385)*

Clinical Note Enlargement of the inguinal lymph nodes (adenopathy) can occur as a result of infections or tumors over a wide area: entire lower limb, perineum, trunk inferior to the umbilicus, and the uterus via vessels accompanying the round ligament.

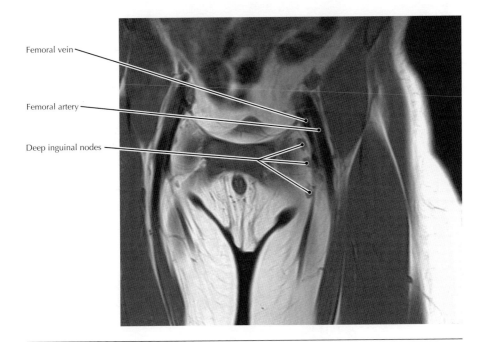

Femoral vein

Femoral artery

Deep inguinal nodes

Coronal T1 MR image of the inguinal region

- Although pathology usually results in lymph node enlargement, even normal-sized nodes can contain malignancy. Newer imaging techniques such as positron emission tomography (PET) scans may be used to identify disease in such nodes.

- Lymph from both the superficial and deep inguinal nodes passes into the pelvis to the iliac nodes and then to the lumbar lymphatic trunks.

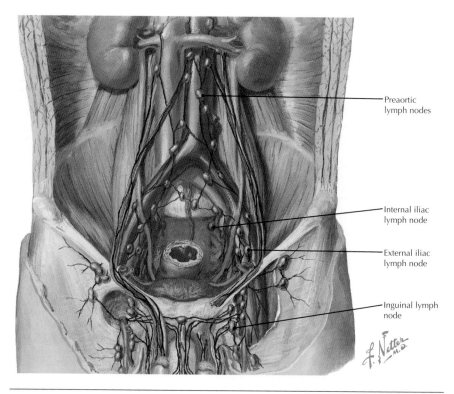

Preaortic
lymph nodes

Internal iliac
lymph node

External iliac
lymph node

Inguinal lymph
node

Lymph nodes *(Atlas of Human Anatomy, 6th edition, Plate 386)*

Clinical Note Tumors in the lymph nodes or damage from radiation treatment can lead to lymphedema in the limb. Because of different lymphatic drainage patterns of gonadal and external genitalia malignancies, tumor staging requires inguinal or preaortic lymph node dissection.

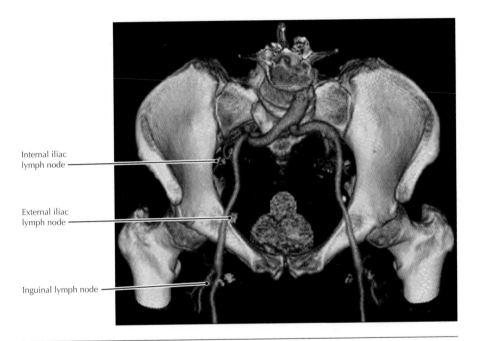

Internal iliac
lymph node

External iliac
lymph node

Inguinal lymph node

MRI-derived lymph node study superimposed on CT data from same patient
(Courtesy Mukesh Harisinghani, MD, Harvard Medical School, Cambridge, Mass.)

- The lymph nodes in the pelvis are in the pathway draining the lower limb.
- Lymphatic drainage from the testes and ovaries goes directly to the preaortic nodes, whereas lymphatic drainage from the external genitalia goes first to inguinal nodes.

Section 6 Upper Limb

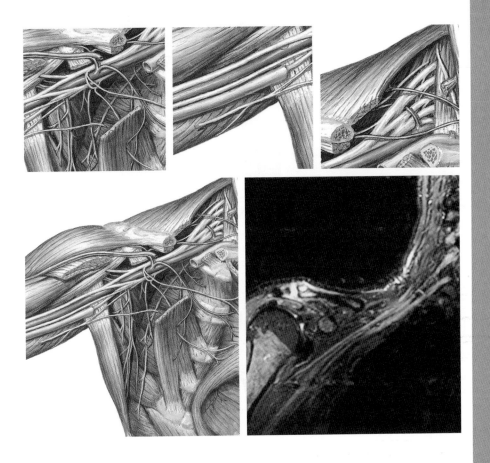

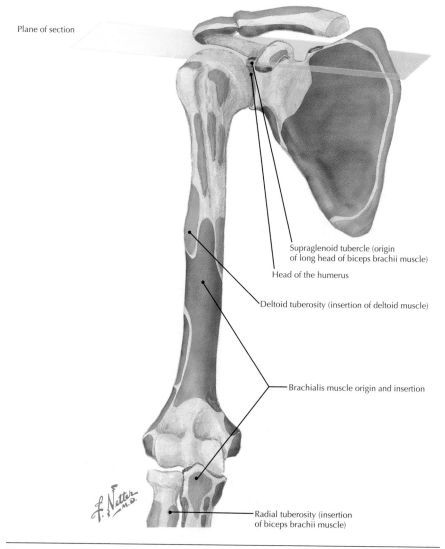

Plane of section

Supraglenoid tubercle (origin of long head of biceps brachii muscle)

Head of the humerus

Deltoid tuberosity (insertion of deltoid muscle)

Brachialis muscle origin and insertion

Radial tuberosity (insertion of biceps brachii muscle)

Muscle origins *(red)*, **insertions** *(blue)* **of the shoulder girdle** *(Atlas of Human Anatomy, 6th edition, Plate 405)*

Clinical Note The glenoid labrum is a fibrocartilaginous ring that surrounds and deepens the glenoid cavity. The long head of the biceps brachii tendon attaches to the top of the labrum at the supraglenoid tubercle (biceps anchor). A superior labrum anterior to posterior (SLAP) tear occurs with overhead activities such as throwing a baseball.

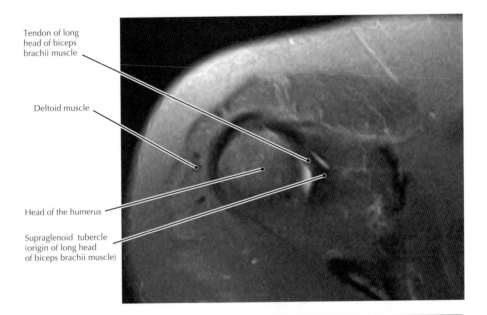

Tendon of long
head of biceps
brachii muscle

Deltoid muscle

Head of the humerus

Supraglenoid tubercle
(origin of long head
of biceps brachii muscle)

Axial FS T1 MR arthrogram of the shoulder

- The tendon of the long head of the biceps brachii muscle, covered by synovial membrane, courses within the fibrous capsule of the glenohumeral joint and is therefore intracapsular but extrasynovial (i.e., outside of the synovial capsule).

- Because of its insertion onto the radial tuberosity, the biceps supinates and flexes the forearm. In contrast, the brachialis is a pure elbow flexor.

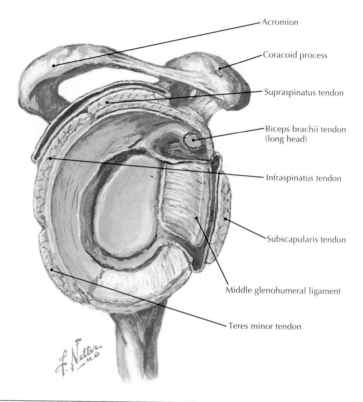

Acromion

Coracoid process

Supraspinatus tendon

Biceps brachii tendon
(long head)

Infraspinatus tendon

Subscapularis tendon

Middle glenohumeral ligament

Teres minor tendon

Lateral view of the glenoid fossa *(Atlas of Human Anatomy, 6th edition, Plate 408)*

Clinical Note Tears of the anterior supraspinatus and superior subscapularis tendons may result in anteromedial dislocation of the tendon of the long head of the biceps brachii.

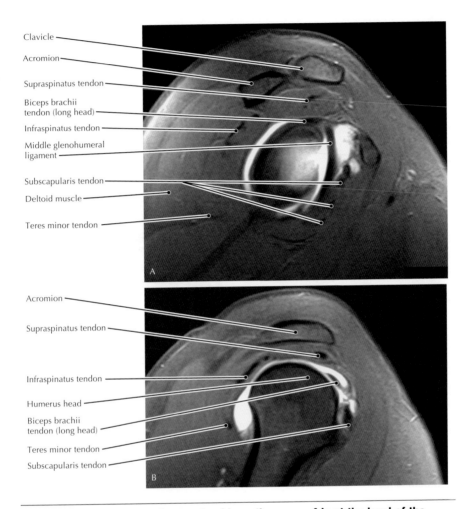

Clavicle

Acromion

Supraspinatus tendon

Biceps brachii tendon (long head)

Infraspinatus tendon

Middle glenohumeral ligament

Subscapularis tendon

Deltoid muscle

Teres minor tendon

Acromion

Supraspinatus tendon

Infraspinatus tendon

Humerus head

Biceps brachii tendon (long head)

Teres minor tendon

Subscapularis tendon

Sagittal FS T1 MR images from a shoulder arthrogram; *A* is at the level of the shoulder joint proper, *B* is more lateral

- In the absence of joint effusion, the intra-articular portion of the long head of the biceps brachii tendon may be difficult to evaluate on routine MRI. However, this tendon is very apparent on an MR arthrogram of the shoulder.

- All of the rotator cuff muscles (supraspinatus, infraspinatus, subscapularis, and teres minor), as well as the long head of the triceps brachii muscle, function to minimize the likelihood of glenohumeral dislocations.

Sternoclavicular Joint

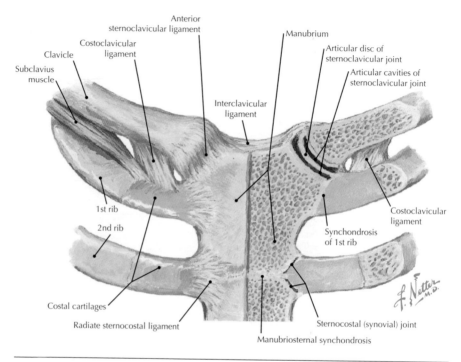

Anterior
sternoclavicular ligament

Costoclavicular
ligament

Clavicle

Subclavius
muscle

Manubrium

Articular disc of
sternoclavicular joint

Articular cavities of
sternoclavicular joint

Interclavicular
ligament

1st rib

2nd rib

Costoclavicular
ligament

Synchondrosis
of 1st rib

Costal cartilages

Radiate sternocostal ligament

Sternocostal (synovial) joint

Manubriosternal synchondrosis

Sternoclavicular joint *(Atlas of Human Anatomy, 6th edition, Plate 404)*

Clinical Note

- The sternoclavicular joint (SCJ) is very strong, so the clavicle often fractures before this joint is dislocated.
- However, a significant force (direct or indirect) to the shoulder can cause a traumatic dislocation of the SCJ.
- The SCJ is subject to a variety of arthritic conditions, usually presenting with pain and swelling due to thickening of periarticular tissues.

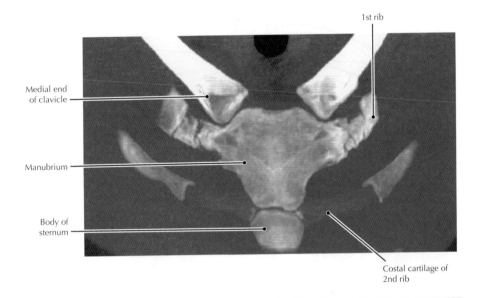

1st rib

Medial end
of clavicle

Manubrium

Body of
sternum

Costal cartilage of
2nd rib

Oblique coronal MIP from chest CT

- The SCJ is a saddle-type joint that enables free movement of the clavicle in nearly all planes. The ability to project the upper limb and shoulder forward requires normal function of this joint.

- The capsule surrounding the SCJ is weakest inferiorly, but it is reinforced on the superior, anterior, and posterior aspects by the interclavicular, anterior and posterior sternoclavicular, and costoclavicular ligaments.

- As shown clearly on the CT scan, less than 50% of the articular surface of the clavicle is actually contained in the bony concavity of the manubrium, and thus it is the capsule and surrounding ligaments that give this joint its stability.

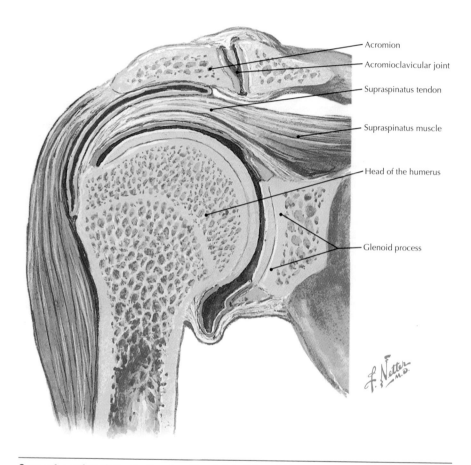

Acromion

Acromioclavicular joint

Supraspinatus tendon

Supraspinatus muscle

Head of the humerus

Glenoid process

Coronal section through the shoulder joint *(Atlas of Human Anatomy, 6th edition, Plate 408)*

Clinical Note The supraspinatus tendon passes through a relatively constrained space between the acromion process and the head of the humerus, and is therefore subject to impingement and subsequent degeneration; such degeneration can lead to rupture.

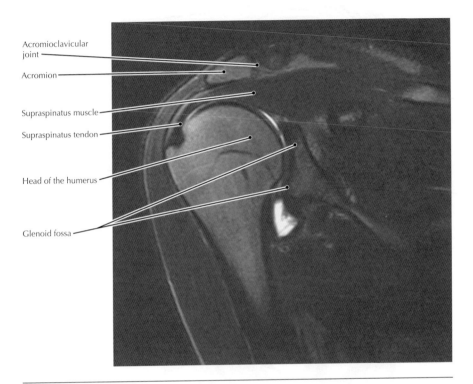

Acromioclavicular joint

Acromion

Supraspinatus muscle

Supraspinatus tendon

Head of the humerus

Glenoid fossa

Oblique coronal MR image of the shoulder

- Note how shallow the glenoid fossa is relative to the humeral head, explaining the ease with which this joint can be dislocated; in most dislocations the humeral head becomes subcoracoid (anterior dislocation).

- Whereas osteoarthritis of the acromioclavicular joint is relatively common, osteoarthritis of the shoulder joint proper (glenohumeral joint) is relatively rare. In osteoarthritis at the acromioclavicular joint, marginal bone spurring may impinge on the supraspinatus tendon.

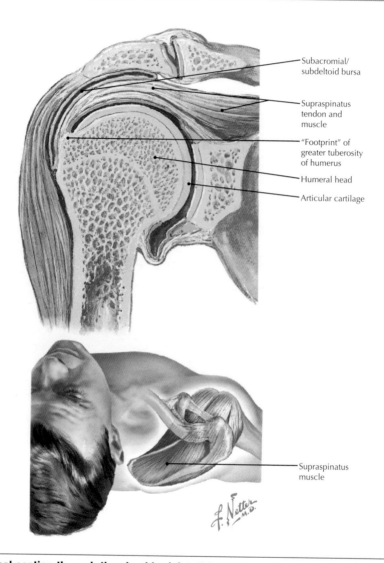

Coronal section through the shoulder joint *(Atlas of Human Anatomy, 6th edition, Plates 408 and 411)*

Clinical Note The most common full-thickness rotator cuff tears involve the supraspinatus tendon. These can be seen on MRI and US. Subacromial/subdeltoid bursitis would result in a sonographically visible fluid collection between the deltoid muscle and the supraspinatus tendon.

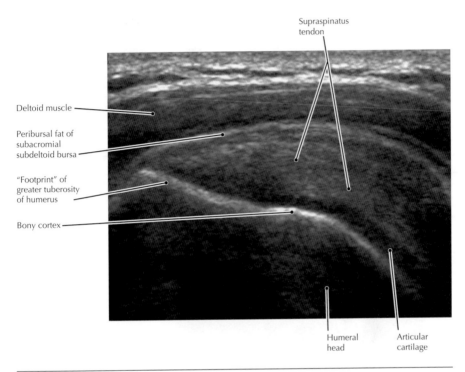

Supraspinatus tendon

Deltoid muscle

Peribursal fat of subacromial subdeltoid bursa

"Footprint" of greater tuberosity of humerus

Bony cortex

Humeral head

Articular cartilage

Oblique coronal ("longitudinal axis") US of distal supraspinatus tendon

- Contraction of the supraspinatus muscle initiates abduction of the arm. The muscle's short lever generates large tensile forces on the tendon; tears of this tendon are common.

- The normal subdeltoid/subacromial bursa is not apparent in the ultrasound image; the thin layers of the bursa are apposed. However, the associated peribursal fat layer is well shown by sonography.

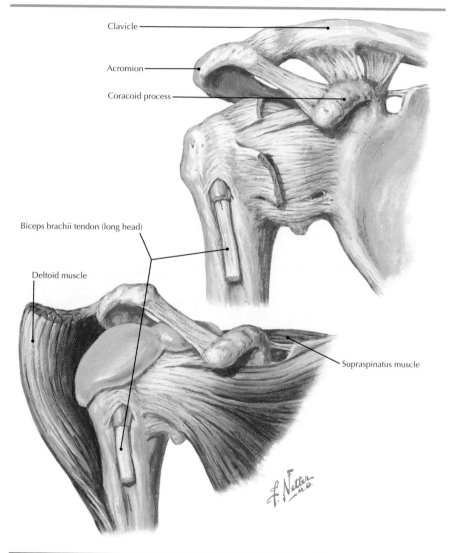

Clavicle

Acromion

Coracoid process

Biceps brachii tendon (long head)

Deltoid muscle

Supraspinatus muscle

The long head of the biceps brachii tendon passing through the shoulder joint capsule *(Atlas of Human Anatomy, 6th edition, Plate 408)*

Clinical Note Inflammation of the long head of the biceps brachii (biceps tendinopathy) is common in sports involving throwing, such as baseball, and is accompanied by shoulder pain. It is rarely seen in isolation. Rather, it occurs with other pathologies of the shoulder such as rotator cuff tendinopathy and tears, shoulder instability, and imbalances in the muscles that stabilize the shoulder.

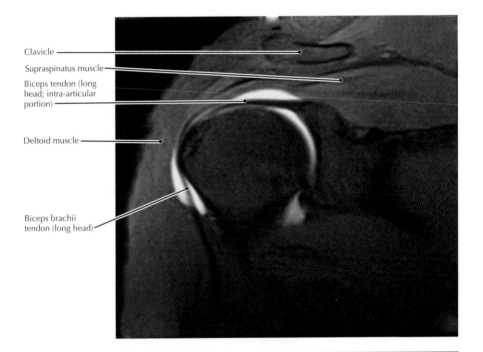

Clavicle

Supraspinatus muscle

Biceps tendon (long
head; intra-articular
portion)

Deltoid muscle

Biceps brachii
tendon (long head)

Coronal FS T1 MR shoulder arthrogram

- The long head of the biceps brachii originates on the supraglenoid tubercle of the
  scapula (biceps anchor). The short head originates from the coracoid process.
  Both heads are innervated by the musculocutaneous nerve.

- Dislocation of the long head of the biceps tendon (anteromedial) or tear of that
  tendon results in an abnormal cranial position of the humeral head and
  impingement of the supraspinatus tendon.

Shoulder Joint, Anterior and Sagittal Views

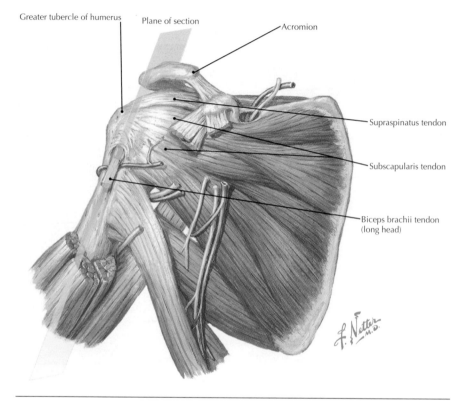

Greater tubercle of humerus

Plane of section

Acromion

Supraspinatus tendon

Subscapularis tendon

Biceps brachii tendon (long head)

Anterior view of the shoulder and axilla *(Atlas of Human Anatomy, 6th edition, Plate 413)*

Clinical Note Avulsion of the lesser tubercle of the humerus occurs infrequently in adolescents due to incomplete fusion of the tubercle to the humerus and may be associated with excessive activity of the subscapularis muscle. Significant disability may occur if this injury is not treated appropriately.

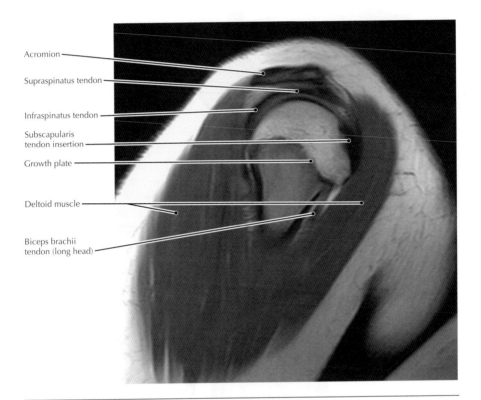

Acromion

Supraspinatus tendon

Infraspinatus tendon

Subscapularis
tendon insertion

Growth plate

Deltoid muscle

Biceps brachii
tendon (long head)

Sagittal FS proton density (PD) MR shoulder arthrogram

- This shoulder MR arthrogram was done on a young patient; note that the growth plate between the epiphysis (humeral head) and diaphysis (humeral shaft) is apparent.

- At the position shown here, the infraspinatus and supraspinatus tendons have fused into a continuous structure forming the cephalad portion of the rotator cuff. This section is just medial to the insertion of this portion of the rotator cuff on the shelf of the greater tuberosity of the humerus.

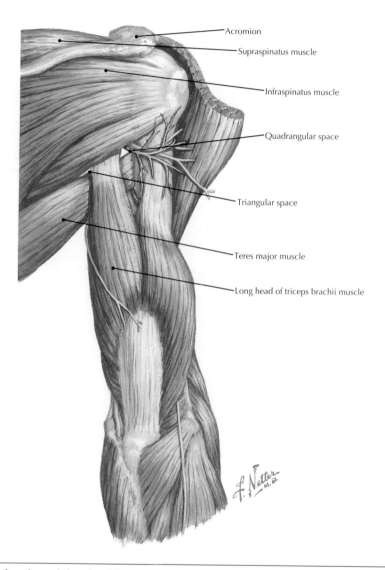

Acromion

Supraspinatus muscle

Infraspinatus muscle

Quadrangular space

Triangular space

Teres major muscle

Long head of triceps brachii muscle

Posterior view of the shoulder and arm *(Atlas of Human Anatomy, 6th edition, Plate 418)*

Clinical Note Compression of the axillary nerve in the quadrangular space is an unusual cause of pain and paresthesia in the upper limb.

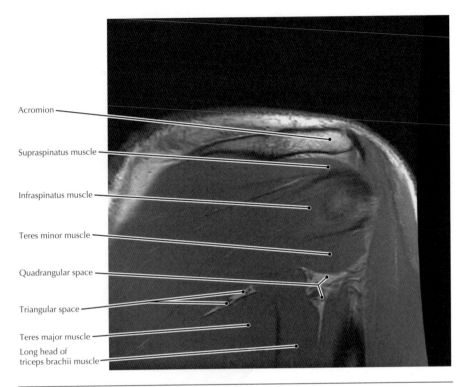

Acromion —

Supraspinatus muscle —

Infraspinatus muscle —

Teres minor muscle —

Quadrangular space —

Triangular space —

Teres major muscle —

Long head of
triceps brachii muscle —

Coronal oblique PD MR image of the shoulder *(From Kassarjian A, Bencardino JT, Palmer WE: MR imaging of the rotator cuff. Radiol Clin North Am 44(4):503-523, 2006)*

- The boundaries of the quadrangular space are the long head of the triceps brachii muscle (medial), shaft of humerus (lateral), teres minor muscle (superior), and teres major muscle (inferior).
- The boundaries of the triangular space are the long head of the triceps brachii (lateral), teres minor muscle (superior), and teres major muscle (inferior).

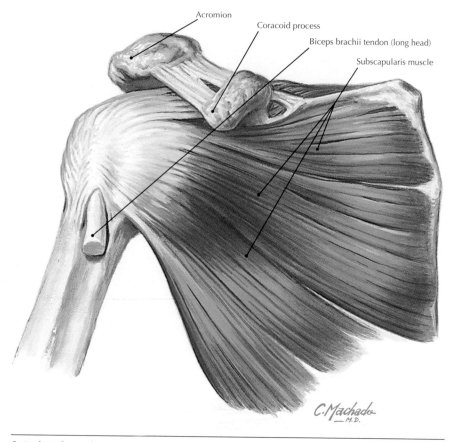

Acromion

Coracoid process

Biceps brachii tendon (long head)

Subscapularis muscle

Anterior view of the subscapularis muscle *(Atlas of Human Anatomy, 6th edition, Plate 411)*

Clinical Note Tears of the subscapularis muscle are less common than tears of the muscles of the more superior aspect of the rotator cuff, and may occur as a result of traumatic or degenerative processes.

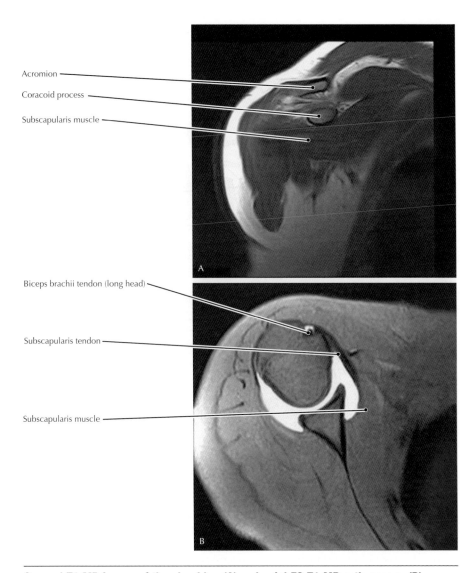

Acromion
Coracoid process
Subscapularis muscle

Biceps brachii tendon (long head)

Subscapularis tendon

Subscapularis muscle

Coronal T1 MR image of the shoulder *(A)* and axial FS T1 MR arthrogram *(B)*

- The subscapularis muscle inserts on the lesser tubercle of the humerus and is the primary medial rotator of the arm.
- Additionally, the subscapularis tendon acts to prevent anterior dislocations of the shoulder joint.

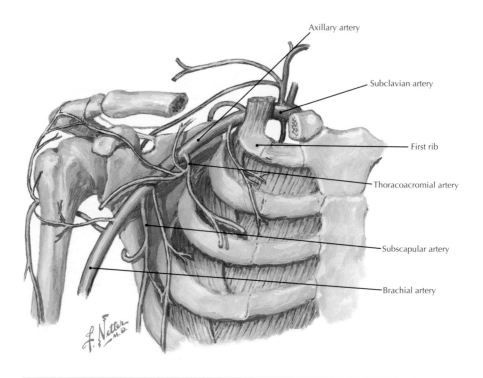

Axillary artery

Subclavian artery

First rib

Thoracoacromial artery

Subscapular artery

Brachial artery

Anterior view of the axilla, demonstrating the axillary artery *(Atlas of Human Anatomy, 6th edition, Plate 414)*

Clinical Note Axillary artery injury may accompany dislocations of the shoulder and fractures of the clavicle. If the axillary artery is damaged, prompt recognition and treatment are necessary to prevent ischemic damage to the involved extremity.

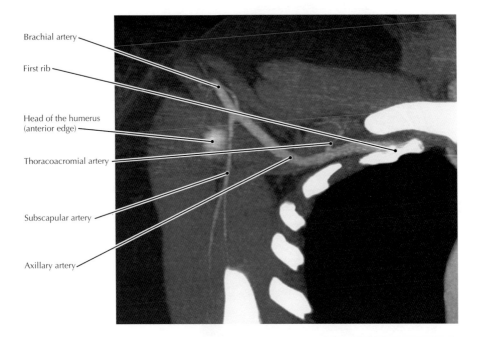

Brachial artery

First rib

Head of the humerus
(anterior edge)

Thoracoacromial artery

Subscapular artery

Axillary artery

Thoracic CTA

- This CT scan was done with arms elevated to optimize image quality in the chest.
- The axillary artery is a continuation of the subclavian after it crosses over the first rib. At the teres major it becomes the brachial artery.
- For descriptive purposes, the axillary artery is divided into three parts: the first part is proximal to the pectoralis minor muscle, the second part is posterior to the pectoralis minor, and the third part is distal to the muscle.

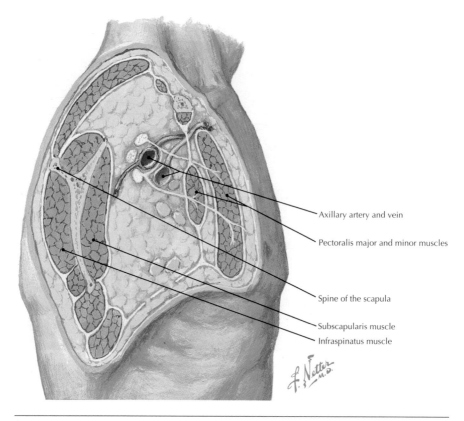

Axillary artery and vein

Pectoralis major and minor muscles

Spine of the scapula

Subscapularis muscle

Infraspinatus muscle

Shoulder and axilla, oblique parasagittal view *(Atlas of Human Anatomy, 6th edition, Plate 412)*

Clinical Note During a regional block of the brachial plexus, the anesthesiologist will frequently aspirate blood from the axillary artery; this serves as a landmark for the cords of the plexus.

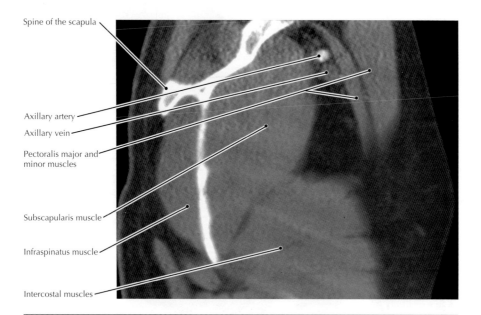

Spine of the scapula

Axillary artery

Axillary vein

Pectoralis major and
minor muscles

Subscapularis muscle

Infraspinatus muscle

Intercostal muscles

Oblique sagittal reconstruction, CT of the chest

- The cords of the brachial plexus are faintly seen surrounding the axillary artery in the CT image.
- Much of the axilla is occupied by fat, which does not stop or scatter many photons and thus has very little CT density (shows up as black on CT imaging).
- The thickness of the subscapularis muscle is exaggerated due to the obliquity of the section.

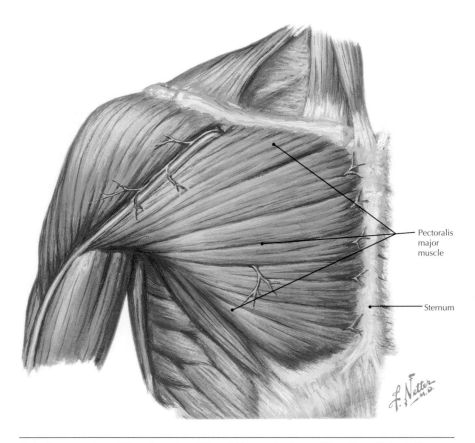

Pectoralis major muscle

Sternum

Anterior muscles of the shoulder *(Atlas of Human Anatomy, 6th edition, Plate 409)*

Clinical Note Poland syndrome is characterized by the unilateral absence of the sternocostal head of the pectoralis major muscle and has an incidence of about 1 per 30,000 live births. Usually there is also webbing of the ipsilateral fingers (cutaneous syndactyly). In females there is unilateral breast hypoplasia.

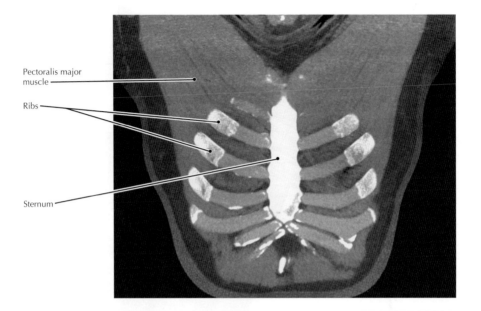

Pectoralis major
muscle

Ribs

Sternum

Curved coronal reconstruction, CT of the chest

- Injuries and deformities of the anterior chest wall are often best depicted by CT images similar to this one.

- The sternocostal head of the pectoralis major muscle is a major extensor of the upper limb and is important in activities such as swimming. The clavicular head, in contrast, can flex the limb.

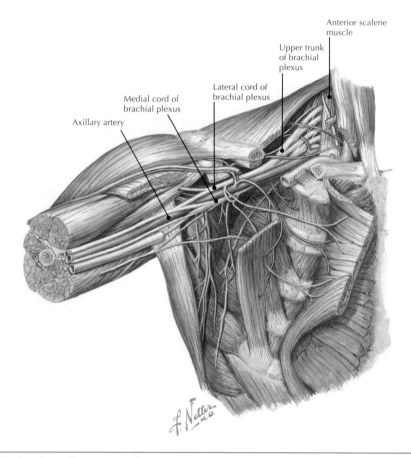

Anterior scalene muscle

Upper trunk of brachial plexus

Lateral cord of brachial plexus

Medial cord of brachial plexus

Axillary artery

Anterior view of structures deep in the axilla, including the brachial plexus *(Atlas of Human Anatomy, 6th edition, Plate 415)*

Clinical Note The brachial plexus courses through the axilla with relatively little protection and therefore is subject to compression, traction, and penetration injuries.

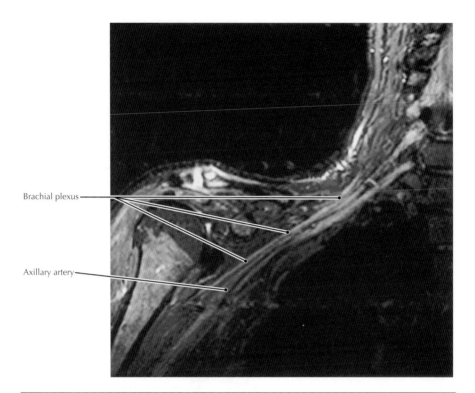

Brachial plexus

Axillary artery

Oblique coronal STIR sequence of the axilla to show the brachial plexus *(From Stone JA: MR myelography of the spine and MR peripheral nerve imaging. Magn Reson Imaging Clin N Am 11(4):543-558, 2003)*

- The axillary artery is surrounded by the cords of the brachial plexus in the axilla.
- Upper lesions of the brachial plexus are known as Erb or Erb-Duchenne palsy and affect the muscles innervated mainly by C5 and C6 ventral rami, which are predominantly in the shoulder. The patient presents with an adducted and medially rotated arm.
- Lower lesions of the brachial plexus are known as Klumpke or Klumpke-Dejerine palsy and affect the muscles innervated mainly by C8 and T1 ventral rami, which are predominantly in the hand. The patient presents with a "claw hand," in which the metacarpophalangeal joints of the fingers are hyperextended and the interphalangeal joints are flexed.

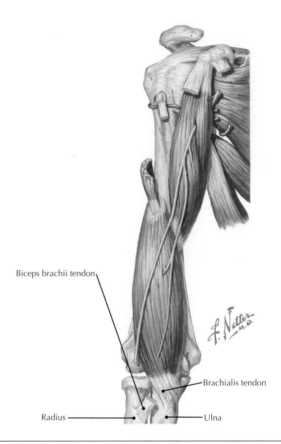

Biceps brachii tendon

Brachialis tendon

Radius

Ulna

Anterior view of the muscles of the arm and proximal forearm *(Atlas of Human Anatomy, 6th edition, Plate 417)*

Clinical Note Ruptures of the proximal and distal tendons of the biceps brachii are more common in patients who are over 50 years old than in younger patients. Ruptures of the long-head tendon occur more commonly than those of the short-head tendon or the distal tendon. Long-head tendon ruptures are often associated with rotator cuff tendinitis, which may cause degeneration that predisposes the tendon to rupture. Repetitive strenuous activity can also lead to ruptures of the long-head tendon.

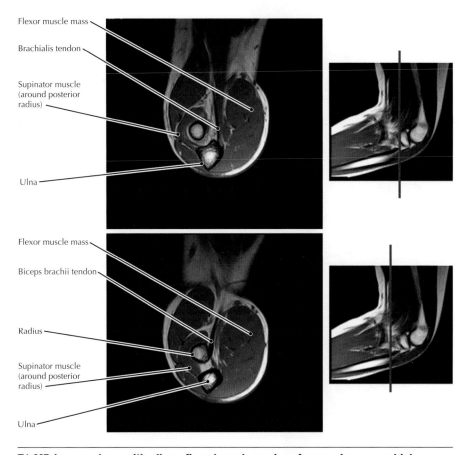

Flexor muscle mass

Brachialis tendon

Supinator muscle
(around posterior
radius)

Ulna

Flexor muscle mass

Biceps brachii tendon

Radius

Supinator muscle
(around posterior
radius)

Ulna

T1 MR images done with elbow flexed as shown in reference images, which illustrate respective planes of section

- The brachialis tendon inserts into the tuberosity of the ulna, and the biceps tendon inserts into the tuberosity of the radius.
- Accordingly, the biceps supinates as it flexes, whereas the brachialis is a pure elbow flexor.

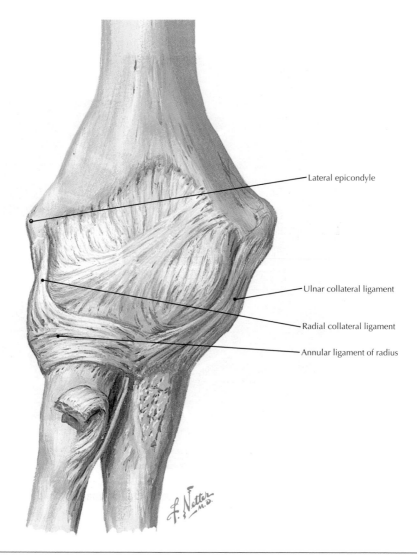

Lateral epicondyle

Ulnar collateral ligament

Radial collateral ligament

Annular ligament of radius

Anterior view of the elbow ligaments (Atlas of Human Anatomy, 6th edition, Plate 424)

Clinical Note Laxity or ruptures of the ulnar or radial collateral ligaments are potential sources of elbow instability.

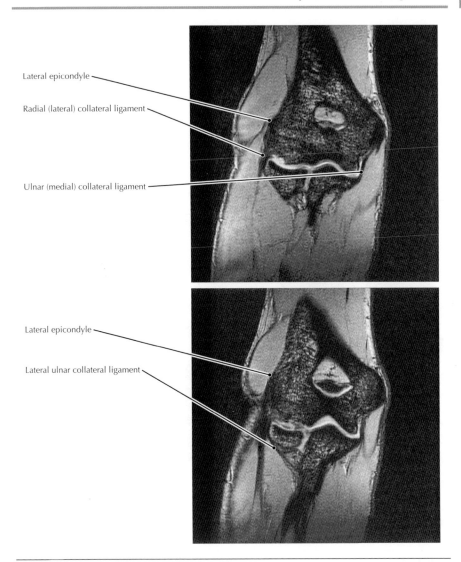

Lateral epicondyle

Radial (lateral) collateral ligament

Ulnar (medial) collateral ligament

Lateral epicondyle

Lateral ulnar collateral ligament

Coronal gradient echo (GRE) MR images of the elbow *(From Kaplan LJ, Potter HG: MR imaging of ligament injuries to the elbow. Radiol Clin North Am 44(4):583-594, 2006)*

- The anterior bundle of the medial collateral ligament is taut in extension and courses from the medial humeral epicondyle to the coronoid process of the ulna, deep to the origin of the pronator teres tendon.
- The lateral ulnar collateral ligament originates on the lateral humeral epicondyle and courses posteriorly around the radial neck to insert on the supinator crest of the ulna.

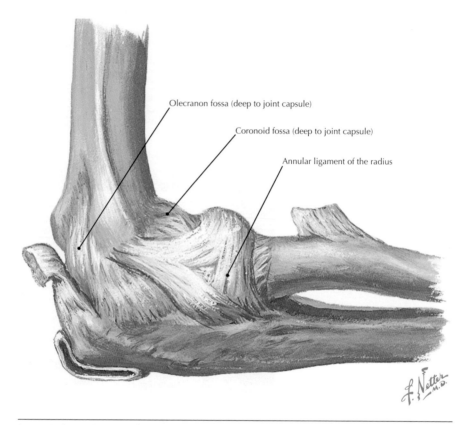

Olecranon fossa (deep to joint capsule)

Coronoid fossa (deep to joint capsule)

Annular ligament of the radius

Lateral view of the elbow *(Atlas of Human Anatomy, 6th edition, Plate 424)*

Clinical Note Young children, especially girls, are vulnerable to transient subluxation of the radial head ("nursemaid's elbow"), which results from a sudden lifting of the limb while pronated. This sudden lifting pulls the head of the radius distal to the annular ligament.

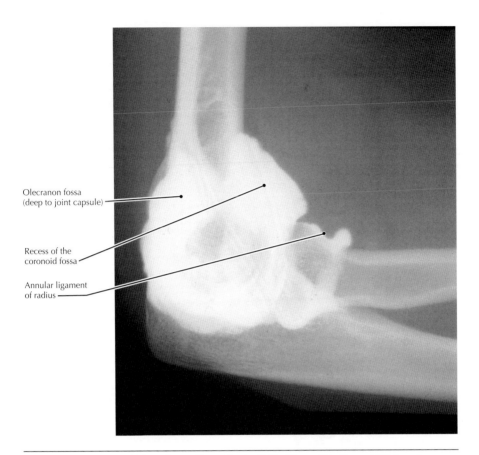

Olecranon fossa
(deep to joint capsule)

Recess of the
coronoid fossa

Annular ligament
of radius

Lateral arthrogram of the elbow *(From Fowler KAB, Chung CB: Normal MR imaging anatomy of the elbow. Radiol Clin North Am 44(4):553-567, 2006)*

- The recess of the coronoid fossa (medial part of the anterior humeral recess) is an anterior pocket within the synovial capsule.
- Note that contrast material within the joint extends distal to the annular ligament.
- Arthrography performed by injecting intra-articular iodinated contrast material followed by CT scanning to produce a CT arthrogram is an alternative modality for patients who cannot undergo MRI because of the presence of, for example, a pacemaker, a spinal stimulator, or an implanted insulin pump.

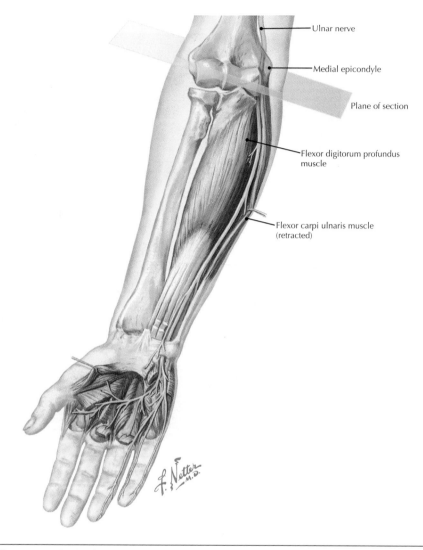

Ulnar nerve

Medial epicondyle

Plane of section

Flexor digitorum profundus muscle

Flexor carpi ulnaris muscle (retracted)

Ulnar nerve in the forearm and hand *(Atlas of Human Anatomy, 6th edition, Plate 464)*

Clinical Note The cubital tunnel is an osseous/fibrous tunnel posterior to the medial epicondyle of the humerus associated with the origin of the flexor carpi ulnaris muscle. It is one of several areas of potential entrapment for the ulnar nerve. Ulnar nerve compression results in loss of intrinsic hand function and paresthesia on the medial aspect of the hand.

Brachioradialis muscle

Radial nerve

Brachialis muscle

Extensor carpi radialis longus muscle

Median nerve

Pronator teres muscle

Medial epicondyle

Olecranon

Ulnar nerve

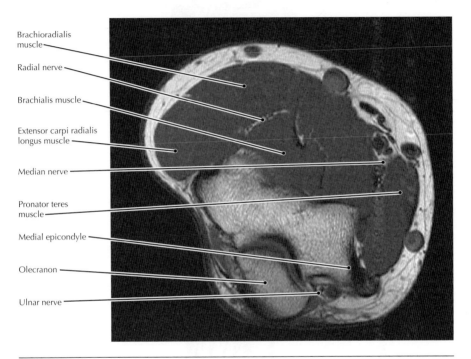

Axial PD MR image through the elbow *(From Hochman MG, Zilberfarb JL: Nerves in a pinch: Imaging of nerve compression syndromes. Radiol Clin North Am 42(1):221-245, 2004)*

- The relatively superficial location of the ulnar nerve posterior to the medial epicondyle results in it being susceptible to externally applied pressure; this can manifest in various paresthesias (i.e., the "funny bone").

- The brachioradialis muscle is innervated by the radial nerve rather than the musculocutaneous nerve, which innervates all the other major forearm flexor muscles.

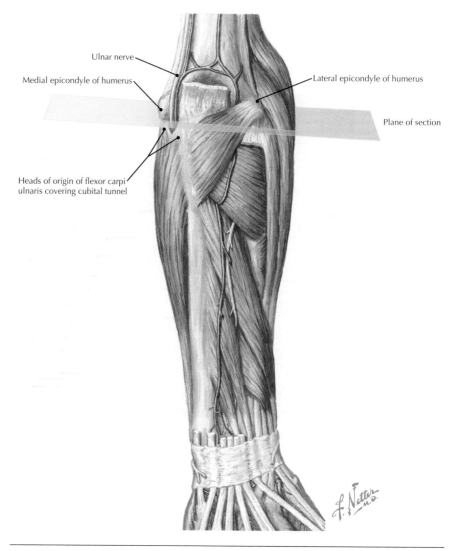

Ulnar nerve

Medial epicondyle of humerus

Lateral epicondyle of humerus

Plane of section

Heads of origin of flexor carpi ulnaris covering cubital tunnel

Posterior view of the elbow and forearm *(Atlas of Human Anatomy, 6th edition, Plate 431)*

Clinical Note The cubital tunnel is a potential site of entrapment of the ulnar nerve, resulting in "cubital tunnel syndrome." Treatment of cubital tunnel syndrome begins with conservative therapy (bracing, exercise) but in severe cases may end with surgical treatments, which include endoscopically performed muscle release, partial removal of the medial epicondyle of the humerus, and transposition of the nerve to anterior of the condyle.

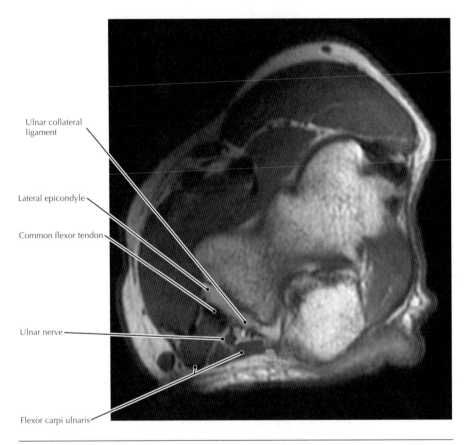

Axial T1 MR image of the cubital tunnel *(From Fowler KAB, Chung CB: Normal MR imaging anatomy of the elbow. Radiol Clin North Am 44(4):553-567, 2006)*

- The floor of the cubital tunnel is composed of the posterior band of the ulnar collateral ligament complex.
- The two heads of the flexor carpi ulnaris arise from the common flexor tendon (curved arrow) and surround the ulnar nerve. The tendinous arch between their origins (Osborne's band, cubital tunnel retinaculum) forms the roof of the tunnel.

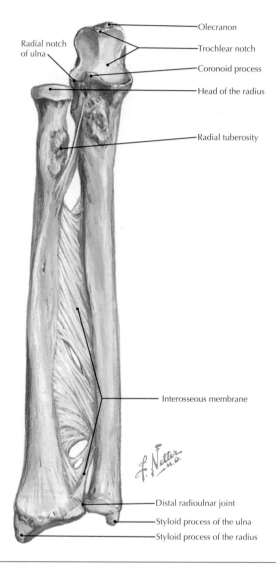

Olecranon

Radial notch of ulna

Trochlear notch

Coronoid process

Head of the radius

Radial tuberosity

Interosseous membrane

Distal radioulnar joint

Styloid process of the ulna

Styloid process of the radius

Radius and ulna with forearm in supination *(Atlas of Human Anatomy, 6th edition, Plate 425)*

Clinical Note A Galeazzi fracture is a fracture of the radial shaft and dislocation of the distal radioulnar joint.

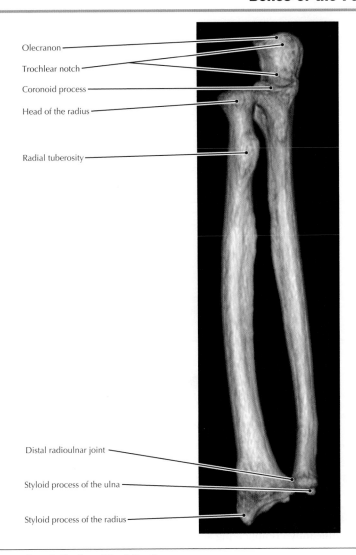

Olecranon

Trochlear notch

Coronoid process

Head of the radius

Radial tuberosity

Distal radioulnar joint

Styloid process of the ulna

Styloid process of the radius

Volume rendered display, CT of the forearm

- The proximal radioulnar joint allows the head of the radius to rotate within a joint formed by the radial notch of the ulna and the annular ligament, whereas at the distal radioulnar joint the radius pivots around the head of the ulna.

- The interosseous membrane forms the middle radioulnar joint, which is a syndesmosis.

- The radius has a larger surface at the wrist, whereas the ulna is larger at the elbow. Forces transmitted through the outstretched hand are more likely to fracture the radius than the ulna.

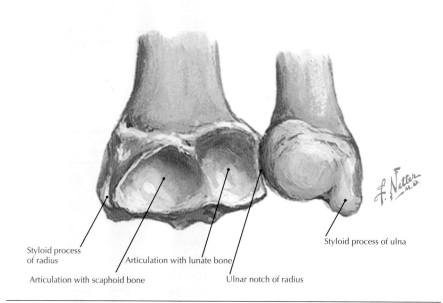

Styloid process
of radius

Articulation with lunate bone

Articulation with scaphoid bone

Ulnar notch of radius

Styloid process of ulna

Distal ends of the radius and ulna *(Atlas of Human Anatomy, 6th edition, Plate 425)*

Clinical Note Fractures at the wrist can involve the articular surface of the radius, significantly complicating surgical repair of the fracture.

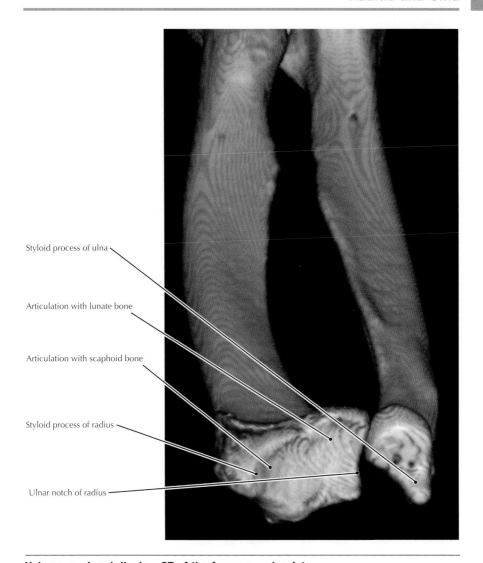

Styloid process of ulna

Articulation with lunate bone

Articulation with scaphoid bone

Styloid process of radius

Ulnar notch of radius

Volume rendered display, CT of the forearm and wrist

- The distal end of the radius articulates with the scaphoid, the lunate, and (when the hand is ulnarly deviated) the triquetrum; the ulna does not directly articulate with any of the carpal bones.
- Fractures of the distal radius (Colles' fracture) are relatively common because they typically result from a fall on an outstretched hand.
- Demonstrating the extent and severity of articular surface fractures is greatly enhanced by volume rendered CT displays.

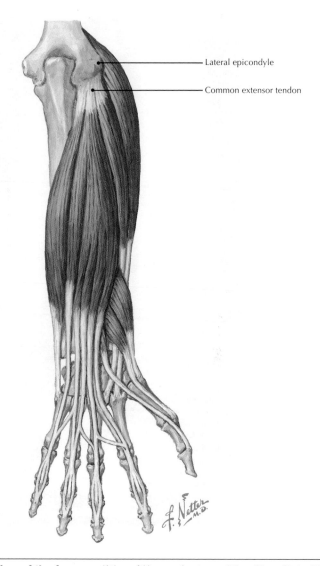

Lateral epicondyle

Common extensor tendon

Posterior view of the forearm *(Atlas of Human Anatomy, 6th edition, Plate 427)*

Clinical Note Chronic pain from the common extensor tendon is called "tennis elbow" (lateral epicondylitis) because it can result from tendon degeneration (inflammation) associated with the use of the backhand swing in tennis. Normal activities and a poor blood supply often hinder healing; surgical intervention is thus sometimes required.

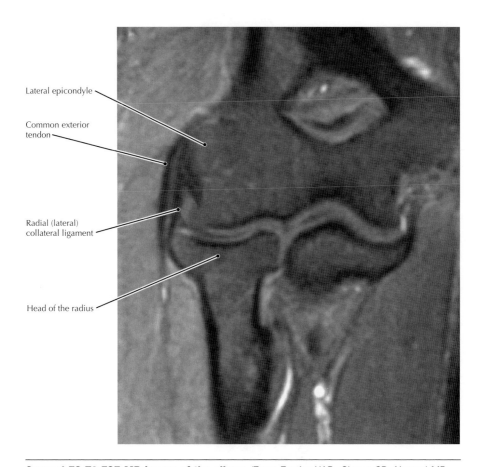

Lateral epicondyle

Common exterior tendon

Radial (lateral) collateral ligament

Head of the radius

Coronal FS T2 FSE MR image of the elbow *(From Fowler KAB, Chung CB: Normal MR imaging anatomy of the elbow. Radiol Clin North Am 44(4):553-567, 2006)*

- The common extensor tendon is composed of the origins of the extensor carpi radialis brevis, extensor digitorum, extensor digiti minimi, and extensor carpi ulnaris.

- The earliest changes associated with lateral epicondylitis (tennis elbow) are found in the more superficial part of the common extensor tendon, associated with the extensor carpi radialis brevis muscle.

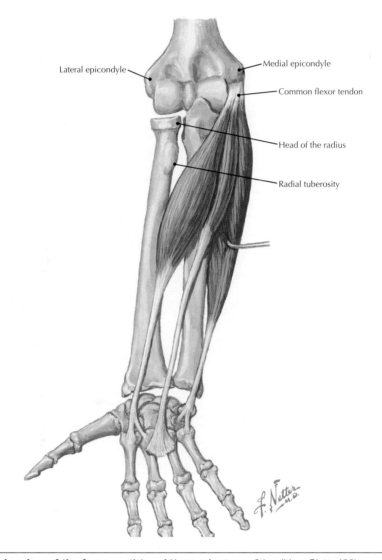

Lateral epicondyle

Medial epicondyle

Common flexor tendon

Head of the radius

Radial tuberosity

Anterior view of the forearm *(Atlas of Human Anatomy, 6th edition, Plate 428)*

Clinical Note Pain from the common flexor tendon is medial epicondylitis, often called "golfer's elbow." Medial epicondylitis is very similar to tennis elbow but on the opposite side of the elbow. It is primarily a degenerative condition affecting the tendon of origin of the wrist and superficial digital flexor muscles from the medial epicondyle of the humerus.

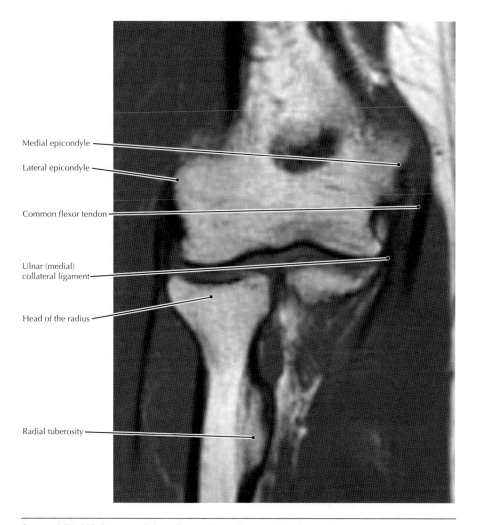

Medial epicondyle

Lateral epicondyle

Common flexor tendon

Ulnar (medial) collateral ligament

Head of the radius

Radial tuberosity

Coronal T1 MR image of the elbow *(From Fowler KAB, Chung CB: Normal MR imaging anatomy of the elbow. Radiol Clin North Am 44(4):553-567, 2006)*

- Tendinosis (degenerative changes in tendons) may be demonstrated by thickenings and increased signal within the common flexor and extensor tendons.
- In prescribing an MR protocol for a specific patient, coronal sequences may be emphasized if the clinical differential diagnosis includes golfer's or tennis elbow.

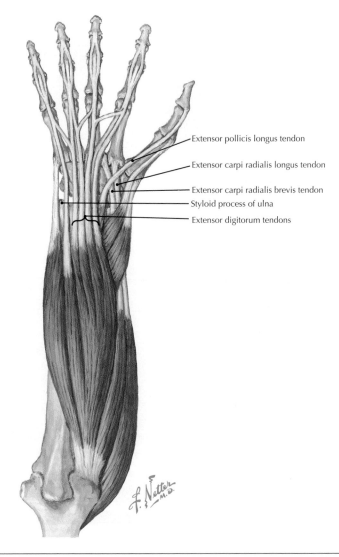

Extensor pollicis longus tendon

Extensor carpi radialis longus tendon

Extensor carpi radialis brevis tendon

Styloid process of ulna

Extensor digitorum tendons

Left forearm muscles, dorsal view *(Atlas of Human Anatomy, 6th edition, Plate 427)*

Clinical Note   All the extensors of the wrist are innervated by the posterior interosseous nerve, which is a terminal branch of the radial nerve. Thus, a midhumeral fracture that lacerates the radial nerve as it traverses the posterior surface of the humerus will result in an inability to extend the wrist, which is referred to as "wrist drop."

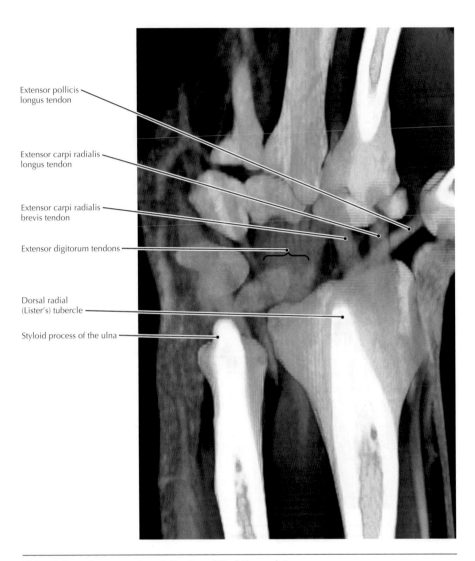

Extensor pollicis longus tendon

Extensor carpi radialis longus tendon

Extensor carpi radialis brevis tendon

Extensor digitorum tendons

Dorsal radial (Lister's) tubercle

Styloid process of the ulna

Thin slab, volume rendered display, CT of the wrist

- The extensor pollicis longus muscle uses the dorsal radial (Lister's) tubercle as a pulley to change its direction of pull.

- As the tendon of the extensor pollicis longus muscle wraps around the tubercle, it is subject to high frictional forces that may cause it to fray or rupture producing a condition known as "drummer's palsy."

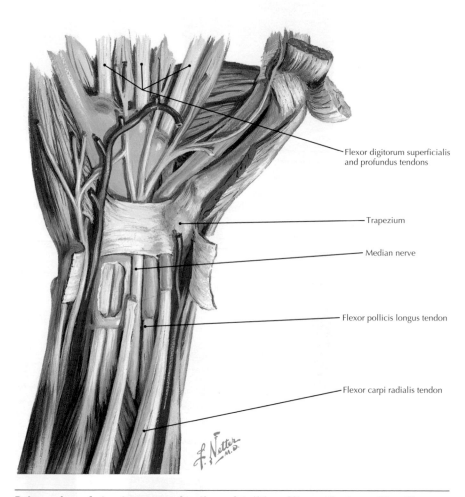

Flexor digitorum superficialis and profundus tendons

Trapezium

Median nerve

Flexor pollicis longus tendon

Flexor carpi radialis tendon

Palmar view of structures crossing the wrist *(Atlas of Human Anatomy, 6th edition, Plate 449)*

Clinical Note Nine tendons pass through the carpal tunnel, surrounded by synovial sheaths. Tenosynovitis of these sheaths can cause carpal tunnel syndrome.

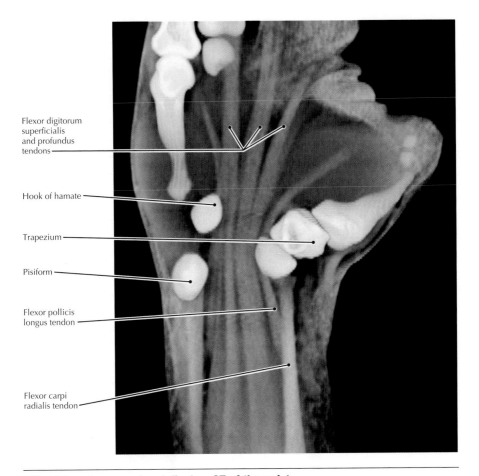

Flexor digitorum
superficialis
and profundus
tendons

Hook of hamate

Trapezium

Pisiform

Flexor pollicis
longus tendon

Flexor carpi
radialis tendon

Thin slab, volume rendered display, CT of the wrist

- Coronal view of the wrist demonstrating tendons passing through the carpal tunnel. The median nerve is palmar to the plane of this image; this nerve is the most superficial structure passing through the carpal tunnel.

- The carpometacarpal joint of the thumb (between the trapezium and the first metacarpal) is the most movable joint of the thumb; it is a saddle-shaped joint that permits opposition of the thumb with the fingers. It is also the hand joint that is most frequently affected by osteoarthritis.

Carpal Bones

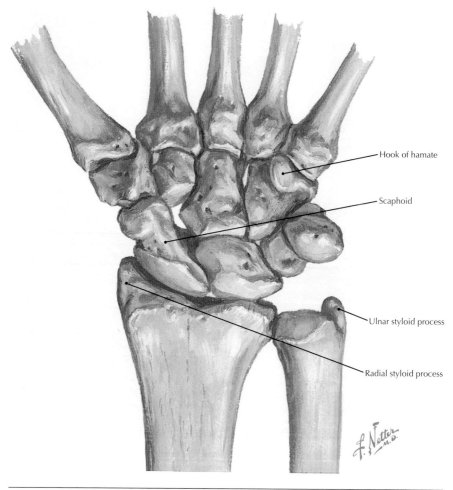

Hook of hamate

Scaphoid

Ulnar styloid process

Radial styloid process

Palmar view of the bones of the wrist *(Atlas of Human Anatomy, 6th edition, Plate 439)*

Clinical Note The hook of the hamate is easily fractured. This injury is most commonly associated with golf ("golfer's wrist"). The fracture is usually a hairline fracture that may be missed on plain radiographs. Symptoms are pain aggravated by gripping and tenderness over the hamate.

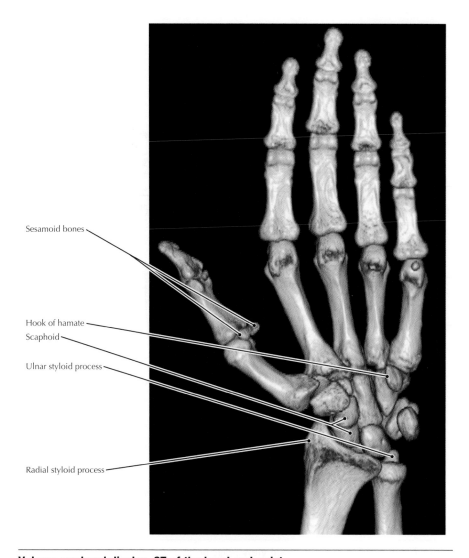

Sesamoid bones

Hook of hamate
Scaphoid

Ulnar styloid process

Radial styloid process

Volume rendered display, CT of the hand and wrist

- The carpal bones are not arranged in two flat rows, but rather form a curved "floor" of the carpal tunnel.

- The sesamoid bones in the tendons of the flexor pollicis brevis can be mistaken for fracture fragments.

- The styloid process of the radius extends further distally than that of the ulna, limiting radial deviation of the hand, relative to ulnar deviation.

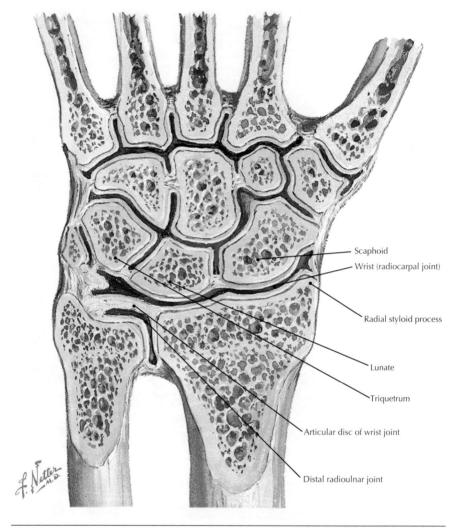

Scaphoid

Wrist (radiocarpal joint)

Radial styloid process

Lunate

Triquetrum

Articular disc of wrist joint

Distal radioulnar joint

Coronal section of the wrist, dorsal view *(Atlas of Human Anatomy, 6th edition, Plate 442)*

Clinical Note The scaphoid is the most frequently fractured carpal bone, often resulting from a fall on the palm with an abducted hand. Pain is felt in the anatomical snuff-box. Because the blood supply to the scaphoid enters the bone distally, midscaphoid lesions may result in avascular necrosis of the proximal segment.

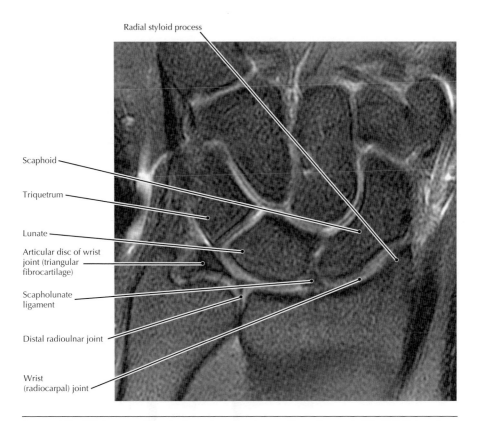

Radial styloid process

Scaphoid

Triquetrum

Lunate

Articular disc of wrist
joint (triangular
fibrocartilage)

Scapholunate
ligament

Distal radioulnar joint

Wrist
(radiocarpal) joint

Coronal T2 MR image of intrinsic wrist structures *(From Ramnath RR: 3T MR imaging of the musculoskeletal system (part II): Clinical applications. Magn Reson Imaging Clin N Am 14(1):41-62, 2006)*

- An intact triangular fibrocartilage complex (TFCC) separates the joint compartments of the radiocarpal joint from the distal radioulnar joint. Therefore when, after an injection of contrast material into one of those compartments, the material appears in the other compartment, the TFCC must be perforated.

- When the scapholunate ligament is torn, plain radiographs may demonstrate a widening of the space between the scaphoid and lunate bones.

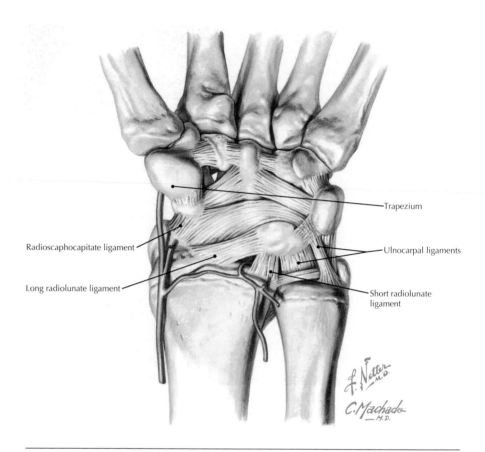

Radioscaphocapitate ligament

Long radiolunate ligament

Trapezium

Ulnocarpal ligaments

Short radiolunate ligament

Ligaments of the palmar wrist *(Atlas of Human Anatomy, 6th edition, Plate 441)*

Clinical Note   The palmar ligaments provide relatively little support for the lunate on the palmar side of the wrist. Thus, when it dislocates, it typically moves in a palmar direction, causing carpal tunnel compression.

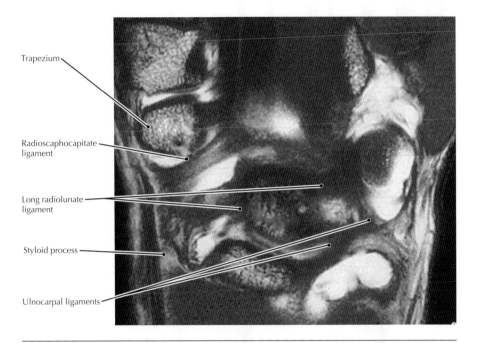

Trapezium

Radioscaphocapitate
ligament

Long radiolunate
ligament

Styloid process

Ulnocarpal ligaments

Coronal MR wrist arthrogram *(From Zlatkin MB, Rosner J: MR imaging of ligaments and triangular fibrocartilage complex of the wrist. Magn Reson Imaging Clin N Am 12(2): 301-331, 2004)*

- Functionally, the palmar carpal ligaments are more important for supporting the integrity of the carpal joints than the dorsal ligaments.
- The radioscaphocapitate ligament creates a strong connection between the radius and the distal carpal row. The radiolunatotriquetral ligament stabilizes the proximal carpal row in relation to the radius.

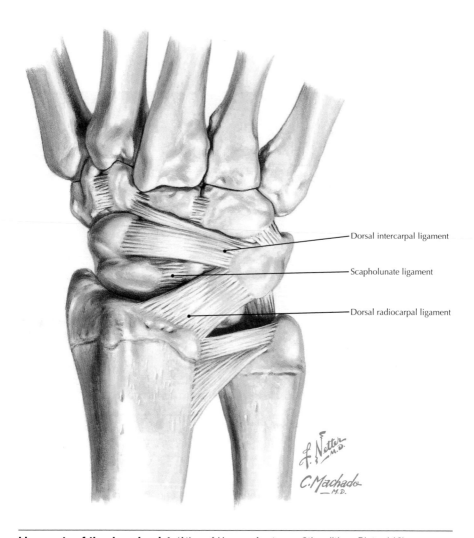

Dorsal intercarpal ligament

Scapholunate ligament

Dorsal radiocarpal ligament

Ligaments of the dorsal wrist *(Atlas of Human Anatomy, 6th edition, Plate 442)*

Clinical Note The dorsal ligaments are less important structurally than the palmar ligaments. However, the dorsal radiocarpal ligament is considered important for stability of the carpal bones during motion.

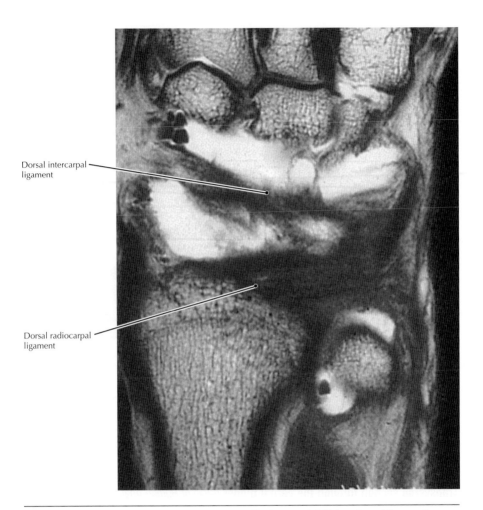

Dorsal intercarpal ligament

Dorsal radiocarpal ligament

Coronal wrist MR arthrogram *(From Zlatkin MB, Rosner J: MR imaging of ligaments and triangular fibrocartilage complex of the wrist. Magn Reson Imaging Clin N Am 12(2): 301-331, 2004)*

- The dorsal radiocarpal ligament originates on the radial styloid process and inserts onto the lunate and triquetrum (there is variability in this structure; the most consistent portion is a radiotriquetral ligament).

- The dorsal intercarpal ligament originates on the triquetrum and extends radially, attaching onto the lunate, the dorsal groove of the scaphoid, and the trapezium.

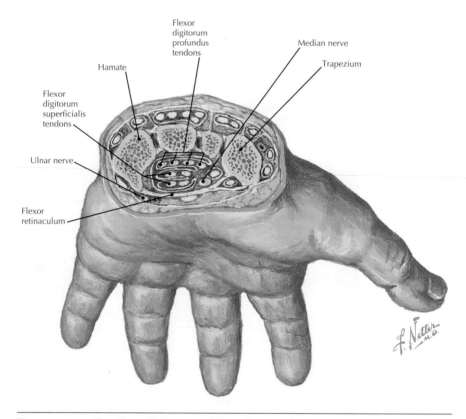

Flexor
digitorum
profundus
tendons

Median nerve

Hamate

Trapezium

Flexor
digitorum
superficialis
tendons

Ulnar nerve

Flexor
retinaculum

Transverse section through the carpal tunnel *(Atlas of Human Anatomy, 6th edition, Plate 449)*

Clinical Note The ulnar nerve does not run within the carpal tunnel (as does the median nerve), so carpal tunnel syndrome does not affect the function of the ulnar nerve.

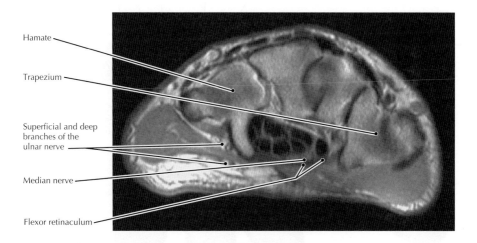

Hamate

Trapezium

Superficial and deep
branches of the
ulnar nerve

Median nerve

Flexor retinaculum

Axial T1 MR image through the carpal tunnel *(From Hochman MG, Zilberfarb JL: Nerves in a pinch: Imaging of nerve compression syndromes. Radiol Clin North Am 42(1):221-245, 2004)*

- The median nerve is seen as a flat ovoid structure immediately deep to the flexor retinaculum. Small, rounded nerve fascicles, uniform in size, can be seen within the nerve.
- The deep and superficial flexor tendons have a low signal and are closely packed.
- The flexor retinaculum may be surgically transected to relieve excessive pressure on the median nerve within the carpal tunnel.

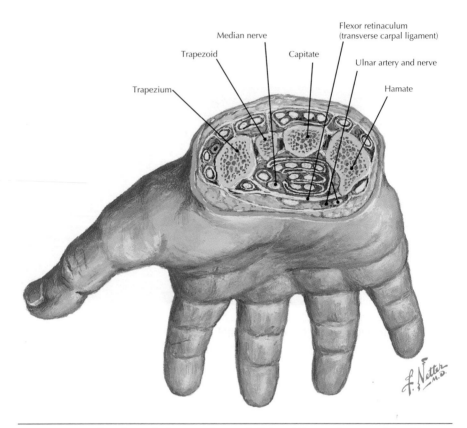

Median nerve

Trapezoid

Trapezium

Capitate

Flexor retinaculum
(transverse carpal ligament)

Ulnar artery and nerve

Hamate

Transverse section through the carpal tunnel *(Atlas of Human Anatomy, 6th edition, Plate 449)*

Clinical Note Any pathology that expands the contents of the tunnel (e.g., tenosynovitis) or diminishes space within the tunnel (e.g., anterior dislocation of a carpal bone) will compress the enclosed median nerve (carpal tunnel syndrome).

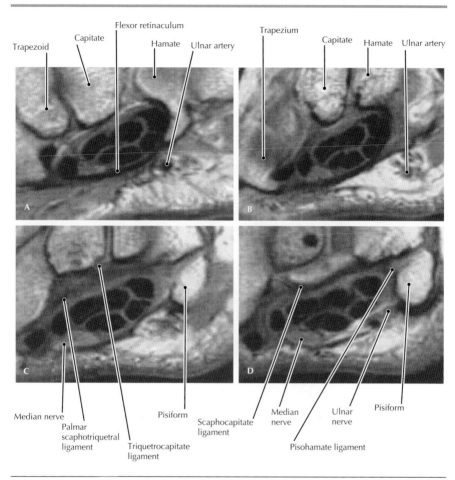

Axial MR images of the carpal tunnel and Guyon's canal (**A** most distal, **D** most proximal) *(From Yu JS, Habib PA: Normal MR imaging anatomy of the wrist and hand. Radiol Clin North Am 44(4):569-581, 2006)*

- The hook of the hamate forms the medial border of the carpal tunnel.
- The median nerve is distinct in MR images of the carpal tunnel as a structure with a higher-intensity signal than the surrounding tendons.
- Guyon's canal (ulnar canal) is a potential space at the wrist between the pisiform and hamate bones through which the ulnar artery and nerve pass into the hand. It is converted into a tunnel by the palmar carpal ligaments (ventrally) and the pisohamate ligament (dorsally). Compression of the ulnar nerve within this space results in a paresthesia in the ring and little fingers. This may be followed by decreased sensation and eventual weakness and clumsiness in the hand as the intrinsic muscles of the hand become involved.

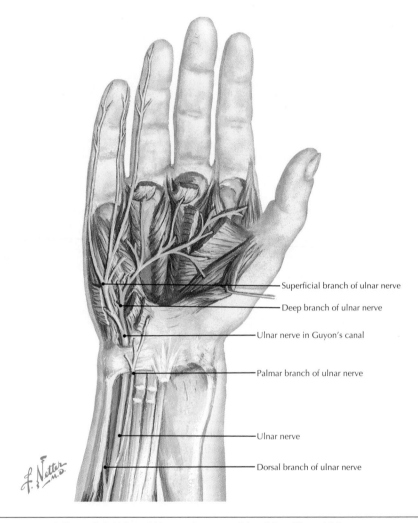

Superficial branch of ulnar nerve

Deep branch of ulnar nerve

Ulnar nerve in Guyon's canal

Palmar branch of ulnar nerve

Ulnar nerve

Dorsal branch of ulnar nerve

Ulnar nerve at the wrist *(Atlas of Human Anatomy, 6th edition, Plate 464)*

Clinical Note The ulnar nerve can be damaged within Guyon's canal. If sensation is intact from the palmar or dorsal branches of the nerve, which are both cutaneous nerves, a lesion proximal to the canal can be ruled out.

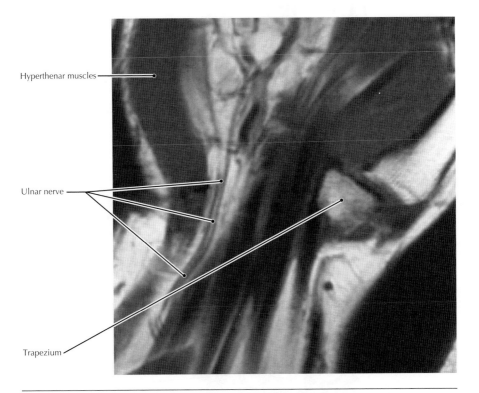

Hyperthenar muscles

Ulnar nerve

Trapezium

Coronal T1 MR image of the ulnar nerve as it travels within Guyon's canal *(From Bordalo-Rodrigues M, Amin P, Rosenberg ZS: MR imaging of common entrapment neuropathies at the wrist. Magn Reson Imaging Clin N Am 12(2):265-279, 2004)*

- The ulnar nerve and artery cross the wrist in a compartment that is separate from the carpal tunnel.
- Within the hand, the ulnar nerve divides into superficial and deep branches, which supply most of the intrinsic muscles of the hand.

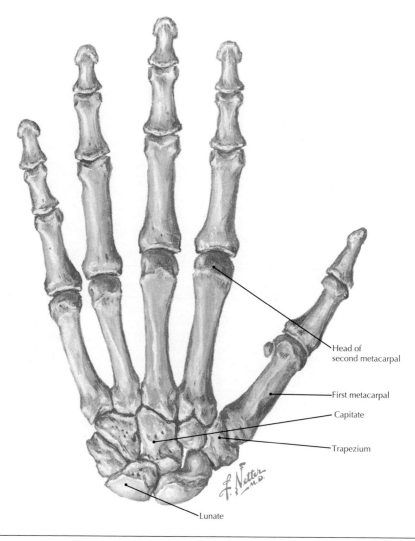

Head of
second metacarpal

First metacarpal

Capitate

Trapezium

Lunate

Dorsal view of the bones of the hand and wrist *(Atlas of Human Anatomy, 6th edition, Plate 443)*

Clinical Note   The capitate is typically well protected by its central location within the wrist, but severe hyperextension can result in fracture of both the scaphoid and capitate (Fenton syndrome).

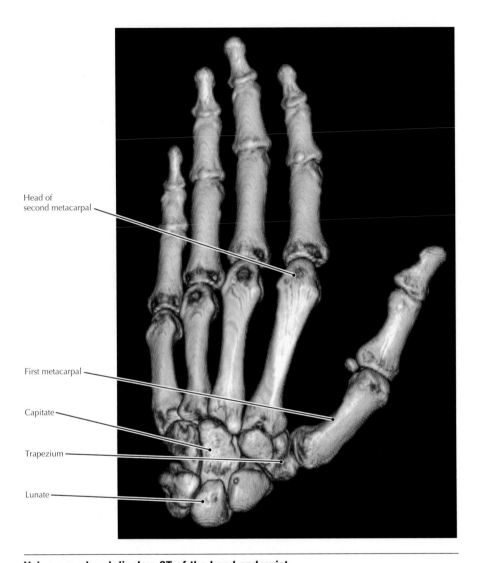

Head of
second metacarpal

First metacarpal

Capitate

Trapezium

Lunate

Volume rendered display, CT of the hand and wrist

- The joint between the trapezium and the first metacarpal is a special configuration referred to as a saddle joint. This joint allows for a wide range of motion, including opposition of the thumb.
- When the metacarpophalangeal joints are flexed, the heads of the metacarpals form the knuckles.

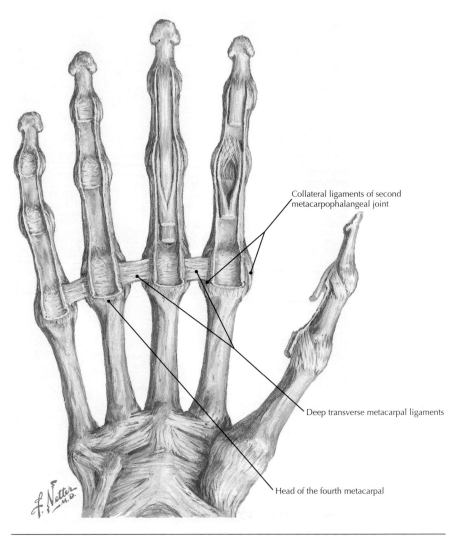

Collateral ligaments of second metacarpophalangeal joint

Deep transverse metacarpal ligaments

Head of the fourth metacarpal

Anterior view of the hand bones and ligaments *(Atlas of Human Anatomy, 6th edition, Plate 445)*

Clinical Note Dorsal dislocations of metacarpophalangeal joints, most commonly of the index finger, are divided into simple and complex, according to whether or not they can be reduced by a closed technique.

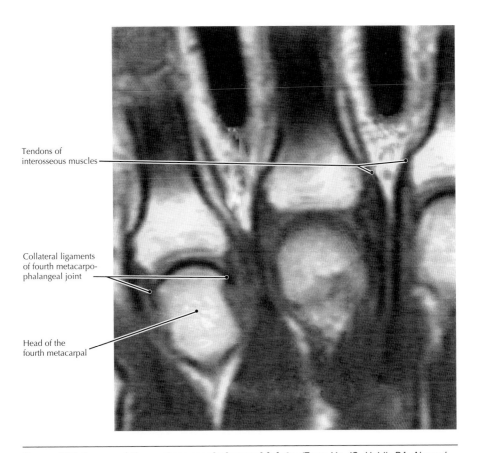

Tendons of
interosseous muscles

Collateral ligaments
of fourth metacarpo-
phalangeal joint

Head of the
fourth metacarpal

Coronal T1 image of the metacarpophalangeal joints *(From Yu JS, Habib PA: Normal MR imaging anatomy of the wrist and hand. Radiol Clin North Am 44(4):569-581, 2006)*

- Tendons of interosseous muscles primarily adduct and abduct the digits.

- This image is at a deep coronal plane so the deep transverse metacarpal ligaments do not appear.

- Tears of the ulnar collateral ligament of the first metacarpophalangeal joint are fairly common and can be demonstrated by MRI ("gamekeeper's thumb").

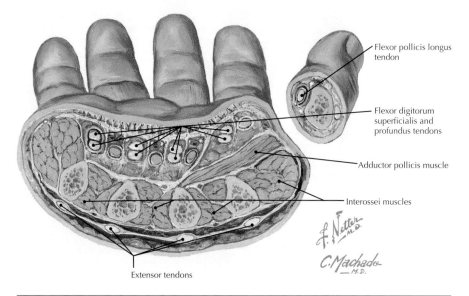

Flexor pollicis longus tendon

Flexor digitorum superficialis and profundus tendons

Adductor pollicis muscle

Interossei muscles

Extensor tendons

Axial section, midpalm of hand *(Atlas of Human Anatomy, 6th edition, Plate 450)*

Clinical Note Trigger or snapping finger (digital tenovaginitis stenosans) occurs when the long digital flexor tendons thicken, preventing smooth movement between a tendon and the overlying fibrous tendon sheaths.

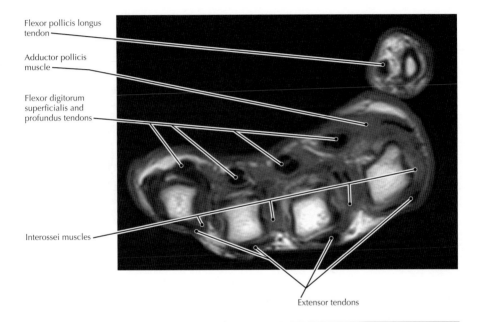

Flexor pollicis longus tendon

Adductor pollicis muscle

Flexor digitorum superficialis and profundus tendons

Interossei muscles

Extensor tendons

Axial PD MR image of the hand

- Complete laceration of a flexor digitorum profundus tendon would eliminate the ability to flex the distal interphalangeal joint of the associated digit.
- A midhumeral fracture that lacerates the radial nerve would paralyze all the extensor muscles of the wrist and digits, producing "wrist drop."

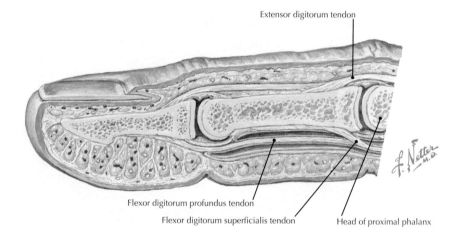

Extensor digitorum tendon

Flexor digitorum profundus tendon

Flexor digitorum superficialis tendon

Head of proximal phalanx

Sagittal view of the distal finger *(Atlas of Human Anatomy, 6th edition, Plate 458)*

Clinical Note Disruption of the extensor digitorum tendon from the distal phalanx is called "mallet finger," and disruption of the flexor digitorum profundus tendon from the distal phalanx is called "jersey finger."

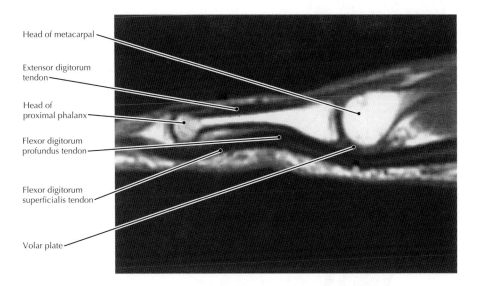

Head of metacarpal

Extensor digitorum tendon

Head of proximal phalanx

Flexor digitorum profundus tendon

Flexor digitorum superficialis tendon

Volar plate

Sagittal MR image of the interphalangeal joints and associated tendons *(From Yu JS, Habib PA: Normal MR imaging anatomy of the wrist and hand. Radiol Clin North Am 44(4):569-581, 2006)*

- The tendons of the flexor digitorum profundus muscle pierce the tendons of the flexor digitorum superficialis muscle to insert on the distal phalanges of the fingers.
- MR images of the fingers are commonly made to determine whether any of the long digital muscle tendons have become avulsed from the phalanges.

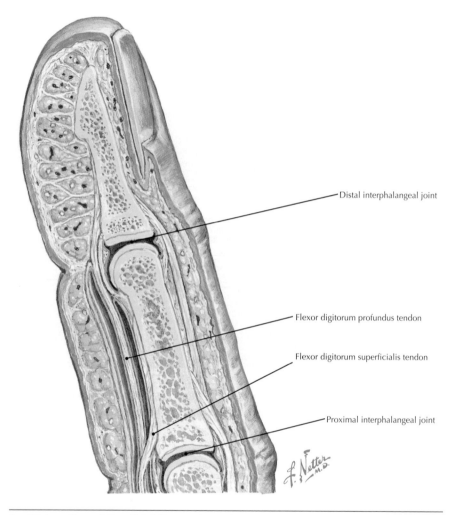

Sagittal section of the distal finger *(Atlas of Human Anatomy, 6th edition, Plate 458)*

Clinical Note   Because the finger tendons are superficial, ultrasound can provide a quick and accurate assessment of the status of the finger joints, fibrous sheaths, and the tendons, although not with the clarity of MRI, as shown in the previous plate.

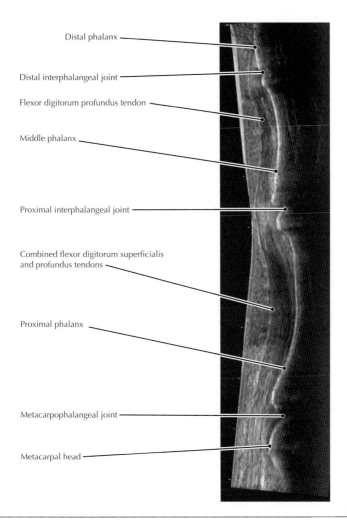

Distal phalanx

Distal interphalangeal joint

Flexor digitorum profundus tendon

Middle phalanx

Proximal interphalangeal joint

Combined flexor digitorum superficialis
and profundus tendons

Proximal phalanx

Metacarpophalangeal joint

Metacarpal head

Sagittal US of the finger

- Bright line shown in US image is the volar cortex of phalanges.
- The flexor tendons of the fingers run along the anterior surface, and these tendons are tethered close to the bones by connective tissue sheaths (pulleys) at eight different locations from the metacarpal-interphalangeal (metacarpophalangeal, MCP) joint to the distal phalanx. Because the tendons are tightly tethered to the bones, their pulling force is more efficient. There are five annular pulleys (A1-A5) and three cruciate pulleys (C1-C3).

Section 7   Lower Limb

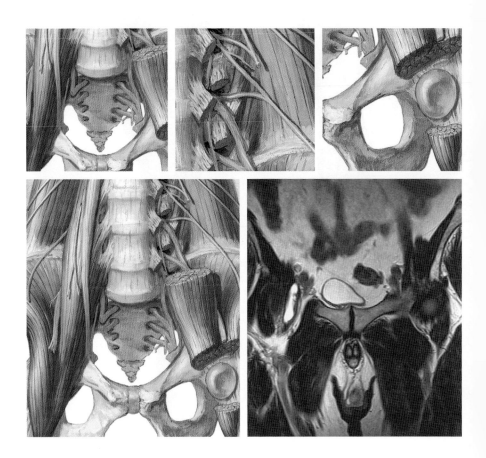

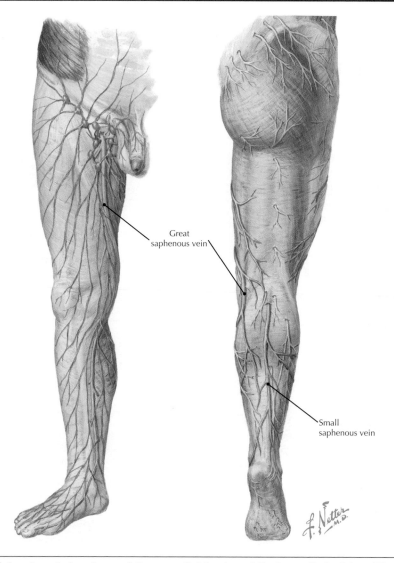

Great
saphenous vein

Small
saphenous vein

Medial and posterior views of the superficial veins of the lower limb *(Atlas of Human Anatomy, 6th edition, Plates 471 and 472)*

Clinical Note The superficial veins of the lower limb, including the saphenous veins, drain to deep veins via perforator veins with valves responsible for unidirectional flow to the deep system. When those valves are incompetent (often damaged by phlebitis), increased pressure in the superficial veins results in varicosities.

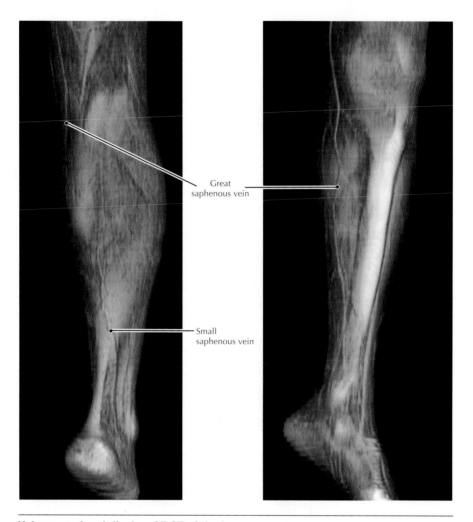

Great
saphenous vein

Small
saphenous vein

Volume rendered display, CE CT of the leg

- The small (lesser) saphenous vein enters the popliteal fossa and joins the popliteal vein.
- The great saphenous vein begins at the anterior margin of the medial malleolus, traverses the medial aspect of the popliteal fossa, and wraps around to the anterior thigh to join the femoral vein.

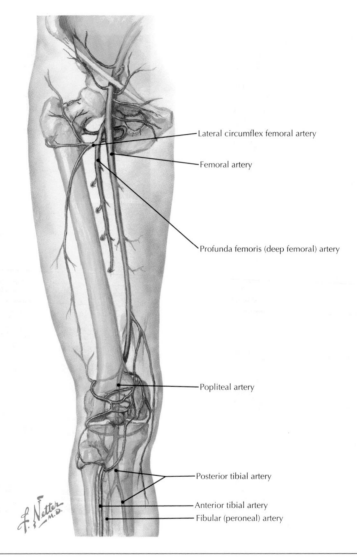

Lateral circumflex femoral artery

Femoral artery

Profunda femoris (deep femoral) artery

Popliteal artery

Posterior tibial artery

Anterior tibial artery

Fibular (peroneal) artery

Arteries of the thigh and knee *(Atlas of Human Anatomy, 6th edition, Plate 499)*

Clinical Note Atherosclerosis can cause narrowing of the arteries of the lower limb, producing peripheral vascular disease (PVD). PVD results in claudication (muscle pain with exertion) due to an inability of the vessels to supply sufficient blood to the muscles during activities (e.g., walking).

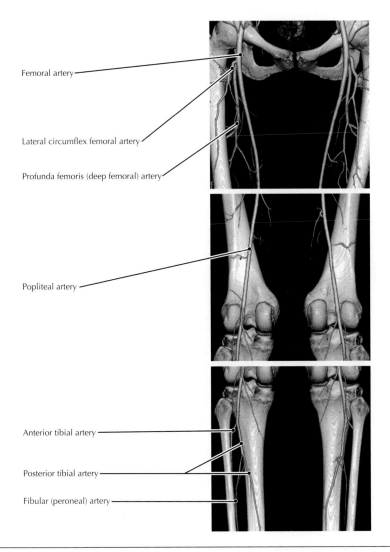

Femoral artery

Lateral circumflex femoral artery

Profunda femoris (deep femoral) artery

Popliteal artery

Anterior tibial artery

Posterior tibial artery

Fibular (peroneal) artery

3-D display from CTA of the normal lower limb *(From Hiatt MD, Fleischmann D, Hellinger JC, Rubin GD: Angiographic imaging of the lower extremities with multidetector CT. Radiol Clin North Am 43(6):1119-1127, 2005)*

- The external iliac artery becomes the femoral artery as it passes posterior to the inguinal ligament.
- The femoral artery becomes the popliteal artery once it traverses the adductor hiatus in the tendon of the adductor magnus muscle.

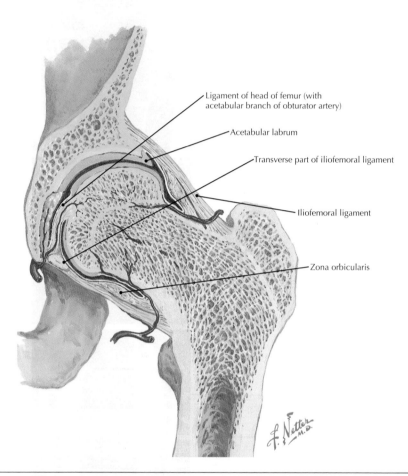

Ligament of head of femur (with acetabular branch of obturator artery)

Acetabular labrum

Transverse part of iliofemoral ligament

Iliofemoral ligament

Zona orbicularis

Coronal view of hip joint *(Atlas of Human Anatomy, 6th edition, Plate 491)*

Clinical Note The acetabulum, with its labrum, extends more than a hemisphere over the head of the femur, which, along with the strong ligaments from the pelvis to the femur, contributes to a very stable hip joint. Fractures (through the neck of the femur) are more common than hip dislocations.

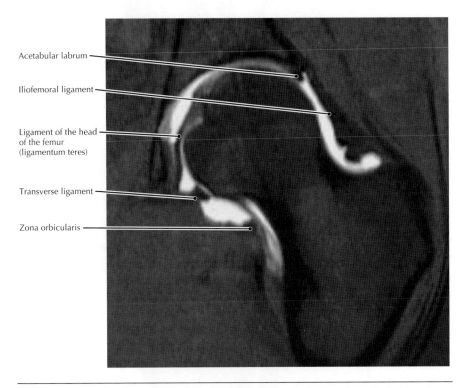

Acetabular labrum

Iliofemoral ligament

Ligament of the head
of the femur
(ligamentum teres)

Transverse ligament

Zona orbicularis

Coronal FS T1 MR arthrogram of the hip joint *(From Chatha DS, Arora R: MR imaging of the normal hip. Magn Reson Imaging Clin N Am 13(4):605-615, 2005)*

- The iliofemoral ligament is the strongest ligament of the hip joint. It is a thickening of the hip joint capsule (intrinsic ligament), as are the ischiofemoral and pubofemoral ligaments.
- If there is clinical suspicion of a labral tear, the preferred imaging procedure is an MR arthrogram of the hip.

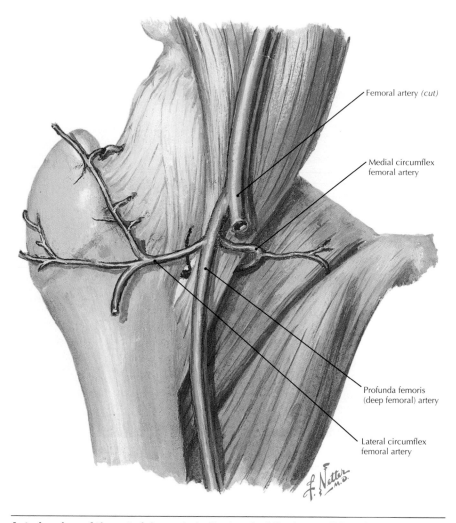

Femoral artery *(cut)*

Medial circumflex femoral artery

Profunda femoris (deep femoral) artery

Lateral circumflex femoral artery

Anterior view of the arterial supply to the head of the femur *(Atlas of Human Anatomy, 6th edition, Plate 491)*

Clinical Note   Most of the blood reaching the head of the femur is supplied by branches of the femoral circumflex arteries (primarily the medial). Because these branches are often compromised in a "fractured hip" (common in elderly women due to osteoporosis), the femoral head commonly undergoes avascular necrosis.

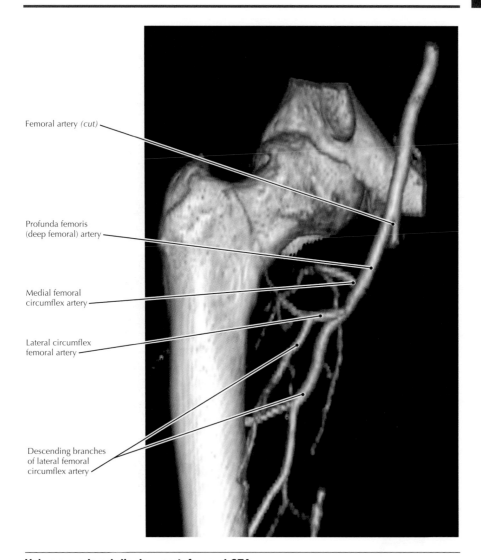

Femoral artery *(cut)*

Profunda femoris
(deep femoral) artery

Medial femoral
circumflex artery

Lateral circumflex
femoral artery

Descending branches
of lateral femoral
circumflex artery

Volume rendered display, aortofemoral CTA

- A small branch of the obturator artery (acetabular) passes through the ligament of the head of the femur (ligamentum teres) to supply the femoral head, but this branch is usually too small to prevent necrosis if the circumflex arteries are torn.
- In cases of avascular necrosis, the femoral head is removed and a prosthetic hip joint is surgically implanted.
- The profunda femoris artery (deep femoral artery) supplies the muscles of the posterior thigh.

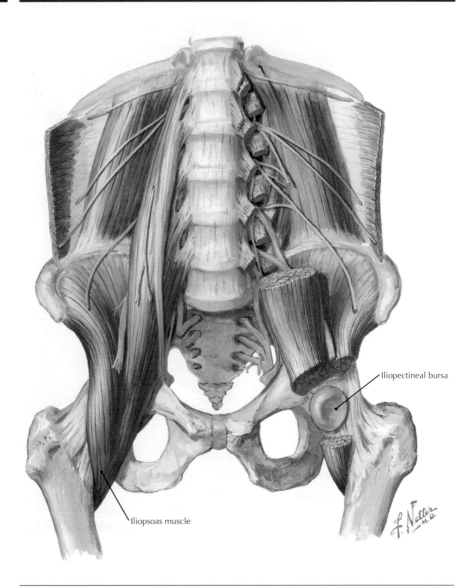

Iliopectineal bursa

Iliopsoas muscle

Psoas and iliacus muscles, and iliopectineal bursa *(Atlas of Human Anatomy, 6th edition, Plate 483)*

Clinical Note The iliopectineal (iliopsoas) bursa is the largest bursa in the body and frequently communicates with the hip joint.

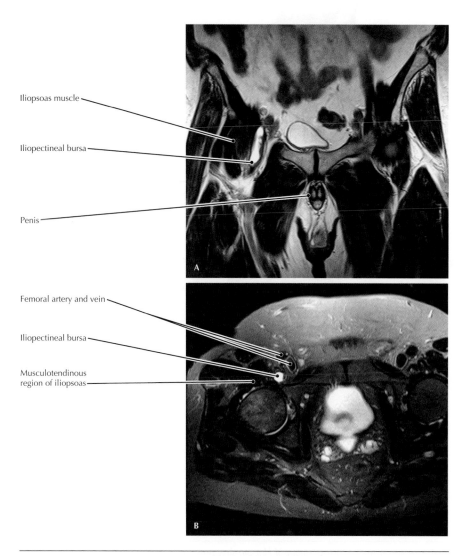

Iliopsoas muscle

Iliopectineal bursa

Penis

A

Femoral artery and vein

Iliopectineal bursa

Musculotendinous
region of iliopsoas

B

(A) Coronal and *(B)* axial FS T2 MR images of the pelvis

- The iliopectineal (iliopsoas) bursa allows the iliopsoas muscle/tendon to move freely over the hip joint as it flexes the thigh. (In the case shown here the normally collapsed bursa is visible because of excess fluid.)

- The iliopsoas tendon (common tendon of iliacus and psoas major muscles) inserts onto the lesser trochanter.

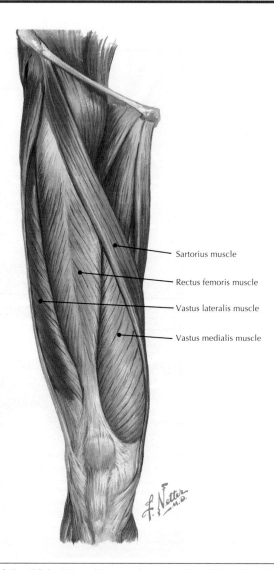

Anterior view of the thigh *(Atlas of Human Anatomy, 6th edition, Plate 479)*

Clinical Note   The quadriceps femoris muscle group (quadriceps femoris, vastus lateralis, vastus medialis, vastus intermedius) is the only extensor of the knee. The rectus femoris is the only head of the quadriceps group that also crosses the hip joint and is thereby a "biarticular" muscle that can flex the hip.

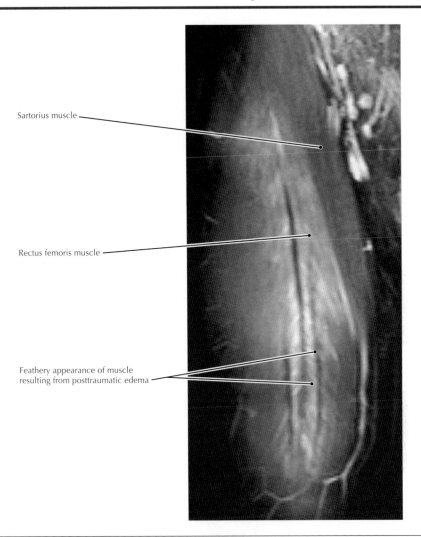

Sartorius muscle

Rectus femoris muscle

Feathery appearance of muscle
resulting from posttraumatic edema

Coronal MR image of the anterior thigh *(From Bordalo-Rodrigues M, Rosenberg ZS: MR imaging of the proximal rectus femoris musculotendinous unit. Magn Reson Imaging Clin N Am 13(4):717-725, 2005)*

- Grade 1 muscle injury is a strain of the muscle without architectural disruption. In Grade 2 muscle injury there is more clearly visible disruption of muscle fibers with hemorrhage. Grade 3 muscle injury is characterized by a complete disruption of the muscle.

- All four parts of the quadriceps femoris muscle group are innervated by the femoral nerve, which is composed of the dorsal divisions of the ventral rami of L2-L4 spinal segments.

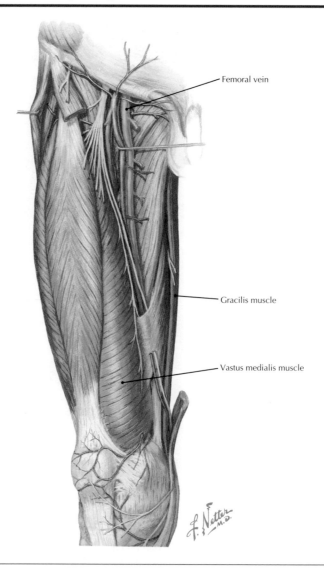

Femoral vein

Gracilis muscle

Vastus medialis muscle

Arteries, nerves, and muscles of the anterior thigh *(Atlas of Human Anatomy, 6th edition, Plate 487)*

Clinical Note The consistent vascular anatomy and nerve supply of the gracilis muscle, plus its relatively small contribution to thigh adduction, allow this muscle to be used as a wound graft when a long vascular leash is not required. Furthermore, it can also be used to reproduce upper limb, lower limb, or facial muscular function.

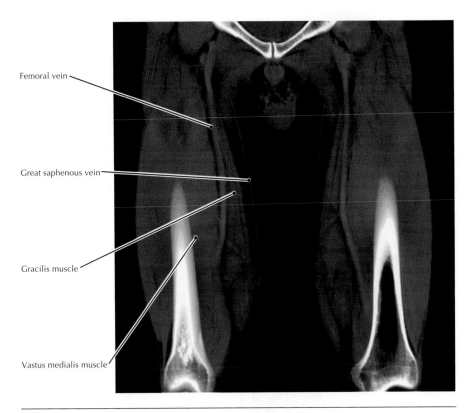

Femoral vein

Great saphenous vein

Gracilis muscle

Vastus medialis muscle

Volume rendered display, low-dose CT scan of the thighs, done shortly after CE CT scan of the chest to rule out pulmonary embolism

- The great saphenous vein has been the vessel of choice for coronary artery grafting for many years, although other vessels (e.g., radial, internal thoracic arteries) are now often used. If the vein is used it must be positioned so that the valves do not impede blood flow.

- Once the popliteal vein passes through the adductor hiatus in the adductor magnus muscle it becomes the femoral vein.

- Clinically suspected pulmonary thromboembolic disease is usually evaluated by a pulmonary CT angiogram to identify or rule out pulmonary emboli. The scan protocol may include a low-dose CT scan of the lower limbs, usually done approximately 2 minutes after the IV contrast injection for the pulmonary artery study. This additional scan may demonstrate popliteal and femoral vein thrombi.

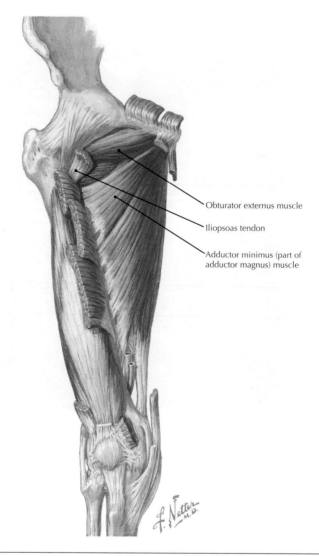

Obturator externus muscle

Iliopsoas tendon

Adductor minimus (part of adductor magnus) muscle

Anterior view of the deep hip muscles *(Atlas of Human Anatomy, 6th edition, Plate 480)*

Clinical Note Clicking or snapping hip (coxa saltans) is a symptom complex characterized by an audible "snap" around the hip on specific movements. It is often painless but may become painful or uncomfortable as chronicity develops. One common cause is the iliopsoas tendon snapping over the iliopectineal eminence or femoral head.

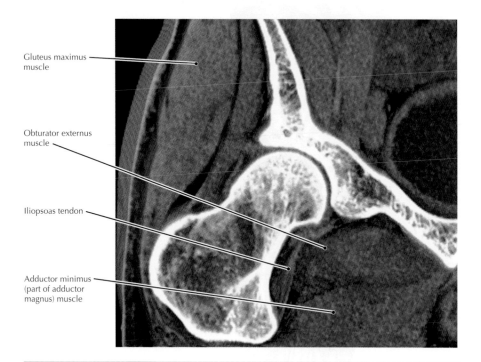

Gluteus maximus muscle

Obturator externus muscle

Iliopsoas tendon

Adductor minimus (part of adductor magnus) muscle

Volume rendered display, CT of the pelvis

- The adductor magnus muscle is actually two muscles that are well blended anatomically, but distinct functionally. The superior part is innervated by the obturator nerve and acts with the other adductors in flexing and adducting the femur. The lower part is innervated by the tibial part of the sciatic nerve and acts with the hamstrings as a hip extensor.

- The obturator externus muscle covers the external surface of the obturator membrane and is a strong lateral rotator of the femur.

- A volume rendered display, such as this image, permits visualization of the posterior relationship between the obturator externus muscle and the femoral neck.

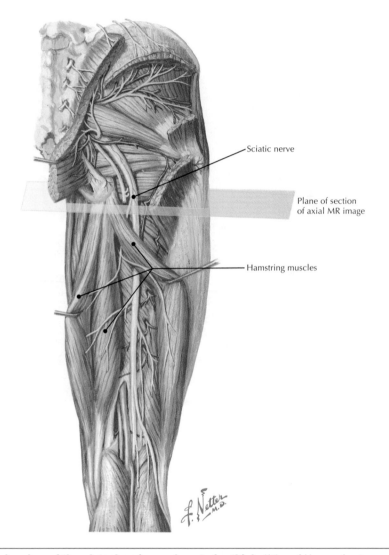

Sciatic nerve

Plane of section of axial MR image

Hamstring muscles

Posterior view of the gluteal region and posterior thigh *(Atlas of Human Anatomy, 6th edition, Plate 489)*

Clinical Note The sciatic nerve can be irritated by tears of the hamstring muscles, producing a type of "sciatica." The resulting pain can be significant and very disproportionate from what might be expected in a hamstring injury that does not involve the nerve.

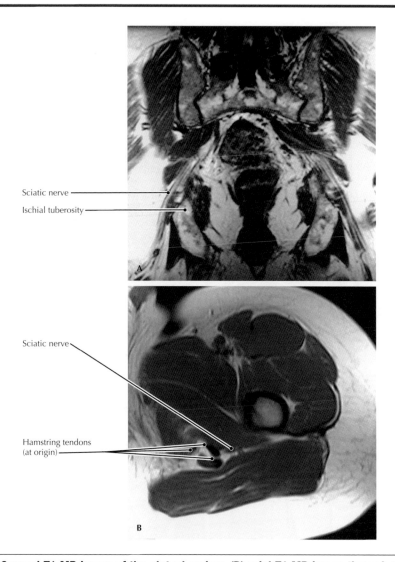

Sciatic nerve

Ischial tuberosity

A

Sciatic nerve

Hamstring tendons
(at origin)

B

(A) **Coronal T1 MR image of the gluteal region;** *(B)* **axial T1 MR image through the gluteal region** *(A, From Stone JA: MR myelography of the spine and MR peripheral nerve imaging. Magn Reson Imaging Clin N Am 11(4):543-558, 2003)*

- The top image is oriented to the long axis of the sciatic nerve as it courses through the greater sciatic foramen; the nerve, which is isointense with muscle, is surrounded by high-signal perineural fat.
- The lower image shows how intragluteal injections placed too far inferiorly and too far medially could injure the sciatic nerve.

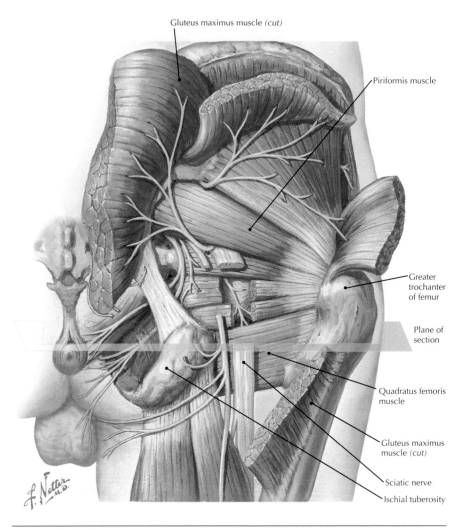

Gluteus maximus muscle *(cut)*

Piriformis muscle

Greater trochanter of femur

Plane of section

Quadratus femoris muscle

Gluteus maximus muscle *(cut)*

Sciatic nerve

Ischial tuberosity

Deep muscles of the posterior thigh *(Atlas of Human Anatomy, 6th edition, Plate 490)*

Clinical Note The proximity of the sciatic nerve to the ischial tuberosity explains how hamstring tears at their origin on the tuberosity can result in sciatic nerve irritation, with symptoms that mimic sciatica.

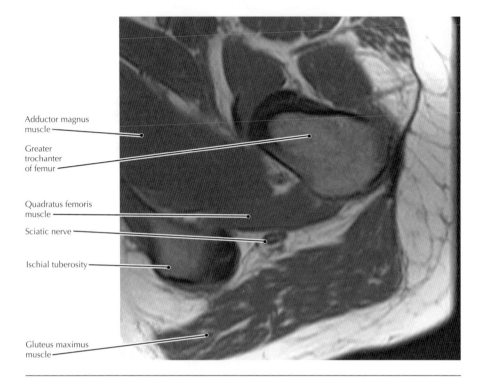

Adductor magnus muscle

Greater trochanter of femur

Quadratus femoris muscle

Sciatic nerve

Ischial tuberosity

Gluteus maximus muscle

Axial T1 MR image, gluteal region

- Although typically the sciatic nerve passes inferior to the piriformis muscle, it may pass through or superior to this muscle.
- The sciatic nerve provides almost all of the motor and sensory innervation of the posterior aspect of the thigh, and the leg and foot.

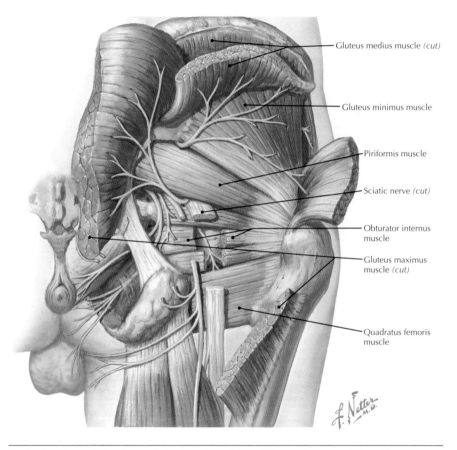

Gluteus medius muscle *(cut)*

Gluteus minimus muscle

Piriformis muscle

Sciatic nerve *(cut)*

Obturator internus muscle

Gluteus maximus muscle *(cut)*

Quadratus femoris muscle

Posterior view of the deep gluteal region *(Atlas of Human Anatomy, 6th edition, Plate 490)*

Clinical Note Tears of the gluteus medius and minimus tendons can mimic symptoms of greater trochanteric bursitis of the hip. However, unlike bursitis, tears of these muscles can be treated surgically.

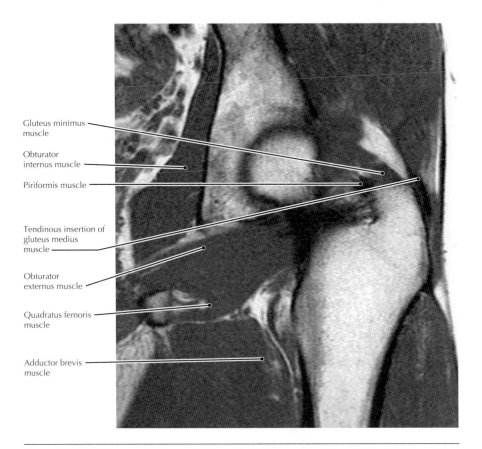

Gluteus minimus muscle

Obturator internus muscle

Piriformis muscle

Tendinous insertion of gluteus medius muscle

Obturator externus muscle

Quadratus femoris muscle

Adductor brevis muscle

Coronal T1 MR image of the posterior gluteal/hip region *(From Chatha DS, Arora R: MR imaging of the normal hip. Magn Reson Imaging Clin N Am 13(4):605-615, 2005)*

- The gluteus medius and minimus are the primary abductors of the hip and are both innervated by the superior gluteal nerve, which also innervates the tensor fascia latae.
- The quadratus femoris is a lateral rotator of the thigh and is sometimes absent.

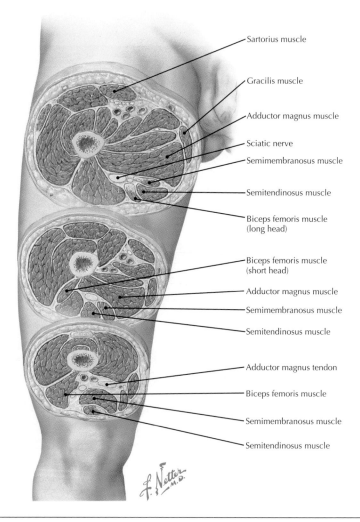

Sartorius muscle

Gracilis muscle

Adductor magnus muscle

Sciatic nerve

Semimembranosus muscle

Semitendinosus muscle

Biceps femoris muscle
(long head)

Biceps femoris muscle
(short head)

Adductor magnus muscle

Semimembranosus muscle

Semitendinosus muscle

Adductor magnus tendon

Biceps femoris muscle

Semimembranosus muscle

Semitendinosus muscle

Axial sections through the thigh *(Atlas of Human Anatomy, 6th edition, Plate 492)*

Clinical Note Hamstring strains (strains of the biceps femoris, semimembranosus, and semitendinosus muscles) are common in patients who participate in running and kicking sports such as baseball, basketball, football, and soccer.

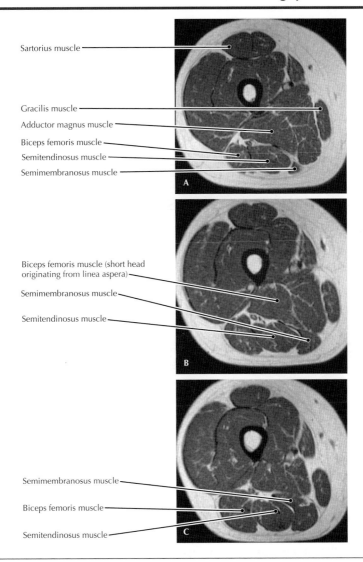

Sartorius muscle

Gracilis muscle
Adductor magnus muscle
Biceps femoris muscle
Semitendinosus muscle
Semimembranosus muscle

A

Biceps femoris muscle (short head originating from linea aspera)
Semimembranosus muscle
Semitendinosus muscle

B

Semimembranosus muscle
Biceps femoris muscle
Semitendinosus muscle

C

Axial T1 MR images of the thigh: *(A)* **proximal,** *(C)* **distal** *(From Chatha DS, Arora R: MR imaging of the normal hip. Magn Reson Imaging Clin N Am 13(4):605-615, 2005)*

- The hamstring muscles (biceps femoris [long head], semimembranosus, semitendinosus) all originate from the ischial tuberosity, insert into the upper tibia or fibula, extend the thigh and flex the knee, and are innervated by the tibial division of the sciatic nerve.

- The short head of the biceps femoris muscle originates from the linea aspera and inserts with the long head onto the head of the fibula. It is innervated by the common fibular division of the sciatic nerve.

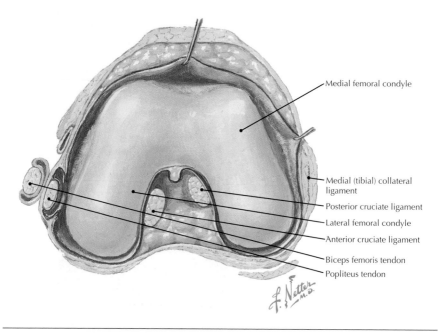

Medial femoral condyle

Medial (tibial) collateral ligament

Posterior cruciate ligament

Lateral femoral condyle

Anterior cruciate ligament

Biceps femoris tendon

Popliteus tendon

Interior knee joint showing superior aspect of the joint *(Atlas of Human Anatomy, 6th edition, Plate 495)*

Clinical Note   Rupture of a cruciate ligament results in anterior-posterior instability of the knee. An anterior cruciate ligament injury occurs more frequently than a posterior cruciate ligament injury and is often surgically repaired. Excessive anterior movement of the tibia relative to the femur (anterior drawer sign) is indicative of an anterior cruciate ligament tear.

Medial (tibial)
collateral ligament

Medial femoral condyle

Posterior cruciate
ligament

Lateral femoral condyle

Anterior cruciate
ligament

Popliteus tendon

Biceps femoris tendon

Popliteal vein

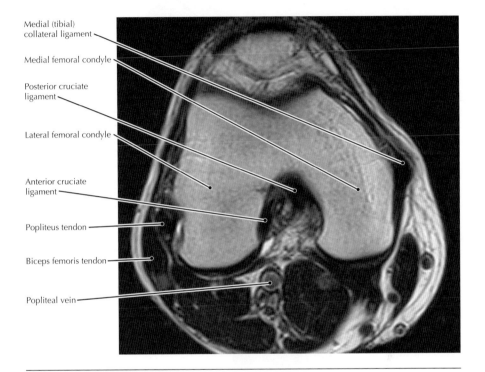

Axial T2 MR image of the knee

- The popliteal vessels may be ruptured in a knee dislocation.
- A tear of the anterior cruciate ligament is often associated with rupture of the medial collateral ligament and tearing of the medial meniscus—the "unhappy triad" (of O'Donoghue).
- The two heads of the gastrocnemius originate on the femoral condyles and therefore flex the knee, as well as plantarflexing the ankle.

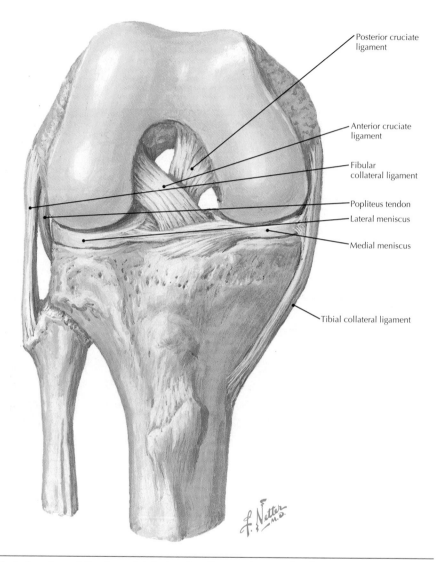

Posterior cruciate ligament

Anterior cruciate ligament

Fibular collateral ligament

Popliteus tendon

Lateral meniscus

Medial meniscus

Tibial collateral ligament

Anterior view of the knee joint showing the cruciate and collateral ligaments, and menisci *(Atlas of Human Anatomy, 6th edition, Plate 496)*

Clinical Note The attachment of the medial meniscus to the medial (tibial) collateral ligament explains why tears of both often occur together, whereas this is not the case for the lateral (fibular) collateral ligament and the lateral meniscus.

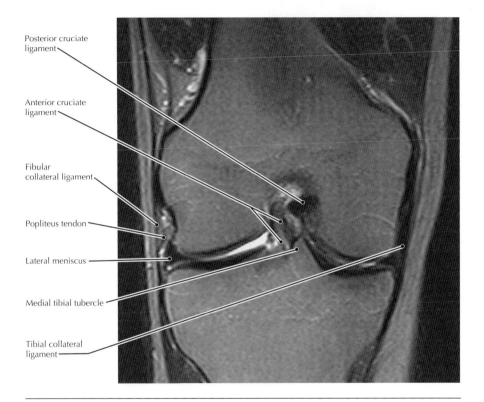

Posterior cruciate ligament

Anterior cruciate ligament

Fibular collateral ligament

Popliteus tendon

Lateral meniscus

Medial tibial tubercle

Tibial collateral ligament

Coronal T1 MR image of the knee

- Tears of the anterior cruciate ligament usually occur when the knee is twisted while the foot is firmly fixed on the ground.

- The popliteus muscle is very important for providing the rotatory movements that "unlock" the extended knee, allowing it to flex.

- In clinical practice, the tibial tubercles are referred to as the tibial spines.

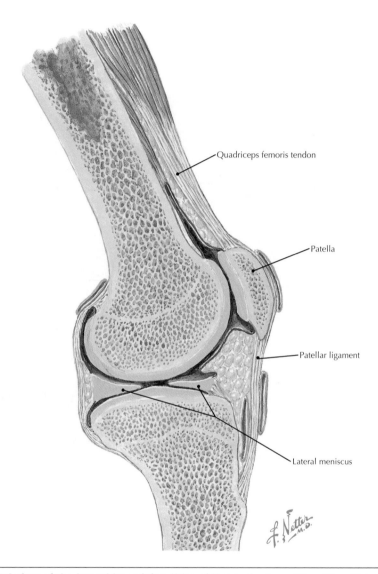

Quadriceps femoris tendon

Patella

Patellar ligament

Lateral meniscus

Sagittal view of the lateral knee joint *(Atlas of Human Anatomy, 6th edition, Plate 498)*

Clinical Note The menisci act as cushions for the joint and are sometimes torn (especially the medial) when the joint is twisted. Patients report pain in the associated knee and a "giving way" of the joint on flexion or extension.

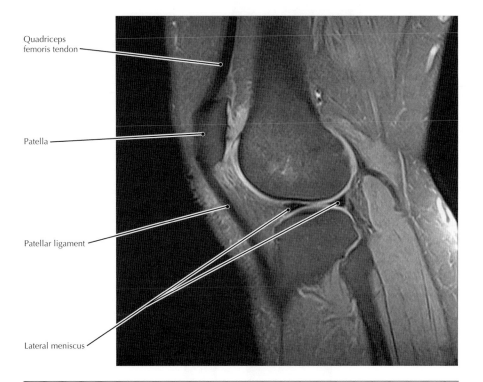

Quadriceps femoris tendon

Patella

Patellar ligament

Lateral meniscus

Sagittal fat-suppressed PD MR image of the lateral knee joint

- The medial meniscus is torn much more frequently than the lateral meniscus, primarily because of its attachment to the medial collateral ligament.
- The patellar ligament is really an extension of the tendons of the quadriceps femoris muscles, which act to extend the knee.

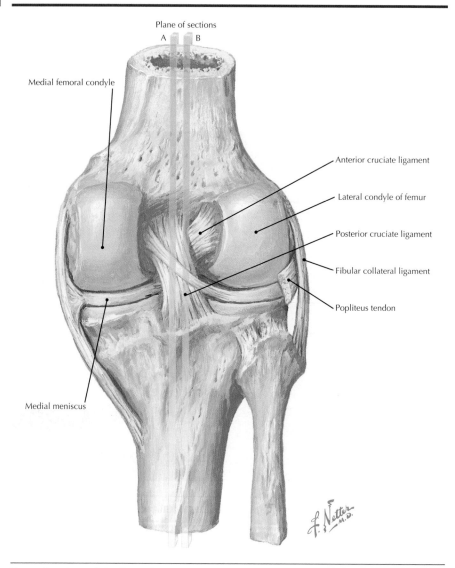

Plane of sections
A   B

Medial femoral condyle

Anterior cruciate ligament

Lateral condyle of femur

Posterior cruciate ligament

Fibular collateral ligament

Popliteus tendon

Medial meniscus

Posterior view of the knee joint showing the cruciate and collateral ligaments, and menisci *(Atlas of Human Anatomy, 6th edition, Plate 496)*

Clinical Note A ruptured anterior cruciate ligament (ACL) is often accompanied by a "popping" sensation. Such ruptures occur at a higher frequency in women athletes than in their male counterparts. This may be explained by anatomic differences between men and women (e.g., wider pelvis, smaller intercondylar notch) and by less powerful muscles in women.

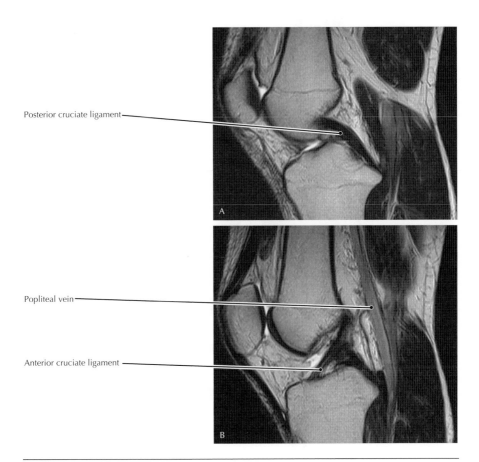

Posterior cruciate ligament

Popliteal vein

Anterior cruciate ligament

Sagittal T2 MR images of the knee; *B* is lateral to *A*

- *Lines A* and *B* on the illustration indicate the sagittal positions of the MR images. However, these images are actually oblique to the sagittal plane in order to maximize the appearance of the ligaments.

- In order to have such oblique images, an MRI technologist must identify the appropriate anatomy on an axial image and then prescribe the appropriate orientation of the sagittal sequences to best show the cruciate ligaments.

- Complete ACL/posterior cruciate ligament (PCL) tears can often be diagnosed clinically, but MRI is used for confirmation and can reveal additional injuries that may not be evident on physical examination.

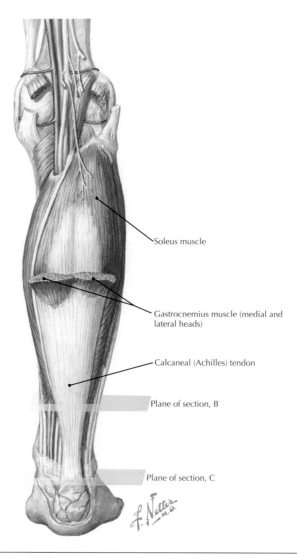

Soleus muscle

Gastrocnemius muscle (medial and lateral heads)

Calcaneal (Achilles) tendon

Plane of section, B

Plane of section, C

Achilles tendon and soleus *(Atlas of Human Anatomy, 6th edition, Plate 504)*

Clinical Note   A ruptured (or torn) Achilles tendon may occur when the tendon has been structurally weakened by tendonitis, or when a healthy tendon is subjected to a sudden, unexpected force. When the tendon tears, people often describe feeling a "pop" at the back of the ankle. The injury is accompanied by pain, swelling, and loss of function.

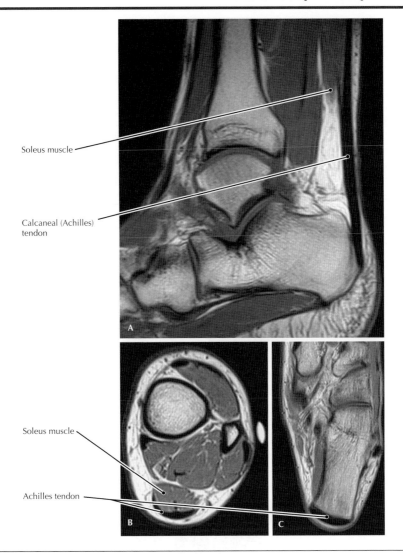

Soleus muscle

Calcaneal (Achilles) tendon

Soleus muscle

Achilles tendon

A

B

C

Sagittal T1 MR image *(A)* and axial PD MR images *(B* and *C)* of the ankle and lower leg

- The gastrocnemius and soleus muscles insert into the calcaneus via the Achilles tendon. The primary action of these muscles is to powerfully plantarflex the ankle using the posterior calcaneus as a lever arm. The gastrocnemius fused with the soleus muscle superior to the axial MR images shown here.

- The remaining ankle plantarflexors, such as the tibialis posterior and fibularis (peroneus) longus muscle, are much weaker plantarflexors than the gastrocnemius and soleus muscles because they wind around the malleoli and lack an extended lever arm.

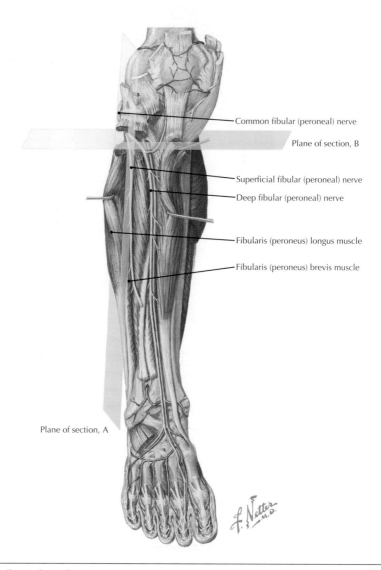

Common fibular (peroneal) nerve

Plane of section, B

Superficial fibular (peroneal) nerve

Deep fibular (peroneal) nerve

Fibularis (peroneus) longus muscle

Fibularis (peroneus) brevis muscle

Plane of section, A

Deep dissection of the anterior leg muscles and nerves *(Atlas of Human Anatomy, 6th edition, Plate 508)*

Clinical Note As it wraps around the neck of the fibula, the common fibular (peroneal) nerve is vulnerable to injury that results in foot drop because all the dorsiflexors of the foot are innervated by its deep branch.

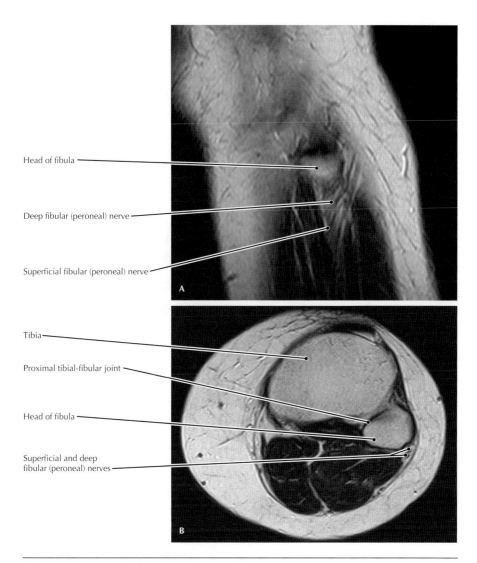

Head of fibula

Deep fibular (peroneal) nerve

Superficial fibular (peroneal) nerve

A

Tibia

Proximal tibial-fibular joint

Head of fibula

Superficial and deep
fibular (peroneal) nerves

B

Sagittal (A) and axial (B) T2 MR image of the upper leg

- The superficial fibular (peroneal) nerve innervates the fibularis (peroneus) longus and brevis, both of which evert and plantarflex the foot.
- Although very little movement occurs between the tibia and fibula, the superior joint is a plane type of synovial joint.

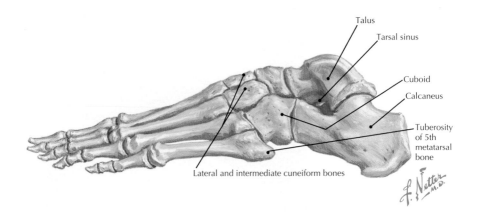

Talus

Tarsal sinus

Cuboid

Calcaneus

Tuberosity of 5th metatarsal bone

Lateral and intermediate cuneiform bones

Lateral view of the osteology of the foot *(Atlas of Human Anatomy, 6th edition, Plate 512)*

Clinical Note Tarsal sinus syndrome is a painful condition of the tarsal sinus that is associated with a sensation of instability in the hindfoot and that may occur after an inversion injury. It often causes lateral ankle pain.

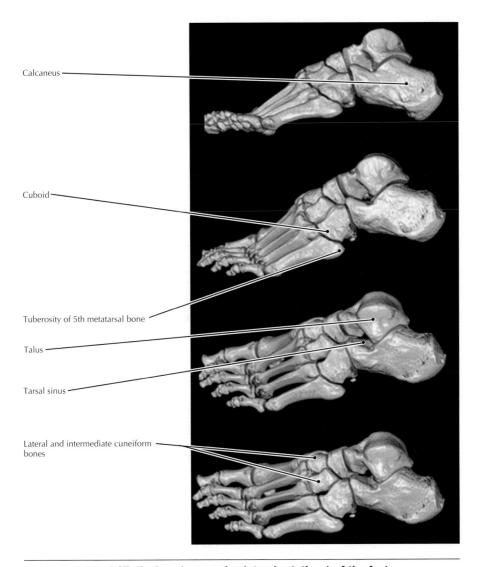

Calcaneus

Cuboid

Tuberosity of 5th metatarsal bone

Talus

Tarsal sinus

Lateral and intermediate cuneiform bones

Volume rendered CT displays (successive lateral rotations) of the foot

- The tarsal sinus is a cone-shaped region located between the inferior aspect of the neck of the talus and the anterosuperior surface of the calcaneus.

- The tuberosity of the fifth metatarsal may be avulsed during excessive eversion by the fibularis (peroneus) brevis tendon, which attaches there.

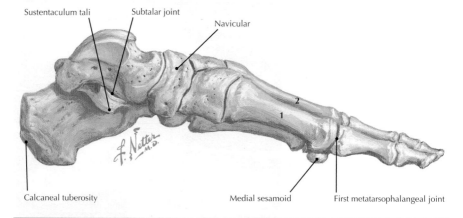

Medial view of the osteology of the foot *(Atlas of Human Anatomy, 6th edition, Plate 512)*

Clinical Note Hallux rigidus is a common painful abnormality associated with osteoarthritis at the first metatarsophalangeal joint.

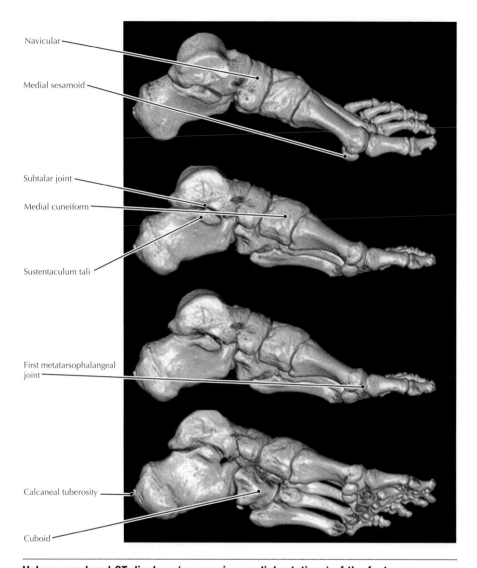

Navicular

Medial sesamoid

Subtalar joint

Medial cuneiform

Sustentaculum tali

First metatarsophalangeal joint

Calcaneal tuberosity

Cuboid

Volume rendered CT displays (successive medial rotations) of the foot

- Rotating volume rendered displays similar to these can clarify many complex fractures of the hindfoot and midfoot that are otherwise very difficult to comprehend with projectional or cross-sectional images.
- The medial and lateral sesamoid bones are located within the tendons of the flexor hallucis brevis and act to increase the leverage of this muscle.

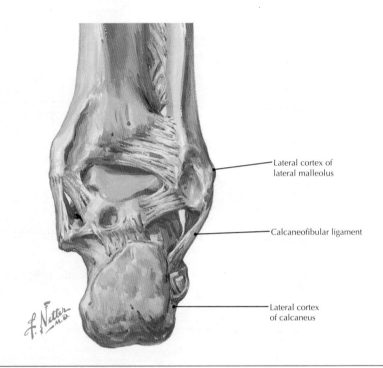

Lateral cortex of
lateral malleolus

Calcaneofibular ligament

Lateral cortex
of calcaneus

Posterior view of the calcaneus, with ligaments *(Atlas of Human Anatomy, 6th edition, Plate 513)*

Clinical Note Inversion injuries of the ankle typically first tear the anterior talofibular ligament and then the calcaneofibular ligament. Inversion ankle sprains present with pain and swelling over the lateral aspect of the ankle. These injuries usually heal with conservative treatment; ankle joint stability is maintained by the syndesmotic tibiofibular ligament, which almost always remains intact in injuries not severe enough to cause fracture.

Medial   Lateral

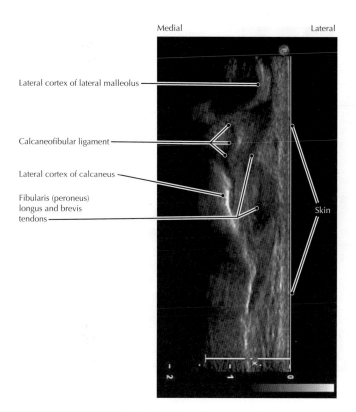

Lateral cortex of lateral malleolus ———

Calcaneofibular ligament———

Lateral cortex of calcaneus ———

Fibularis (peroneus)
longus and brevis
tendons ———

Skin

US of calcaneofibular ligament

- This image is made by placing the transducer in a coronal orientation at the lateral ankle.
- The calcaneofibular is one of the lateral ligaments of the ankle; the other two are the anterior and posterior talofibular ligaments.

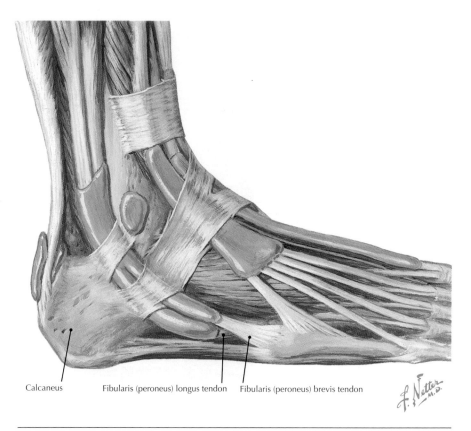

Calcaneus   Fibularis (peroneus) longus tendon   Fibularis (peroneus) brevis tendon

Tendons of the lateral ankle *(Atlas of Human Anatomy, 6th edition, Plate 516)*

Clinical Note   Peroneal (fibular) tendon tears (ruptures) are associated with excessive inversion injuries to the ankle joint and cause lateral ankle pain.

Fibularis
(peroneus)
longus
tendon

Fibularis
(peroneus)
brevis tendon

Tuberosity of
fifth metatarsal

Fifth metatarsal

Calcaneus

Fibularis
(peroneus)
longus
tendon

Cuboid
bone

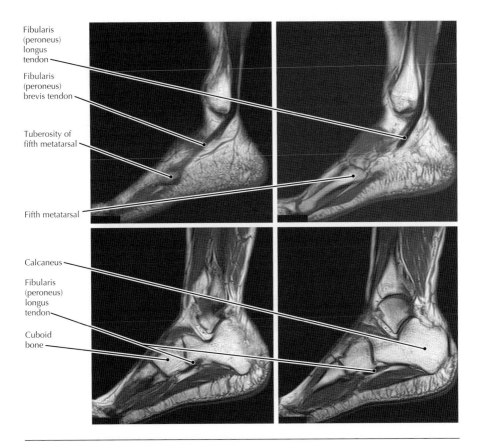

Sagittal T1 MR images of the lateral foot

- The peroneus (fibularis) longus tendon traverses and supports the transverse arch of the foot to insert on the base of the first metatarsal and the medial cuneiform.
- The fibularis (peroneus) brevis tendon inserts on the base of the fifth metatarsal, at the tuberosity.

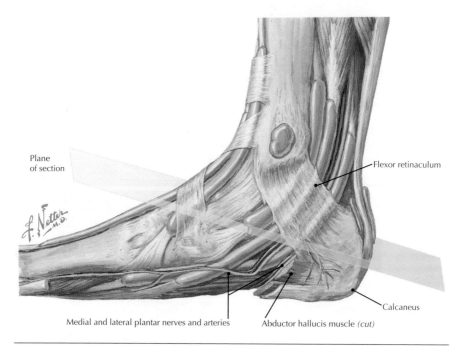

Plane of section

Flexor retinaculum

Calcaneus

Medial and lateral plantar nerves and arteries

Abductor hallucis muscle *(cut)*

Medial view of the tendons and neurovasculature (tarsal tunnel) at the ankle
(Atlas of Human Anatomy, 6th edition, Plate 516)

Clinical Note As the tibial nerve divides into the medial and lateral plantar nerves, it passes deep to the flexor retinaculum. This area, known as the tarsal tunnel, is a potential site for entrapment of these nerves and the accompanying posterior tibial vessels.

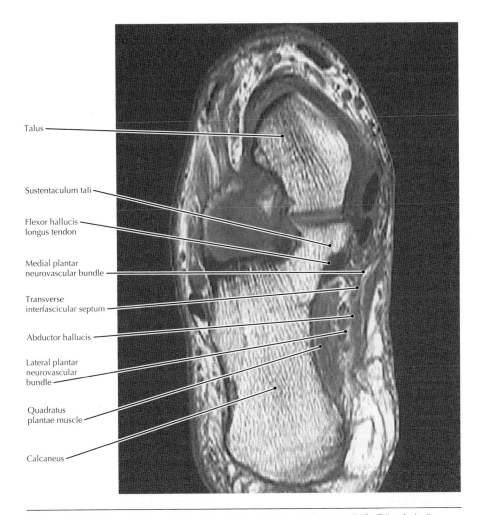

Talus

Sustentaculum tali

Flexor hallucis
longus tendon

Medial plantar
neurovascular bundle

Transverse
interfascicular septum

Abductor hallucis

Lateral plantar
neurovascular
bundle

Quadratus
plantae muscle

Calcaneus

Oblique T1 MR image through the tarsal tunnel *(From Hochman MG, Zilberfarb JL: Nerves in a pinch: Imaging of nerve compression syndromes. Radiol Clin North Am 42(1):221-245, 2004)*

- The sustentaculum tali is a projection of the calcaneus that supports the talus along the medial side of the hindfoot.

- Talocalcaneal coalition, which is a fusion of the talus and calcaneus, is a cause of chronic pain and is very difficult to appreciate on plain radiographs.

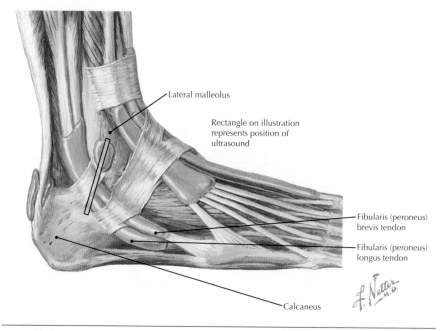

Lateral malleolus

Rectangle on illustration represents position of ultrasound

Fibularis (peroneus) brevis tendon

Fibularis (peroneus) longus tendon

Calcaneus

Lateral ankle tendons and tendon sheaths *(Atlas of Human Anatomy, 6th edition, Plate 516)*

Clinical Note Chronic lateral ankle pain is often caused by disease of the fibularis tendons. Ultrasound may reveal a fluid-distended tendon sheath in a patient with tenosynovitis and can demonstrate tendon tears.

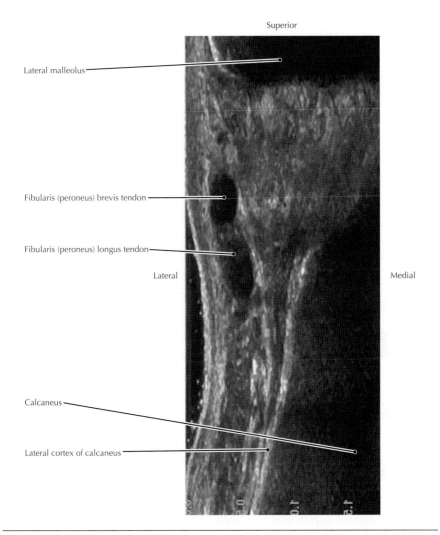

Superior

Lateral malleolus

Fibularis (peroneus) brevis tendon

Fibularis (peroneus) longus tendon

Lateral   Medial

Calcaneus

Lateral cortex of calcaneus

Coronal US images of peroneal tendons adjacent to lateral malleolus

- The fibularis longus tendon is posterior to the fibularis brevis tendon superior to the malleolus, but inferior to the peroneus longus tendon inferior to the malleolus.

- The fibularis longus and fibularis brevis muscles are the only muscles innervated by the superficial fibular (peroneal) nerve.

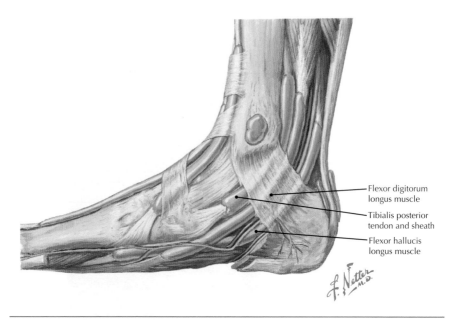

Flexor digitorum longus muscle

Tibialis posterior tendon and sheath

Flexor hallucis longus muscle

Medial ankle tendons and tendon sheaths *(Atlas of Human Anatomy, 6th edition, Plate 516)*

Clinical Note   Ultrasound of the medial ankle offers a convenient and inexpensive imaging modality for assessing the musculature and neurovascular structures located in the tarsal tunnel. However, sonography requires extensive experience for reliable interpretation because of the inherent, relatively low image quality of US compared with CT and MRI.

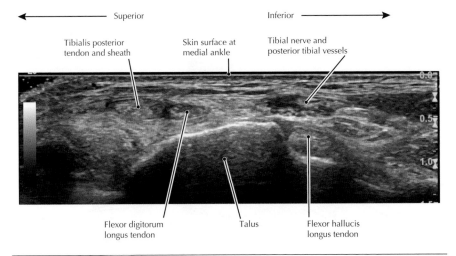

Superior   Inferior

Tibialis posterior
tendon and sheath

Skin surface at
medial ankle

Tibial nerve and
posterior tibial vessels

Flexor digitorum
longus tendon

Talus

Flexor hallucis
longus tendon

Axial US at medial ankle

- Medical students learn the order of the tendons passing along the medial side of the ankle from anterior to posterior as "Tom, Dick, and Harry": **t**ibialis posterior, flexor **d**igitorum longus, and flexor **h**allucis longus.

- The neurovascular structures are found between the flexor digitorum longus and flexor hallucis longus tendons. Note how the cortical bone of the talus has a bright linear echo.

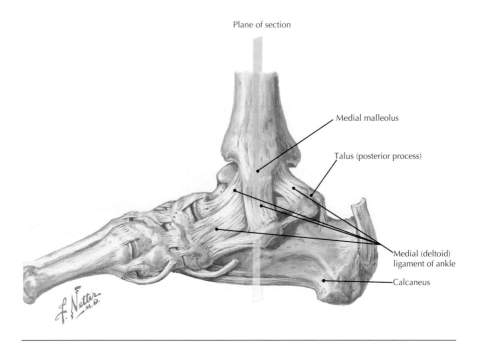

Plane of section

Medial malleolus

Talus (posterior process)

Medial (deltoid) ligament of ankle

Calcaneus

Medial view of the ligaments of the ankle and foot *(Atlas of Human Anatomy, 6th edition, Plate 514)*

Clinical Note Sprains or tears of the deltoid ligament are associated with excessive ankle eversion. A significant eversion injury may result in a bimalleolar (Pott's) fracture in which the distal fibula and medial malleolus are fractured in addition to the tear in the deltoid ligament.

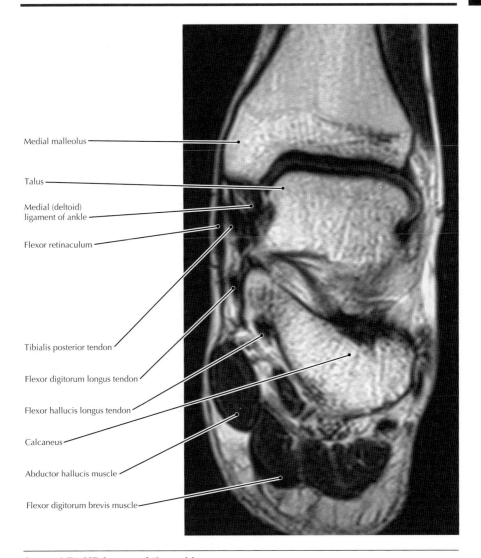

Medial malleolus

Talus

Medial (deltoid)
ligament of ankle

Flexor retinaculum

Tibialis posterior tendon

Flexor digitorum longus tendon

Flexor hallucis longus tendon

Calcaneus

Abductor hallucis muscle

Flexor digitorum brevis muscle

Coronal T1 MR image of the ankle

- The deltoid ligament has four components: anterior and posterior tibiotalar, tibionavicular, and tibiocalcaneal ligaments.
- A more severe injury than the bimalleolar (Pott's) fracture is a "trimalleolar" fracture involving the posterior corner of the tibia, as well as the distal fibula and medial malleolus.
- Tendinopathy of the tibialis posterior and flexor hallucis longus is a frequent cause of medial ankle pain.

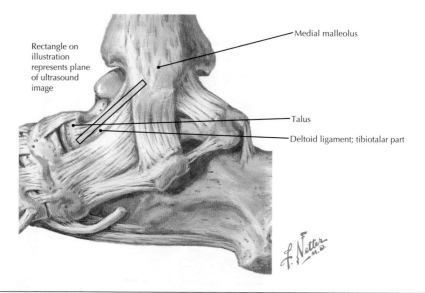

Rectangle on illustration represents plane of ultrasound image

Medial malleolus

Talus

Deltoid ligament; tibiotalar part

Medial view of the ligaments of the ankle *(Atlas of Human Anatomy, 6th edition, Plate 514)*

> **Clinical Note** Most ankle sprains are inversion injuries that tear the lateral ligaments, beginning with the anterior talofibular ligament. Eversion injuries can result in a tear of the deltoid ligament. Eversion injuries may also result in an avulsion fracture of the medial malleolus rather than a tear of the deltoid ligament.

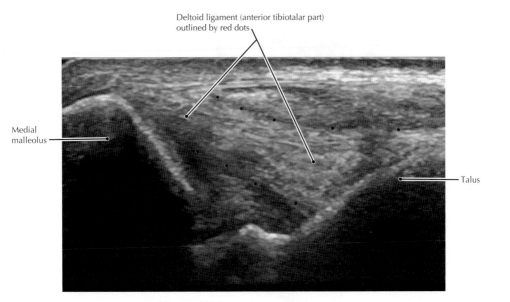

Deltoid ligament (anterior tibiotalar part) outlined by red dots

Medial malleolus

Talus

US of anterior tibiotalar part of the deltoid ligament

- The deltoid ligament is a strong, flat ligament that consists of four parts (see page 467). The anterior tibiotalar (deep part) attaches to the tip of the medial malleolus.

- The deltoid ligament's name comes from its resemblance to the Greek letter delta (Δ).

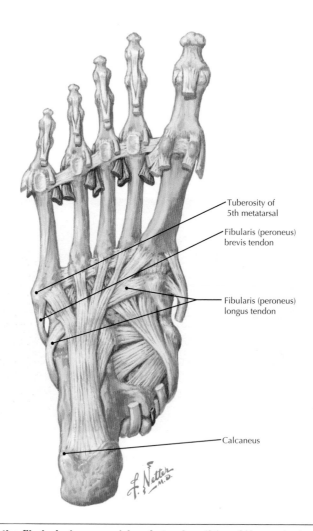

Tuberosity of
5th metatarsal

Fibularis (peroneus)
brevis tendon

Fibularis (peroneus)
longus tendon

Calcaneus

Insertion of the fibularis (peroneus) brevis tendon *(Atlas of Human Anatomy, 6th edition, Plate 515)*

Clinical Note   An inversion injury of the foot may result in an avulsion fracture of the tuberosity at the base of the fifth metatarsal by the peroneus brevis tendon, called a pseudo-Jones fracture. A true Jones fracture is at the junction of the metaphysis and diaphysis of the fifth metatarsal, approximately 1.5 cm distal to the tuberosity, and is predisposed to nonunion.

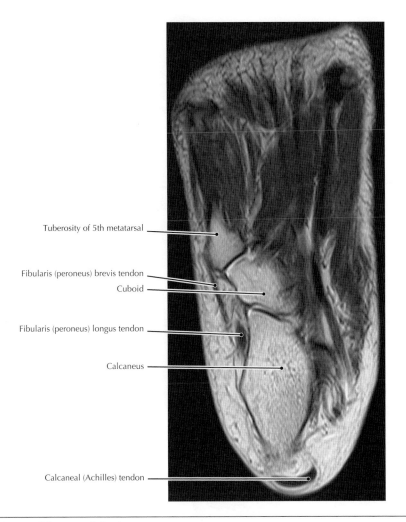

Tuberosity of 5th metatarsal

Fibularis (peroneus) brevis tendon

Cuboid

Fibularis (peroneus) longus tendon

Calcaneus

Calcaneal (Achilles) tendon

Oblique MR image of the foot

- This plane of section shows the articulations between the calcaneus and cuboid and between the cuboid and the fifth metatarsal.

- The calcaneocuboid joint forms the lateral component of the transverse tarsal joint.

- The peroneus tendons are essentially parallel structures at the level of the lateral malleolus cephalad to this image. At this level, the peroneus tendons diverge to their respective insertion sites.

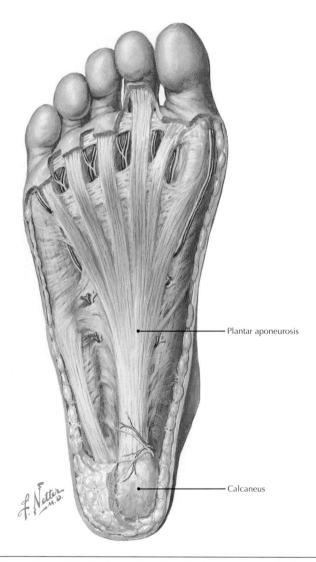

Plantar aponeurosis

Calcaneus

Superficial dissection of the foot showing the plantar aponeurosis *(Atlas of Human Anatomy, 6th edition, Plate 519)*

Clinical Note Inflammation of the plantar aponeurosis at its attachment to the calcaneus results in plantar fasciitis, a painful condition in which the pain is typically felt on the undersurface of the heel. This pain is often the most severe after awakening in the morning.

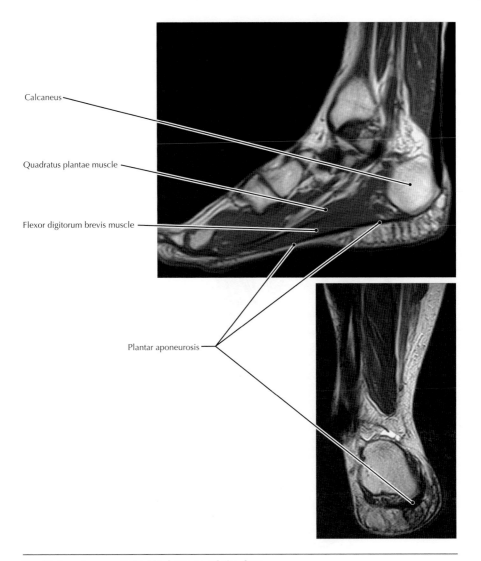

Calcaneus

Quadratus plantae muscle

Flexor digitorum brevis muscle

Plantar aponeurosis

Sagittal and coronal T1 MR images of the foot

- A bone spur may develop in association with plantar fasciitis at the junction between the plantar aponeurosis and the calcaneus; this spur may be associated with increased pain during walking.

- The plantar aponeurosis acts as a structural support tie beam, maintaining the integrity of the components of the foot skeleton and especially supporting the longitudinal arch of the foot.

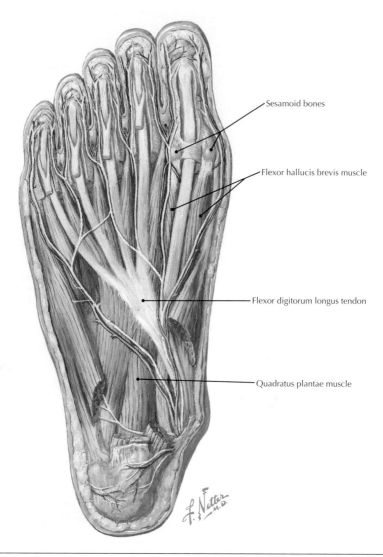

Sesamoid bones

Flexor hallucis brevis muscle

Flexor digitorum longus tendon

Quadratus plantae muscle

View of the sole of the foot, with the first of four muscle layers removed *(Atlas of Human Anatomy, 6th edition, Plate 521)*

Clinical Note Hallux valgus is a lateral deviation of the great toe (mnemonic: relate the "L" in valgus to "lateral") causing inflammation and pain at the first metatarsophalangeal joint. This is called a bunion.

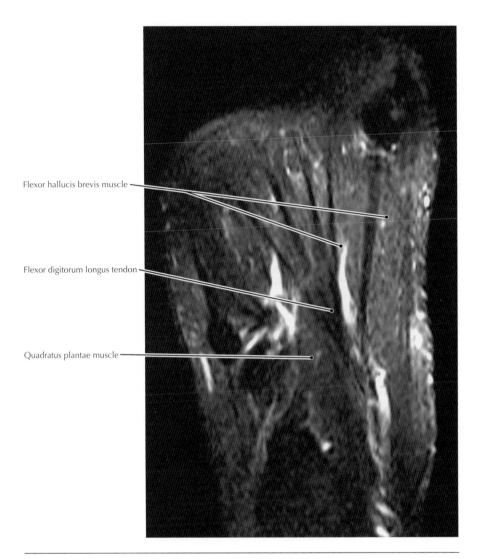

Flexor hallucis brevis muscle

Flexor digitorum longus tendon

Quadratus plantae muscle

FS T2 MR image tangent to the plantar surface of the foot

- The flexor digitorum longus tendon corresponds to the flexor digitorum profundus tendon in the upper limb and accordingly inserts into the terminal phalanges of the lateral four digits.

- The quadratus plantae muscle inserts into the tendons of the flexor digitorum longus tendon and aligns the pull of that muscle with the long axis of the foot.

Glossary and Abbreviations

Angiography Imaging of vessels. Lymphangiography and venography have become relatively uncommon. Therefore, when angiography is used, it most often refers to the imaging of arteries, or arteriography.

Arthrography Imaging of a joint enhanced by the intra-articular injection of contrast material. It is widely understood that "magnetic resonance shoulder arthrography" is done with an intra-articular injection, but that "contrast-enhanced MRI of the shoulder" is done with an intravenous injection.

Computed tomographic angiography (arteriography) (CTA) A contrast-enhanced CT scan done with the intravenous injection and scan timing protocol optimized for vascular visualization. Most commonly, the protocol is optimized for arterial visualization. In addition to review of the axial images, MIP and 3-D displays are commonly used for diagnosis.

Computed tomography (CT) Sectional imaging technology using x-rays. See Introduction to Medical Imaging for more discussion.

Contrast enhanced (CE) Generally understood to refer to the intravenous injection of iodinated contrast material in CT or the gadolinium-based intravenous contrasts in MRI.

IMA Inferior mesenteric artery.

IVC Inferior vena cava.

LAD Left anterior descending coronary artery.

Magnetic resonance angiography (arteriography) (MRA) MRI sequence, done with or without contrast enhancement, which optimizes visualization of vessels, usually arteries.

Magnetic resonance imaging (MRI) An imaging technology utilizing magnetic fields and radiofrequency energy. See Introduction to Medical Imaging for more discussion.

Maximum intensity projection (MIP) The two-dimensional image resulting from displaying only those values from CT or magnetic resonance above a specified threshold value, along a particular linear coordinate. This results in a projectional image that is somewhat analogous to a radiographic projection. When the intensity of each pixel in a MIP display is modified by the volume of tissue that is above a density threshold and/or by distance from a certain viewpoint, it is referred to as a

VIP display. A minimum intensity projection display (MinIP) emphasizes for display those CT densities below a set threshold; it is often very useful for inspecting airways and lung parenchyma.

MRI pulse sequences   The technical explanation of even the simplest MRI pulse sequences is very far beyond the scope of this anatomy atlas. For details about the specifics of the gradient magnetic and radiofrequency pulses within the large number of available MRI sequences, there are many physics and MRI texts available.

Following is an abbreviated list of MRI pulse sequences mentioned in the atlas:

> **Fast spin echo (FSE)**   A common MRI sequence that may be T1 or T2 weighted and can be done with or without fat suppression.
>
> **Fluid-attenuated inversion recovery (FLAIR) sequence**   Sequence in which water or serous fluid has very low MR signal, but fluid with high protein content, and edematous tissue (tissue with high water content) has high signal.
>
> **Gradient echo (GRE) image**   A common MRI sequence that may be T1 or T2 weighted and can be done with or without fat suppression. Can provide volume acquisition and rapid "breath hold" images. Often used for CE MRI angiography.
>
> **Proton density MRI**   Image obtained with a short signal echo (TE) as in a T1-weighted image but a long repetition time (TR) as in a T2-weighted image.
>
> **Short tau inversion recovery (STIR) sequence**   A common fat-suppressed sequence with high sensitivity for detecting fluid signal.
>
> **Spin echo (SE) sequence**   A basic MRI pulse sequence that uses a 90° RF pulse and one or more 180° refocusing pulses.
>
> **T1-weighted MRI sequence**   Sequence that uses a short repetition time (TR) between RF pulses and short time interval for acquiring the signal echo (TE). In this sequence, fluid has low signal, shown on grayscale images as a relatively dark shade.
>
> **T2-weighted MR image**   Image that uses longer repetition time (TR) and signal echo (TE) intervals than T1 images and has fluid with high signal, shown on grayscale images as a relatively bright shade.

Multiplanar reformatting (MPR)   In CT scanning, although an imaging data set is considered to be an acquisition of a volume, it consists of a series of thin axial sections. Therefore, reconstruction of images into any plane other than axial, whether sagittal, oblique, or coronal, is considered to be reformatting of the image. These reconstructions display the geometric form of specific organs and tissues and can be rotated in any plane to provide a circumferential perspective. MPR also refers to the multiplanar displays created from a 3-D, or volume, acquisition in MRI.

PCA   Phase contrast angiography.

RF   Radiofrequency; the pulses of radio energy used in MRI.

SMA   Superior mesenteric artery.

SVC   Superior vena cava.

TRUS   Transrectal ultrasonography.

US   Ultrasound.

Volume rendered display   This reconstruction displays the geometric form of specific organs and tissues and can be rotated in any plane to provide a circumferential perspective. In addition, this image is often colorized, with tissues of various CT density ranges assigned different colors that enable them to appear lifelike.

Index